UPDATES IN HEMODIALYSIS

Edited by **Hiromichi Suzuki**

Updates in Hemodialysis
http://dx.doi.org/10.5772/58667
Edited by Hiromichi Suzuki

Contributors

Akihiro Yamashita, Eirini Grapsa, Konstantinos Pantelias, Dr. Pornanong Aramwit, Roland E. Winkler, M.B.A., Kosaku Nitta, Guy Rostoker, David Johnson, Eric Chou, David Mudge, Carmel Hawley, Ross Francis, Shu Wakino, Shozo Yano, Paulo Roberto Santos, Hiromichi Suzuki, Shyam Dheda, Fumitaka Koga, Elitsa Deliverska, Angelina Kisselova, Maria Dencheva, Asya Zaharieva Krasteva, Jordan Galabov

Published by InTech

Janeza Trdine 9, 51000 Rijeka, Croatia

Publishing Process Manager Iva Simcic

Technical Editor InTech DTP team

Cover InTech Design team

First published September, 2015

Printed in Croatia

Additional hard copies can be obtained from orders@intechopen.com

Updates in Hemodialysis, Edited by Hiromichi Suzuki

p. cm.

ISBN 978-953-51-2162-6

For EU product safety concerns:
IN TECH d.o.o., Prolaz Marije Krucifikse Kozulić 3, 51000 Rijeka, Croatia,
info@intechopen.com or visit our website at intechopen.com.

Meet the editor

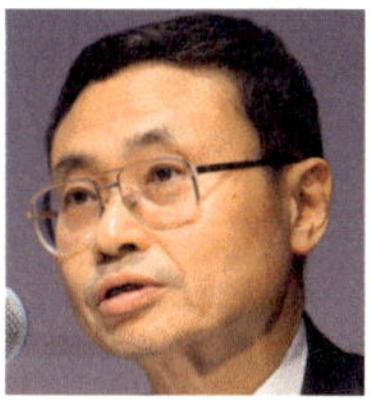

Dr. Suzuki graduated from Hokkaido University school of Medicine in 1975 and received the residency program of internal medicine in Keio University Hospital. He spent 4 years as clinical fellow in Nephrology and Endocrinology, Keio University Hospital from 1977 to 1982. After that, he studies as a Research Fellow of Basic Nephrology and Hypertension in Cleveland Clinic Foundation, Ohio, USA from 1982 to 1984. Coming back to Japan, he became an assistant and then associate professor, Department of Internal Medicine, Keio University, School of Medicine and carried out these professor ship until 1995. He became a professor, Department of Nephrology, Saitama Medical University and continued this job until the present time. He is involved in clinical nephrology including dialysis and hypertension and published more than 400 peer-reviewed articles. His recent focus on clinical and research is home dialysis.

Contents

Preface

Population which needs dialysis therapy is rapidly growing in the world, especially in the Asian countries. In line with these trends, recent advances in methodology and technology for dialysis therapy have been remarkable and astonishing. This book is intended to satisfy people working in the dialysis field. We call extinguish researchers as well as younger ambitious scholar for submitting recent review of their specialties. In 2013, InTech inaugurated book entitled "Hemodialysis", which gained a remarkable reputation in this field. This book is online with free access and numerous people accessed chapters of this book, indicating that this type of book is very helpful for the young people working in the field of hemodialysis. From these reviews, the reader will gain precious hints and suggestions in every day practice. I appreciate tremendous efforts of the authors to complete this special issue. Lastly, I thank Ms Iva Simcic, who carried out an exceptional secretarial task of collecting and editing the manuscripts.

Prof. Hiromichi Suzuki
Professor of Department of Nephrology,
Head of Community Health Science Center
Director of Library
Saitama Medical College
Japan

Section 1

Complications

Chapter 1

Vascular Calcification in Patients with End-Stage Renal Disease

Kosaku Nitta

Additional information is available at the end of the chapter

http://dx.doi.org/10.5772/59403

1. Introduction

Chronic kidney disease (CKD)-mineral and bone disorder (CKD-MBD) becomes an important issue in CKD management [1]. CKD patients show a bone and mineral disorder as follows: (i) laboratory abnormal metabolisms of calcium, phosphate, and vitamin D; (ii) evidence of calcified tissue disturbance; (iii) and arterial calcification. Arterial calcification is known to be related to numerous worse symptomatic outcomes, such as ischemic cardiovascular attacks and death [2]. The pathogenesis of vascular calcification in CKD is complex, and instead of occurring by a simple process of calcium and phosphate precipitation, it is produced by an active process in which vascular smooth muscle cells (VSMCs) undergo apoptosis and vesicle formation and are transformed into osteoblast-like cells that induce matrix formation and attract local factors that are involved in the mineralization process [3] (Fig. 1).

The pathogenesis of the multifactorial interactions between aging and progression of vascular calcification remains uncertain. However, there is no doubt that end-stage renal disease (ESRD) patients are at high risk of and have a common finding of vascular calcification due to multiple confounders that promote the differentiation of VSMCs to osteoblast-like cells, which are able to enhance the tissue calcium deposition process [4]. Vascular calcification has recently reported to be associated with many traditional risk factors, aging, high blood pressure, diabetes, and hyperlipidemia, and with nontraditional risk factors, including elevated serum phosphate level, hyperparathyroidism, and high-dose prescription of calcium [5]. Vascular calcification causes a decrease in vascular elasticity, an increase in pulse wave velocity [6], an induction of cardiomyopathy [7], a decrease in coronary artery flow, and an ischemic change (Fig. 2).

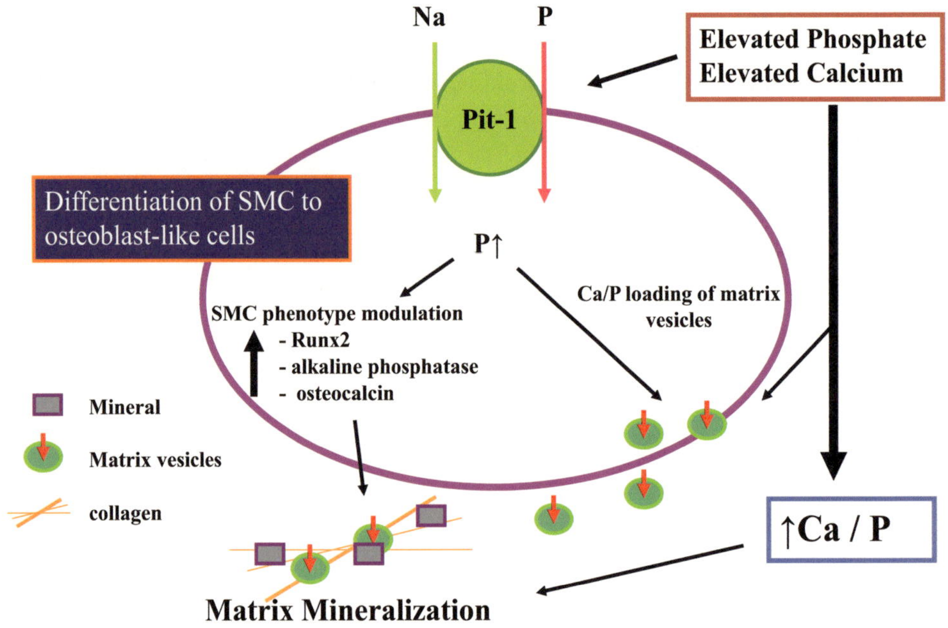

Figure 1. Relationship between calcium and phosphorus and vascular calcification.

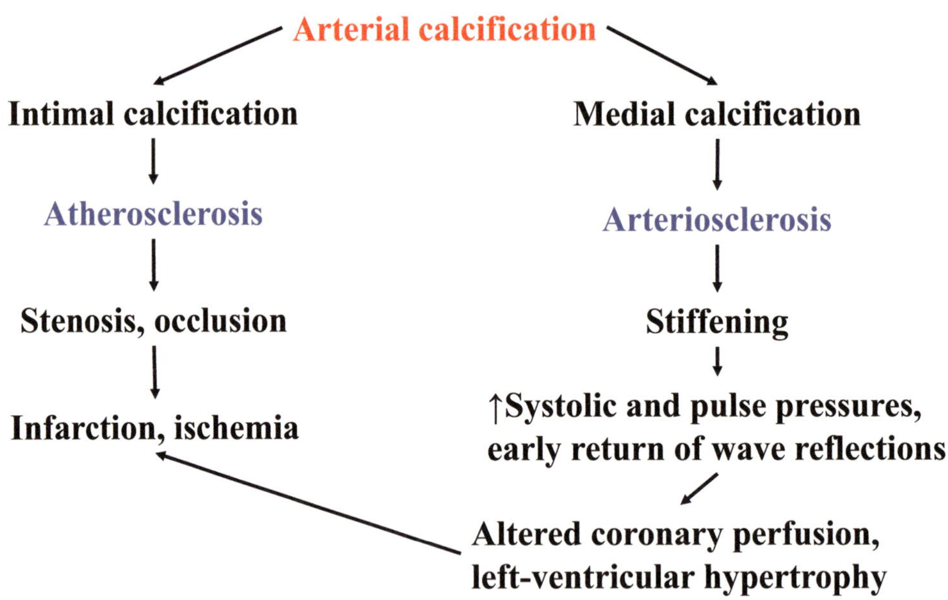

Figure 2. Schematic representation of the clinical effects of arterial intimal and medial calcification.

Recent therapeutic regimens that are performed to suppress vascular calcification are concentrated on the control of metabolic markers of skeletal disorder, including phosphate, and vitamin D. The antiosteoporosis drugs such as bisphosphonates [8] have shown therapeutic possibility, but more additional clinical trials are needed. The ADVANCE study has recently shown that cinacalcet and low-dose vitamin D reduce vascular and cardiac valve calcification in hemodialysis (HD) patients with secondary hyperparathyroidism (SHPT) [9]. This review article describes recent progress in terms of the pathogenic mechanisms and methods of assessing and managing vascular calcification in ESRD patients.

2. Pathophysiology and bone-associated proteins

The pathophysiology of vascular disorder in HD patients is recently recognized as different from the pathophysiology of atherosclerotic alterations in healthy subjects [10]. Vascular calcification progresses in association with aging, and deposition of calcium in the media is > 30-times more in the thoracic aorta at 90 years old than those at 20 years old [11]. Age-associated medial calcinosis in arteries is also related to hypertension, diabetes, and hyperlipidemia [12], and it is specific for arteries and does not affect other soft tissues in normal subjects. Vascular calcification was previously considered as a passive finding, but it has recently been recognized as an active process [13–15].

Two patterns of vascular calcification have been reported. One appears in the intimal layer and the other occurs in the medial layer of the vessel wall which is known as in Monckeberg's calcification [16], and both types are related to increased mortality of HD patients [17]. Intimal calcification is found to be related to chronic inflammatory changes and the occurrence of plaques and occlusive lesions. This intimal type of calcification is a predictor of the advanced atherosclerosis and is found to be seen in the aorta and coronary arteries. Medial calcification is identified with diffuse calcium deposition and can occur independent of atherosclerosis, and it is frequently shown in conduit arteries, including the femoral and tibial arteries [13, 16].

There are well-known changes in the arterial wall, such as intimal thickening, calcification of elastic lamellae, an increased extracellular matrix, and deposition of collagen and a relatively small elastic fiber content, and these findings are associated with arterial remodeling in CKD patients [17]. Numerous bone-related proteins, including osteopontin, osteocalcin, and osteoprotegerin (OPG), and bone morphogenetic proteins (BMPs) are associated with the vascular remodeling, and they are found to be appeared in the calcified lesions and are known to be related to vascular calcification [18]. VSMCs are the main component of the arterial media, and they can transform to osteoblast-like cells in association with up-regulation of transcription factors, such as Runt-related transcription factor 2 (Runx2) and Msh homeobox 2 (Msx2), which are important factors for normal bone formation [19]. This phenotypic differentiation may be related to the deposition of calcium in the layer of VSMCs that is similar to bone development, indicating that this type of vascular calcification is ectopic ossification. In addition, uremic condition has been found to induce transformation of VSMCs into osteoblast-like cells and suppresses the transformation of macrophages into osteoclasts [20]. The arteries of HD patients demonstrate up-regulation of alkaline phosphatase activity and enhanced expression of Runx2, which is predictor of osteogenic differentiation of VSMCs [21].

3. Dysregulation of calcium and phosphate metabolism

Traditional risk factors, such as aging, hypertension, diabetes, and hyperlipidemia, and various nontraditional factors, including low serum calcium levels, high serum phosphate levels, high-dose prescription of $CaCO_3$, chronic inflammation, and malnutrition, have been observed in ESRD patients [22]. Patients with advanced CKD demonstrate hyperphosphatemia followed by reduced renal phosphate excretion. Vascular calcification is obviously related to impaired serum calcium and phosphate concentrations [16, 21, 23]. Elevated serum phosphate concentration is found to be recognized as an arterial injury factor [24], and when phosphate control had been poorest, vascular calcification had rapidly progressed in CKD patients [25].

There are two different mechanisms of vascular calcification that are proposed to verify the relationship between abnormal calcium and phosphate metabolism and vascular calcification. Previous studies have shown that calcium is a key element in the initiation of vascular calcification by promoting calcium deposition in VSMCs under normal phosphate metabolism [26], and when the phosphate levels are increased, this calcium deposition has been enhanced additionally [27]. Hyperphosphatemia may directly cause vascular injury, and it indirectly promotes osteoblastic differentiation via a type III sodium-dependent phosphate cotransporter (PiT-1). A previous report [28] demonstrated that an increased intracellular phosphate concentration may directly enhance VSMCs to differentiate to calcifying cells by activating genes. In addition, El-Abbadi et al. [29] has shown an experimental model of CKD-related vascular calcification in which severe arterial calcification progresses only after the mice are treated with a high-phosphate diet, indicating that hyperphosphatemia is a powerful stimulator of arterial calcification. These results suggest that high-dose phosphate and calcium prescription is the most important risk factor in vascular calcification.

It is recognized that secondary hyperparathyroidism (SHPT) is common in ESRD patients and appears even in the early stage of CKD. Mineral metabolism disorders, such as hyperphosphatemia, is associated with the progression of CKD stage, leading to the occurrence of SHPT, which is detected by elevated serum parathyroid hormone (PTH) concentrations and parathyroid gland hyperplasia [30]. Increased PTH concentration is critical for the proliferation and activation of osteoclasts and important for the enhanced bone resorption in these patients. A remarkable reduction in serum 1,25-dihydroxyvitamin D [1,25(OH)2D] concentration is detected in the early stage of CKD [31], and the decrease in 1,25(OH)2D level is associated with renal and nonrenal mediators, such as decreased sun light exposure, reduced synthesis of the 25(OH) D precursor, and decreased dietary injection [32]. Reduced vitamin D production occurs in parallel with CKD progression and stimulates parathyroid gland enlargement, followed by SHPT [30].

Decreased 25(OH)D concentrations influenced survival independently of vascular calcinosis and increased arterial stiffness, indicating that 25(OH)D may affect mortality of CKD patients through additional mechanisms that require to be expected [33]. Active vitamin D promotes intestinal uptake of calcium and phosphate and stimulates osteoblastic transformation of VSMCs. Furthermore, 1,25(OH)2D has been known to play a role as a negative modulator of

http://dx.doi.org/10.5772/59403

the renin–angiotensin axis, which acts an important key element in the cardiovascular system by controlling extracellular volume and electrolyte metabolism [34]. Even though high-dose of 1,25(OH)2D promotes arterial calcinosis [35], normal doses have been reported to inhibit arterial calcinosis in experimental models of CKD [36].

4. Fibroblast growth factor 23 and vascular calcification

Fibroblast growth factor 23 (FGF-23) is a new regulator produced by osteoblasts, which is associated with the regulation of phosphate and vitamin D metabolism [37]. FGF-23 has been shown to reduce the synthesis and promote the degradation of 1,25(OH)2D. Actually, recombinant FGF-23 suppresses renal 25-hydroxyvitamin D-1α-hydroxylase mRNA within 1 h in mice [38]. The enhanced degradation of 1,25$(OH)_2$D by 24-hydroxylase may be related to this phenomenon. In addition, a phosphaturic effect of FGF-23 contributes to decreased phosphate uptake in the kidney. FGF-23 has been shown to down-regulate types IIa and IIc sodium-phosphate cotransporters on the apical area of proximal epithelial cells [38, 39].

Klotho has been reported as a 130-kDa β-glucuronidase that catalyzes the hydrolysis of steroid β-glucuronides [40]. The Klotho gene is mainly expressed in the kidneys, and its mutation induces many aging-associated diseases [41]. Since the phenotype of FGF-23-knockout (KO) mice is similar to those of Klotho-KO mice [42, 43], a common signaling pathway has been proposed, FGF-23 receptors (FGF-Rs). FGF-23 acts via FGF receptors (FGF-Rs) in a Klotho-dependent manner since a Klotho/FGF-R complex binds to FGF-23 with higher affinity than FGF-R or Klotho only [44]. FGF-23 has lower affinity for its receptors, and the combination with circulating Klotho is important to enhance the binding of FGF-23 to FGF-Rs [45]. Taken together, the activation of FGFRs needs not only circulating FGF-23 as a ligand but also Klotho as a specific activator those affinity attributes the selectivity on target organs.

Klotho is mainly present in the kidneys, whereas FGF-23 secretes from bone cells, and this bone–kidney interaction is essential for physiological and pathological mechanism. According to recent information, it is likely that this axis exerts a fundamental regulation of calcium metabolism with Klotho and to show a more specific effect on phosphate homeostasis via the presence of FGF-23. Both Klotho and FGF-23 affect synthesis of active vitamin D and PTH, indicating that FGF-23 may control PTH secretion in the parathyroid glands. In support of this mechanism, results obtained *in vitro* suggest that FGF-23 suppresses PTH mRNA transcription and protein secretion in a dose-dependent manner [46]. On the other hand, PTH promotes FGF-23 production by osteoblasts because increased FGF-23 concentrations in animals with primary HPT occur, which is decreased by parathyroidectomy [47].

5. Inhibitors of vascular calcification

Fetuin-A is originally synthesized in the liver, and circulating fetuin-A concentrations fall during the inflammatory process [48]. Fetuin-A is an extracellular calcium-regulatory factor that functions as a new inhibitor of calcium-phosphate deposition [49], suppresses calcinosis by binding hydroxyapatite [50], and protects VSMCs from the harmful effects of calcium overload and subsequent calcification [51]. Fetuin-A suppresses VSMC apoptosis through death-signaling pathways: (i) it is internalized by VSMCs, concentrated in intracellular vesicles, and secreted via vesicle release from apoptotic and living VSMCs; (ii) fetuin-A in vesicles suppresses their ability to nucleate calcium phosphate; and (iii) fetuin-A increases phagocytosis of vesicles by VSMCs. These results confirm finding that the internalization of fetuin-A into VSMCs is a key finding in the inhibition of vesicle-mediated VSMC calcification [51]. In *in vitro* experiments, fetuin-A has been reported to antagonize the action of TGF-β1 (transforming growth factor-β1) and inhibit osteogenesis and calcium-containing matrix deposition in dexamethasone-treated rat bone marrow cells [49]. Moreover, fetuin-A-KO mice show severe ectopic calcinosis in the myocardium, kidney, lung, tongue, and skin [49]. A recent study [49] demonstrated that ESRD patients who had lower serum fetuin-A concentrations showed a lower survival rate from cardiovascular diseases, indicating that fetuin-A is related to the mechanism of the accelerated extraskeletal calcinosis.

Matrix Gla protein (MGP) is a matrix protein that was firstly discovered from bone [52], and it is an important modulator of vascular calcification. To exert its biological activity, MGP requires to be activated through interaction with vitamin K [53]. The calcification of cartilage and blood vessels has been found to be inhibited by MGP [54]. MGP affects on vascular calcification directly by reducing calcium crystal formation and indirectly by modulating transcription factors that suppress VSMC transformation to the osteoblast-like cells [55]. Moreover, MGP is an important factor capable of transformation of VSMCs [58]. A decrease in glomerular filtration rate has been shown to result in a reduction in uncarboxylated MGP level which is related to vascular calcification [56].

The receptor activator of nuclear factor κ-light-chain-enhancer of activated B-cells (RANK), and RANK ligand (RANKL), and osteoprotegerin (OPG) might be associated with the mechanism of vascular calcification. RANKL functions are inhibited by OPG that acts as a decoy receptor to inhibit RANKL/RANK relationships [57]. This system may be related to the imbalance of bone–vascular calcification interactions and could be a predictor of the grade of vascular calcification. A recent study [58] demonstrated that coronary arterial calcification (CAC) is significantly associated with plasma OPG values in CKD patients. The serum OPG levels >757.7 pg/ml in CKD patients were indicator of CAC. These results are compatible with those reported in our previous study [59]. The relationship between serum OPG concentrations and CAC is unclear. The functional role of circulating OPG has been found to be modulated by several factors, including the relevant association of different tissue sources and the contribution of various comorbidities. OPG has been reported to have protective effect against vascular calcium deposition in experimental models [60]. Interestingly, higher OPG concentrations have been shown in patients with vascular injury, indicating that an elevated OPG concentration may be attribute to a compensatory self-defense mechanism that stimulates vascular calcification [61].

http://dx.doi.org/10.5772/59403

6. Evaluation of vascular calcification

Several types of noninvasive methods are useful for screening of the detection of vascular calcification: plain X-rays for visible calcification of the aorta and peripheral arteries; two-dimensional ultrasound for detecting calcification of the carotid arteries and femoral arteries; and echocardiography for the evaluation of valvular calcification; and computer tomography (CT) is considered to be the gold standard for quantification of coronary artery and aorta calcification.

Electron-beam CT (EBCT) and multislice CT (MSCT) are relatively sensitive methods for quantitative assessment of vascular calcification, such as CAC, which utilize an electrocardiographic trigger capable of the evaluation of the heart in diastolic phase, thereby prohibiting moving artifacts [62]. These methods can be usually used to assess the presence of vascular calcifications, the evaluation of longitudinal vascular calcification, and the effect of various treatments on vascular calcification [63]. EBCT is not available in every hospital, although most hospitals have MSCT equipment and, with software applications to enable gated imaging, the new MSCT can evaluate vascular calcification. However, there have been conflicting reports concerning the relationship between the grade of CAC estimated by EBCT and the prevalence of cardiovascular events in ESRD patients [64, 65]. The conflicting results could be confirmed by the evidence that the arterial calcification score evaluated by MSCT is a combination of both medial and intimal calcification, and the finding that is a limitation of the CT-based assessment. MSCT can be used to evaluate aortic calcification [66, 67]. Conventional CT could be used to estimate noncoronary vascular calcification, such as aortic calcification. The area of the aortic circumference that is calcified can be estimated as an aortic calcification index (ACI). It is likely that conventional CT is relatively inexpensive and applicable for screening of vascular calcification. A previous study [72] utilized the conventional CT to estimate aortic calcification in diabetic HD patients. The ACI could not be applicable to evaluate the medial/intimal calcification.

Plain lateral-abdominal X-ray is an inexpensive method for detecting the presence of vascular calcification in CKD patients, but it is semiquantitative, and longitudinal alterations of vascular calcification may not be confirmed. Lateral abdominal X-ray could be utilized as an alternative to CT [69]. The presence of vascular calcification observed on plain X-rays may give some information concerning the pattern of the arterial wall calcification. Kauppila et al. [70] showed the application of lateral lumbar X-rays to confirm the pattern of aortic calcification, in the area responsible to the part of the first to the fourth lumbar vertebrae. This semiquantitative method is a more applicable and less expensive technique for showing arterial calcification and could be utilized for cardiovascular risk management.

We have shown a simple method to study the grade of aortic arch calcification (AoAC) using plain chest X-ray in HD patients [71]. AoAC score (AoACS) was evaluated as a percentage of the proportion of calcified aortic arch, and the mean AoACS was 5.0% ± 4.5% ranging from 0% to 15%. Older age and longer dialysis duration were significant factors in the patients with AoAC. The grade of AoAC was significantly associated with the AoAC volume measured by MSCT. We suggest that screening HD patients for AoAC is a cost-effective method to find patients at the highest risk of cardiovascular diseases and of identifying therapy by inhibiting vascular calcification.

7. Applicable therapy of vascular calcification

Hyperphosphatemia is associated with SHPT and contributes to cardiovascular and all-cause mortality. The phosphate binders are recently utilized to treat hyperphosphatemia, including sevelamer, lanthanum, and the calcium-based phosphate binders (CBPBs) such as $CaCO_3$. Sevelamer is a calcium-free phosphate binder that does not increase serum calcium concentrations, enables better serum phosphate management than CBPBs, reduces the extent of aortic calcification in ESRD patients, and improves serum lipid profile because it decreases low-density lipoprotein cholesterol (LDL-C) and induces the increase in high-density lipoprotein cholesterol (HDL-C) [72]. In a clinical study consisting of 200 HD patients, Chertow et al. [73] showed that sevelamer had significantly reduced the extent of coronary and aortic calcification compared with CBPBs after 1 year of therapy. These results were reevaluated by other investigators [74], who demonstrated that sevelamer significantly reduced the progression of vascular calcification when compared with $CaCO_3$. One of the possible mechanism is a strong phosphate-binding ability of sevelamer in the intestine, without calcium overload. In the Renagel in New Dialysis study including HD patients with pretreatment CAC scores of 30 or higher, no significant difference was detected in the rate of CAC progression up to 18 months of follow-up between the sevelamer group and CBPB group [75]. *In vitro* experimental studies have demonstrated that acetylated LDL-C induces calcium deposition, whereas HDL-C reduces it in cultured VSMCs [76]. In *in vivo* human studies, sevelamer has been shown to decrease LDL-C and to increase HDL-C concentrations. This improved lipid profile may be associated with the lowering grade of vascular calcification found after sevelamer therapy. These findings were confirmed with the evidence that intensive LDL-C-lowering therapy with atorvastatin in the Calcium Acetate Renagel Evaluation-2 study demonstrated similar effects on the extent of CAC in HD patients treated with sevelamer and those treated with calcium acetate [77].

The calcium-sensing receptor (CaR) is a G protein-coupled receptor that binds calcium ions and makes it possible to respond to changes in the extracellular calcium ion levels [78]. CaR expression in the arterial wall has been found to be profoundly decreased in HD patients compared with normal subjects [79]. These results are compatible with those reported by Alam et al. [80], who showed lower expression CaR in the calcified human arteries compared with those without calcification. These findings indicate that CaR expression was closely associated with vascular calcification in the vessel wall. Ivanovski et al. [81] showed finding of direct suppression of phosphate-stimulated calcium deposition in cultured human VSMC *in vitro* by a calcimimetic R-568, through local CaR activation. Lopez et al. [82] examined the effect of the R-568 alone and in combination with calcitriol on the induction of vascular calcification in a uremic rat model with SHPT. The results of the experiment indicated that the R-568 decreased serum PTH concentrations without induction of vascular calcification, suppressed calcitriol-stimulated calcium deposition on vasculature, and reduced mortality rate related to supplementation of calcitriol. They concluded that R-568 suppresses increased serum PTH concentrations in uremic rats and inhibits calcitriol-stimulated calcium deposition in arterial tissues.

Bisphosphonates might play a possible role in the treatment of vascular calcification because these agents have been found to eliminate vascular calcification in experimental animal models. Tamura et al. [83] previously reported that etidronate suppressed calcitriol-stimulated aortic calcium deposition in uremic rats. They showed that 2 mg/kg of etidronate was not effective but that 5–10 mg/kg of etidronate inhibited calcium deposition in the aorta. In another experimental study using cultured bovine VSMCs, pamidronate reduced arterial calcium deposition [84]. In clinical studies, etidronate has been found to suppress and even reverse the CAC progression in some of HD patients [8, 85], but the mechanism is unclear. Bisphosphonates suppress bone resorption, with decreased efflux of calcium and phosphate, limiting their deposition in the vascular tissues, or may affect the function of the sodium/phosphate cotransporter in VSMCs [86].

There are a few prospective randomized trials available in the literature with therapeutic interventions aimed at controlling vascular calcification and improving survival in patients with advanced CKD. Since there is an association between CKD-MBD, vascular calcification and mortality, mineral balance abnormalities became an obvious target for therapeutic interventions. Unfortunately, no additional data have been published to change the perspective in the KDIGO guidelines [69]. The EVOLVE trial in 3883 HD patients was conducted to test the hypothesis that treatment with cinacalcet would reduce the risks of death and nonfatal cardiovascular events [87]. However, no benefit was demonstrated from using the calcimimetic agent.

8. Conclusion

Vascular calcification is highly prevalent in ESRD and independently predictive of future cardiovascular events and mortality. Calcification occurs in both the intimal and medial layers of vasculature, but medial calcification is the major form in ESRD patients. Medial calcification increases arterial stiffness and pulse pressure, induces left ventricular hypertrophy, reduces perfusion of the coronary arteries, and ultimately promotes increased cardiovascular mortality. Vascular calcification results not from a passive deposition of calcium and phosphate but rather is an active cell-mediated process involving vascular smooth muscle cell apoptosis and vesicle release; muscle cell differentiation forms a contractile to osteoblast-like phenotype. Cutting-edge scientific research on the mechanisms underlying vascular calcification is increasingly being undertaken, and further insight into the mechanisms may lead to the development of several types of therapeutic agents that will improve the cardiovascular outcome in ESRD patients.

Author details

Kosaku Nitta

Address all correspondence to: knitta@kc.twmu.ac.jp

Department of Medicine, Kidney Center, Tokyo Women's Medical University, Tokyo, Japan

References

[1] Moe SM, Drueke T, Lameire N, Eknoyan G. Chronic kidney disease-mineral-bone disorder: a new paradigm. Adv Chronic Kidney Dis 2007; 14; 3–12.

[2] Goldsmith D, Covic A, Sambrook P, Ackrill P. Vascular calcification in long-term haemodialysis patients in a single unit: a retrospective analysis. Nephron 1997; 77: 37–43.

[3] Moe SM, Chen NX. Mechanisms of vascular calcification in chronic kidney disease. J Am Soc Nephrol 2008; 19: 213–6.

[4] Shroff RC, Shanahan CM. The vascular biology of calcification. Semin Dial 2007; 20: 103–9.

[5] Chertow GM, Raggi P, Chasan-Taber S, et al. Determinants of progressive vascular calcification in haemodialysis patients. Nephrol Dial Transplant 2004; 19: 1489–96.

[6] Raggi P, Bellasi A, Ferramosca E, Islam T, Muntner P, Block GA. Association of pulse wave velocity with vascular and valvular calcification in hemodialysis patients. Kidney Int 2007; 71: 802–7.

[7] Nitta K, Akiba T, Uchida K, et al. Left ventricular hypertrophy is associated with arterial stiffness and vascular calcification in hemodialysis patients. Hypertens Res 2004; 27: 47–52.

[8] Nitta K, Akiba T, Suzuki K, et al. Effects of cyclic intermittent etidronate therapy on coronary artery calcification in patients receiving long-term hemodialysis. Am J Kidney Dis 2004; 44: 680–8.

[9] Raggi P, Chertow GM, Torres PU, et al. The ADVANCE study: a randomized study to evaluate the effects of cinacalcet plus low-dose vitamin D on vascular calcification in patients on hemodialysis. Nephrol Dial Transplant 2010; 26: 1327–39.

[10] Kalantar-Zadeh K, Block G, Humphreys MH, Kopple JD. (2003) Reverse epidemiology of cardiovascular risk factors in maintenance dialysis patients. Kidney Int 2003; 63: 793–808.

http://dx.doi.org/10.5772/59403

[11] Elliott RJ, McGrath LT. Calcification of the human thoracic aorta during age. Calcif Tissue Int 1994; 54: 268–73.

[12] Atkinson J. Age-related medial elastocalcinosis in arteries: mechanisms, animal models, and physiological consequences. J Appl Physiol 2008; 105: 1643–51.

[13] Shanahan C, Cary N, Salisbury J, Proudfoot D, Weissberg P, Edmonds M. (1999) Medial localization of mineralization-regulating proteins in association with Monckeberg's sclerosis: evidence for smooth muscle cell-mediated vascular calcification. Circulation 1999; 100: 2168–76.

[14] Shioi A, Taniwaki H, Jono S, Okuno, Y., Koyama, H., Mori, K. and Nishizawa, Y. Monckeberg's medial sclerosis and inorganic phosphate in uremia. Am J Kidney Dis 2001; 38: S47–9.

[15] Wexler L, Brundage B, Crouse J, Detrano R, et al. Coronary artery calcification: pathophysiology, epidemiology, imaging methods, and clinical implications. A statement for health professionals from the American Heart Association. Circulation 1996; 94:1175–92.

[16] London G, Marchais S, Guerin A, Metivier F, Adda H. Arterial structure and function in end-stage renal disease. Nephrol Dial Transplant 2002; 17: 1713–24.

[17] Dhore CR, Cleutjens JP, Lutgens E, et al. Differential expression of bone matrix regulatory proteins in human atherosclerotic plaques. Arterioscler Thromb Vasc Biol 2001; 21: 1998–2003.

[18] Chillon JM, Mozar A, Six I, et al. Pathophysiological mechanisms and consequences of cardiovascular calcifications: role of uremic toxicity. Ann Pharm Fr 2009; 67: 234–40.

[19] Shroff RC, McNair R, Figg N, et al. Dialysis accelerates medial vascular calcification in part by triggering smooth muscle cell apoptosis. Circulation 2008; 118: 1748–57.

[20] Chen NX, Duan D, O'Neill KD, et al. The mechanisms of uremic serum-induced expression of bone matrix proteins in bovine vascular smooth muscle cells. Kidney Int 2006; 70: 1046–53.

[21] Speer MY, Yang HY, Brabb T, et al. Smooth muscle cells give rise to osteochondrogenic precursors and chondrocytes in calcifying arteries. Circ Res 2009; 104: 733–41.

[22] Cannata-Andia JB, Rodriguez-Garcia M, Carrillo-Lopez N, Naves-Diaz M, Diaz-Lopez B. Vascular calcifications: pathogenesis, management, and impact on clinical outcomes. J Am Soc Nephrol 2006; 17 (12 Suppl 3): S267–73.

[23] Raggi P, Boulay A, Chasan-Taber S, et al. Cardiac calcification in adult hemodialysis patients. A link between end-stage renal disease and cardiovascular disease? J Am Coll Cardiol 2002; 39: 695–701.

[24] Kanbay M, Goldsmith D, Akcay A, Covic A. Phosphate: the silent stealthy cardiorenal culprit in all stages of chronic kidney disease: a systematic review. Blood Purif 2009; 27: 220–30.

[25] Kestenbaum B, Sampson JN, Rudser KD, et al. Patterson, D. J., Seliger, S. L., Young, B., Sherrard, D. J. and Andress, D. L. (2005) Serum phosphate levels and mortality risk among people with chronic kidney disease. J Am Soc Nephrol 2005; 16: 520–8.

[26] Yang H, Curinga G, Giachelli, C. Elevated extracellular calcium levels induce smooth muscle cell matrix mineralization in vitro. Kidney Int 2004; 66: 2293–9.

[27] Reynolds JL, Joannides AJ, Skepper JN, et al. Human vascular smooth muscle cells undergo vesicle-mediated calcification in response to changes in extracellular calcium and phosphate concentrations: a potential mechanism for accelerated vascular calcification in ESRD. J Am Soc Nephrol 2004; 15: 2857–67.

[28] Jono S, McKee M, Murry C, et al. Phosphate regulation of vascular smooth muscle cell calcification. Circ Res 2000; 87: E10–17.

[29] El-Abbadi MM, Pai AS, Leaf EM, et al. Phosphate feeding induces arterial medial calcification in uremic mice: role of serum phosphorus, fibroblast growth factor-23, and osteopontin. Kidney Int 2009; 75: 1297–307.

[30] Eknoyan G, Levin A, Levin NW. Bone metabolism and disease in chronic kidney disease. Am J Kidney Dis 2003; 42: S1–201.

[31] Levin A, Bakris G, Molitch M, et al. Prevalence of abnormal serum vitamin D, PTH, calcium, and phosphorus in patients with chronic kidney disease: results of the study to evaluate early kidney disease. Kidney Int 2007; 71: 31–8.

[32] Holick M. Vitamin D deficiency. N Engl J Med 2007; 357: 266–81.

[33] Barreto DV, Barreto FC, Liabeuf S, et al. Vitamin D affects survival independently of vascular calcification in chronic kidney disease. Clin J Am Soc Nephrol 2009; 4: 1128–35.

[34] Li Y, Kong J, Wei M, Chen Z, Liu S, Cao L. 1,25-Dihydroxyvitamin D3 is a negative endocrine regulator of the renin–angiotensin system. J Clin Invest 2002; 110: 229–38.

[35] Henley C, Colloton M, Cattley RC, et al. 1,25-Dihydroxyvitamin D3 but not cinacalcet HCl (Sensipar/Mimpara) treatment mediates aortic calcification in a rat model of secondary hyperparathyroidism. Nephrol Dial Transplant 2005; 20: 1370–7.

[36] Mathew S, Lund R, Chaudhary L, Geurs T, Hruska K. Vitamin D receptor activators can protect against vascular calcification. J Am Soc Nephrol 2008; 19: 1509–19.

[37] Shimada T, Kakitani M, Yamazaki Y, et al. Targeted ablation of Fgf23 demonstrates an essential physiological role of FGF23 in phosphate and vitamin D metabolism. J Clin Invest 2004; 113: 561–8.

[38] Shimada T, Hasegawa H, Yamazaki Y, et al. FGF23 is a potent regulator of the vitamin D metabolism and phosphate homeostasis. J Bone Miner Res 2004; 19: 429–35.

[39] Segawa H, Kawakami E, Kaneko I, et al. Effect of hydrolysis-resistant FGF23-R179Q on dietary phosphate regulation of the renal type II Na/Pi transporter. Pflugers Arch 2003; 446: 585–92.

[40] Kuro-o M, Matsumura Y, Aizawa H, et al. Mutation of the mouse Klotho gene leads to a syndrome resembling ageing. Nature 1997; 390: 45–51.

[41] Tsujikawa H, Kurotaki Y, Fujimori T, et al. Klotho, a gene related to a syndrome resembling human premature ageing, functions in a negative regulatory circuit of vitamin D endocrine system. Mol Endocrinol 2003; 17: 2393–403.

[42] Razzaque MS, Sitara D, Taguchi T, et al. Premature aging-like phenotype in fibroblast growth factor 23 null mice is a vitamin D-mediated process. FASEB J 2006; 20: 720–2.

[43] Nakatani T, Sarraj B, Ohnishi M, et al. In vivo genetic evidence for Klotho-dependent, fibroblast growth factor 23 (Fgf23)-mediated regulation of systemic phosphate homeostasis. FASEB J 2009; 23: 433–41.

[44] Kurosu H, Ogawa Y, Miyoshi M, et al. Regulation of fibroblast growth factor-23 signaling by Klotho. J Biol Chem 2006; 281: 6120–3.

[45] Mohammadi M, Olsen SK, Ibrahimi OA. Structural basis for fibroblast growth factor receptor activation. Cytokine Growth Factor Rev 2005; 16: 107–37.

[46] Krajisnik T, Björklund P, Marsell R, et al. Fibroblast growth factor-23 regulates parathyroid hormone and 1-hydroxylase expression in cultured bovine parathyroid cells. J Endocrinol 2007; 195: 125–31.

[47] Kawata T, Imanishi Y, Kobayashi K, et al. Parathyroid hormone regulates fibroblast growth factor-23 in a mouse model of primary hyperparathyroidism. J Am Soc Nephrol 2007; 18: 2683–8.

[48] Ketteler M, Vermeer C, Wanner C, Westenfeld R, Jahnen-Dechent W, Floege J. Novel insights into uremic vascular calcification: role of matrix Gla protein and α-2-Heremans Schmid glycoprotein/fetuin. Blood Purif 2002; 20: 473–6.

[49] Ketteler M, Wanner C, Metzger T, et al. Deficiencies of calcium-regulatory proteins in dialysis patients: a novel concept of cardiovascular calcification in uremia. Kidney Int 2003; Suppl 84: S84–7.

[50] Schafer C, Heiss A, Schwarz A, et al. The serum protein α2-Heremans-Schmid glycoprotein/fetuin-A is a systemically acting inhibitor of ectopic calcification. J Clin Invest 2003; 112: 357–66.

[51] Reynolds JL. Multifunctional roles for serum protein fetuin-A in inhibition of human vascular smooth muscle cell calcification. J Am Soc Nephrol 2005; 16: 2920–30.

[52] Price P, Williamson M. Primary structure of bovine matrix Gla protein, a new vitamin K-dependent bone protein. J Biol Chem 1985; 260: 14971–5.

[53] Cancela L, Hsieh CL, Francke U, Price PA, (1990) Molecular structure, chromosome assignment, and promoter organization of the human matrix Gla protein gene. J Biol Chem 1990; 265: 15040–8.

[54] Luo G, Ducy P, McKee M, et al. Spontaneous calcification of arteries and cartilage in mice lacking matrix GLA protein. Nature 1997; 386: 78 81.

[55] Bostrom K, Tsao D, Shen S, Wang Y, Demer L. Matrix GLA protein modulates differentiation induced by bone morphogenetic protein-2 in C3H10T1/2 cells. J Biol Chem 2001; 276: 14044–52.

[56] Parker B, Ix J, Cranenburg E, Vermeer C, Whooley M, Schurgers L. (2009) Association of kidney function and uncarboxylated matrix Gla protein: data from the Heart and Soul Study. Nephrol Dial Transplant 2009; 24: 2095–101.

[57] Collin-osdoby P. Regulation of vascular calcification by osteoclast regulatory factors RANKL and osteoprotegerin. Circ Res 2004; 95: 1046–57.

[58] Morena M, Dupuy AM, Jaussent I, et al. A cut-off value of plasma osteoprotegerin level may predict the presence of coronary artery calcifications in chronic kidney disease patients. Nephrol Dial Transplant 2009; 24: 3389–97.

[59] Nitta K, Akiba T, Uchida K, et al. Serum osteoprotegerin levels and the extent of vascular calcification in haemodialysis patients. Nephrol Dial Transplant 2004; 19: 1886–9.

[60] Bennet BJ, Scatena M, Kirk EA, et al. Osteoprotegerin inactivation accelerates advanced atherosclerotic lesion progression and calcification in older $ApoE^{-/-}$ mice. Arterioscler Thromb Vasc Biol 2006; 26: 2117–24.

[61] Schoppet M, Sattler AM, Schaefer JR, Herzum M, Maisch B, Hofbauer LC. (2003) Increased osteoprotegerin serum levels in men with coronary artery disease. J Clin Endocrinol Metab 2003; 88: 1024–8.

[62] Salazar H, Raggi P. Usefulness of electron-beam computed tomography. Am J Cardiol 2002; 89: 17B-22B.

[63] Chertow GM, Raggi P, Chasan-Taber S, Bommer J, Holzer H, Burke SK. (2004) Determinants of progressive vascular calcification in haemodialysis patients. Nephrol Dial Transplant 2004; 19: 1489–96.

[64] Sharples E, Pereira D, Summers S, et al. Coronary artery calcification measured with electron-beam computerized tomography correlates poorly with coronary artery angiography in dialysis patients. Am J Kidney Dis 2004; 43: 313–9.

[65] Haydar A, Hujairi N, Covic A, Pereira D, Rubens M, Goldsmith D. Coronary artery calcification is related to coronary atherosclerosis in chronic renal disease patients: a

http://dx.doi.org/10.5772/59403

study comparing EBCT-generated coronary artery calcium scores and coronary angiography. Nephrol Dial Transplant 2004; 19: 2307–12.

[66] Moe SN, O'Neill KD, Fineberg N, Persohn S, Ahmed S, Garrett P, Meyer CA. Assessment of vascular calcification in ESRD patients using spiral CT. Nephrol Dial Transplant 2003; 18: 1152–1158

[67] Nitta K, Akiba T, Suzuki K, et al. Assessment of coronary artery calcification in hemodialysis patients using multi-detector spiral CT scan. Hypertens Res 2004; 27: 527–33.

[68] Taniwaki H, Ishimura E, Tabata T, et al. Aortic calcification in haemodialysis patients with diabetes mellitus. Nephrol Dial Transplant 2005; 20: 2472–8.

[69] Kidney Disease: Improving Global Outcomes (KDIGO) CKD-MBD Work Group. KDIGO clinical practice guideline for the diagnosis, evaluation, prevention, and treatment of chronic kidney disease-mineral and bone disorder (CKD-MBD). Kidney Int 2009; Suppl 113: S1–S130.

[70] Kauppila LI, Polak JF, Cupples LA, Hannan MT, Kiel DP, Wilson PW. New indices to classify location, severity and progression of calcific lesions in the abdominal aorta: a 25-years follow-up study. Atherosclerosis 1997; 132: 245–50.

[71] Ogawa T, Ishida H, Matsuda N, et al. Simple evaluation of aortic arch calcification by chest radiography in hemodialysis patients. Hemodial Int 2009; 13: 301–6.

[72] Chertow GM, Burke SK, Dillon MA, Slatopolsky E. Long-term effects of sevelamer hydrochloride on the calcium × phosphate product and lipid profile of hemodialysis patients. Nephrol Dial Transplant 1999; 14: 2907–14.

[73] Chertow GM, Burke SK, Raggi P. Sevelamer attenuates the progression of coronary and aortic calcification in hemodialysis patients. Kidney Int 2002; 62: 245–52.

[74] Cozzolino M, Staniforth ME, Liapis H, et al. Sevelamer hydrochloride attenuates kidney and cardiovascular calcifications in long-term experimental uremia. Kidney Int 2003; 64: 1653–61.

[75] Block GA, Spiegel DM, Ehrlich J, et al. Effects of sevelamer and calcium on coronary artery calcification in patients new to hemodialysis. Kidney Int 2005; 68: 1815–24.

[76] Proudfoot D, Davies JD, Skepper JN, Weissberg PL, Shanahan CM. Acetylated low-density lipoprotein stimulates human vascular smooth muscle cell calcification by promoting osteoblastic differentiation and inhibiting phagocytosis. Circulation 2002; 106: 3044–50.

[77] Qunibi W, Moustafa M, Muenz LR, et al. A 1-year randomized trial of calcium acetate versus sevelamer on progression of coronary artery calcification in hemodialysis patients with comparable lipid control: the Calcium Acetate Renagel Evaluation-2 (CARE-2) study. Am J Kidney Dis 2008; 51: 952–65.

[78] Brown EM, MacLeod RJ. Extracellular calcium sensing receptors as integrators of multiple metabolic signals. Cell Calcium 2004; 35: 209–16.

[79] Molostvov G, James S, Fletcher S, et al. Extracellular calcium-sensing receptor is functionally expressed in human artery. Am J Physiol Renal Physiol 2007; 293: F946–55.

[80] Alam MU, Kirton JP, Wilkinson FL, et al. Calcification is associated with loss of functional calcium-sensing receptor in vascular smooth muscle cells. Cardiovasc Res 2009; 81: 260–8.

[81] Ivanovski O, Nikolov IG, Joki N, et al. The calcimimetic R-568 retards uremia-enhanced vascular calcification and atherosclerosis in apolipoprotein E deficient (apoE(–/–)) mice. Atherosclerosis 2009; 205:55–62.

[82] Lopez I, Aguilera-Tejero E, Mendoza FJ, et al. Calcimimetics R-568 decreases extraosseous calcifications in uremic rats treated with calcitriol. J Am Soc Nephrol 2006; 17: 795–804.

[83] Tamura K, Suzuki Y, Matsushita M, Fujii, H., Miyaura, C., Aizawa, S. and Kogo, H. (2007) Prevention of aortic calcification by etidronate in the renal failure rat model. Eur J Pharmacol 2007; 558: 159–66.

[84] Saito E, Wachi H, Sato F, Sugitani H, Seyama Y. Treatment with vitamin k2 combined with bisphosphonates synergistically inhibits calcification in cultured smooth muscle cells. J Atheroscler Thromb 2007; 14: 317–24.

[85] Hashiba H, Aizawa S, Tamura K, Kogo H. Inhibition of the progression of aortic calcification by etidronate treatment in hemodialysis patients: long-term effects. Ther Apher Dial 2006; 10: 59–64.

[86] Persy V, De Broe M, Ketteler M. Bisphosphonates prevent experimental vascular calcification: Treat the bone to cure the vessels? Kidney Int 2006; 70: 1537–8.

[87] Chertow GM, Block GA, Correa-Rotter R, et al. Effect of cinacalcet on cardiovascular disease in patients undergoing dialysis. N Engl J Med 2012; 367: 2482–94.

Chapter 2

Uremic Pruritus; Its Prevalence, Pathophysiology and Management

Pornanong Aramwit and Ouppatham Supasyndh

Additional information is available at the end of the chapter

http://dx.doi.org/10.5772/59352

1. Introduction

Pruritus is a nociceptive sensation transmitted centrally from the periphery by the unmyelinated, large, slowly conductive C fibers [1]. Pruritus is the dominant symptom of skin disease and a frequent manifestation of systemic disease. Of all of the systemic disorders, uremia is certainly the most important cause of pruritus [2]. The association between uremia and pruritus was first reported more than a century ago. Patients with severe chronic renal failure may be predisposed to the development of xerosis, hyperpigmentation, uremic roseola, calcinosis cutis, acquired perforating dermatosis, bullous dermatosis of hemodialysis, half and half nails and pruritus [3,4]. However, pruritus is often the most difficult to manage [5] and also related to mortality of end-stage renal disease (ESRD) patients. Aside from kidney transplantation, which is the only definitive treatment, therapeutic approaches for the treatment of pruritus have largely been empirical. The main goal of therapy remains to minimize the severity of pruritus and improve the quality of life, especially among those who are not transplantation candidates or are waiting for surgery.

Uremic pruritus (UP) may not be associated with the initiation of hemodialysis therapy, or symptoms may first become apparent with it [6]. A global study reported a 42% prevalence of moderate or extreme UP, which was strongly associated with sleep disturbance, depression, impaired quality of life and mortality [7]. Another study noted a higher percentage of pruritus in patients with more advanced chronic kidney disease (CKD): 18% of stage 3, 26% of stage 4, 42% of stage 5 and 58% of stage 5 CKD on maintenance hemodialysis for 1 month or greater [8] experienced UP. Once pruritus manifests itself, it often persists [6]. Pruritus can be a temporary condition lasting only a few months, but more commonly, it affects patients for more than 1 year. About one quarter of patients suffer from it only during or soon after hemodialysis, whereas others find this period a time of pruritus symptomatic exacerbation [9,10]. The intensity of pruritus was described as mild in 22- 52.6%, moderate in 22.6- 40% and severe in 8- 40% of patients [10-12]. About half of UP patients suffer from continuous itch, while the others experience it only occasionally with episodes of exacerbation. UP affects quality of life because of serious discomfort, anxiety, depression and sleeping disorders, especially because it is usually worse at night [13]. Pruritus may increase in intensity during the summer months, possibly due to the rising skin temperature reducing the threshold for the perception of UP, as occurs in other types of pruritus [14]. For that reason, external heat, sweat and stress can aggravate UP, and cold or hot showers can alleviate the symptoms [15]. The skin may appear normal or display different types of lesions, mostly related to scratching (e.g., lichen simplex, prurigo nodularis or keratosis papules) [13].

UP may be localized or generalized. Generalized itching is evident in about half of the patients [6]. Pruritus in dialysis patients is most commonly localized to the back, followed by the forearm with an arterio-venous fistula (perhaps due to frequent washing and traumatization of this region), abdomen, or head [16]. It has been reported that patient age, sex, underlying renal disease or dialysate solution used for hemodialysis (bicarbonate-based or acetate-based) have no influence on UP [6,10]. However, using less permeable and less biocompatible dialysis membranes show higher incidence of pruritus [6,10]. Moreover, patients with longer period of hemodialysis (> 3 months) may have high tendency to experience UP [13], possibly due to the accumulation of undefined pruritogenic cytokines or other substances [10].

Different scoring systems were used to quantify the severity of UP in clinical trials. The most commonly used include the visual analogue score (VAS) [17-19], a 4-point pruritus score [20] and a comprehensive validated questionnaire that was developed based on a short form of the McGill pain questionnaire [17,21]. This questionnaire was found to be reliable and provided valid data on the sensory, affective and overall intensity of UP and may provide a basis for future cross-cultural studies of itching [17] and for other study-specific scales [22].

Clinical appearance of UP can be observed by secondary changes such as atrophy of adnexal structures, microangiopathy with necrosis of endothelial cells, changes of sebaceous glands, lesions or lichen complex chronicus, excoriations and prurigo nodularis [23]. Although hemodialysis and continuous ambulatory peritoneal dialysis (CAPD) seem to be associated with a similar incidence of UP [24,25], some have found its incidence with CAPD was 10% [4] to 14% [26] lower, possibly due to a more effective elimination of possible pruritogenic substances by the peritoneum than by artificial membranes [27].

Due to the effect of UP which can cause serious discomfort, severe anxiety or even depression and sleeping disorders, it really affect patients' quality of life. Since sleeping disorders are related to chronic fatigue, it has strong influence on mental and physical health of patients [15]. Recently, studies demonstrated an association between UP and an increased risk of mortality [7,19].

2. Pathophysiology

The pathophysiology for this condition is not well understood. Known risk factors that predispose patients to UP are male gender [19], although some studies showed a higher prevalence in females [22,28], high levels of blood urea nitrogen and elevated calcium, phosphorus and β_2-microglobulin [22,29]. Other contributing factors include hypervitaminosis

A [20], high aluminum levels [30], anemia, erythropoietin insufficiency, elevated ferritin, low transferrin, low albumin, peripheral neuropathy [31] and secondary hyperparathyroidism with elevated divalent ions such as calcium, phosphate and magnesium ions [22]. Xerosis, which is very frequent in uremic patients as a result of a decrease in sweat volume as well as atrophy of the sebaceous glands and dehydration of the stratum corneum, may indeed play a role in UP.

It is hypothesized that UP is caused by the metabolic disequilibrium of CKD [32]. Some studies mentioned that it involves cutaneous nerve proliferation, pruritogenic cytokines or other chemicals, mast cell proliferation and secondary hyperparathyroidism. [5] Others propose that a poorly dialyzable substance is responsible for UP due to its systemic accumulation but that this resolves with renal transplantation [32]. UP has also been proposed to be a manifestation of multisystem dysfunction that is comorbid with renal failure. Proinflammatory mediators such as T-helper (Th)-1 cytokine and interleukin (IL)-2 may play a role in pruritus. Hypercalcemia and hyperphosphatemia with secondary deposition of calcium phosphate crystals in the skin may also contribute to itch [32]. Some biochemical parameters have been reported to be associated with the development of UP including magnesium [33], intact-parathyroid hormone (iPTH) [34], phosphate [33] and calcium [35]. While uremia may cause pruritus, other etiologies of pruritus must also be ruled out. Patients must be evaluated for endocrine disorders, atopic dermatitis, infestations, psychiatric disorders (e.g., delusions parasitosis), contact dermatitis and allergic reactions to the dialysate [23].

In UP, the stimulation of free nerve endings or dermal itch receptors generate impulses via C-fibers to the spinal cord and further to thalamus and finally reach cerebrum [36]. It is believed that substance P, which is a type of neurotransmitter, is a key to transmit the sensation of itch [3].

The physical appearances of skin in patients with chronic renal failure are totally difference from healthy people. Microangiopathy, thickening of basement membrane, epidermal atrophy or atrophy of sebaceous glands are normally found in hemodialysis patient [37,38,39]. Due to the lower levels of fat and water content on stratum corneum of skin with chronic kidney diseases, pruritus is normally found [40]. Reduction of sweat is another factor related to UP since the amount of electrolytes, lactate, urea, protein, lipids and amino acid elimination are normally decreased [40]. There is a positive correlation between xerosis and pruritus [11,25], but no correlation between cutaneous water content or transepidermal water loss and pruritus has been found [41,42]. However, the stratum corneum layers on the skin of dialysis patients are significantly less hydration compared to healthy skin [43].

There are several reports indicated that serum levels of divalent ions such as magnesium, calcium, aluminum and phosphate are related to UP [3,10,40,44]. Magnesium can stimulate neuron or activate histamine releasing from mast cells [45] while calcium and phosphate can induce itch receptors and cause metastatic cutaneous calcification [10,30]. An elevated serum aluminum concentration in chronic hemodialysis patients with UP was also reported as a possible etiology [30].

Secondary hyperparathyroidism has been proposed as a possible cause of UP, and normally, end-stage renal disease (ESRD) patients develop secondary hyperparathyroidism [3,46]. However, UP is relieved after parathyroidectomy [46]. Although hyperparathyroidism in UP is frequently associated with pruritus [47], a positive correlation was not confirmed [3]. Intact parathyroid hormone is not related to UP while mid-region parathyroid hormone (m-PTH) shows some correlation [6]. In patients with UP, the large amounts of inactive carboxy-terminal metabolites of parathyroid hormone is normally found in serum [6].

Mast cell accumulation and degranulation may play a role in UP [10,48,49]. Parathyroid hormone is known to stimulate mast cell production and accumulation in various organs [49]. Some studies have shown an increased number of cutaneous mast cells in uremic patients compared with healthy subjects [10,38], but very few reports show the correlation between mast cells and pruritus [47,50]. Very numerous, degranulated mast cells with diffusely distribution within dermis are normally found in patients with UP while mast cells in healthy subjects are mainly localized and intact in the upper dermis [10,51].

Mediators of inflammation may also be important. Histamine, a well-known mediator of pruritus in dermatologic disease, is elevated in the plasma of patients with ESRD as a result of histamine retention in renal insufficiency [52]. Histamine is released from mast cells in response to substance P and is thought to be implicated in UP. The number of mast cells is increased in patients with CKD, and increased plasma levels of tryptase and histamine have been reported in patients with severe UP [53]. In addition, prostaglandins are thought to modulate pruritus by lowering the threshold for histamine-induced pruritus [54]. There is a correlation between plasma histamine levels and pruritus [52,55]. It is found that histamine levels in patients with UP is significant higher compared to nonpruritic subjects [52,55] but specific differences in plasma histamine levels in subjects with and without UP cannot be found [26,56]. Since antihistamine has been widely used but ineffective for the treatment of UP, histamine should not have a significant role for this symptom [57].

It is possible that there are unknown pruritogenic cytokines produced by activated cells in some itching dermatoses [36]. Nitric oxide was also postulated to have a possible role in the development of UP [58], as it can be synthesized from cells under inflammatory stimulants including tumor necrosis factor-α (TNF-α), interferon-γ (IFN-γ) and IL-1β, and it has cytotoxic effects that can be involved in inflammatory dermatoses. During hemodialysis, several cytokines, including IL-1, are released following contact between plasma and the dialysis membrane [59]. IL-1 has been postulated to induce the release of inflammatory and potentially pruritogenic substances [6].

The two newest hypotheses that were proposed to explain the underlying pathophysiological mechanisms of UP are the immune hypothesis and the opioid hypothesis [22]. The immune hypothesis considers UP to be an inflammatory systemic disease [21] with over-activation of $CD4^{+}$TH1 lymphocytes and overproduction of IL-2, IFN-γ and TNF-α. IL-2 is released during hemodialysis secondary to the contact of blood and dialysis membranes [60], and it is known to be pruritogenic when injected into the skin. The increased serum levels of inflammatory biomarkers such as C-reactive protein and IL-6 confirms the inflammatory nature of the disease [61]. For the opioid hypothesis, it is well known that opioids play a role in modulating the sensation of pruritus both centrally and peripherally. Endogenous opioids are known to play a role in cholestatic prutitus [22], but it was also postulated that they have a role in UP secondary to the overexpression of opioid μ-receptors in dermal cells and lymphocytes, and concomitant down-regulation of opioid κ-receptors caused by the increase in serum β-endorphin to endorphin A ratio that is observed in patients with CKD [62]. Despite all these mechanisms, the certain pathophysiology of UP remains unknown.

3. Treatment

Despite high prevalence and life-altering comorbidities, UP remains poorly characterized and lacks effective treatment [63]. Because the pathophysiological mechanisms of UP are poorly understood, the treatments have largely been empirical, and no treatment has been shown to have sufficient efficacy and safety [64]. Moreover, no drugs have been approved by the U.S. Food and Drug Administration for this problem. Before considering the treatment of UP, an evaluation should be performed to define whether pruritus in a specific patient is caused by uremia (which needs adequate dialysis) or is related to dermatologic or systemic disease such as hyperparathyroidism, hyperphosphatemia and anemia that may require a different approach [2]. Once the etiology of pruritus has been established, several therapies can potentially be adopted. Treatments can be classified as topical, physical or systemic applications.

In order to control UP in dialysis patients, several factors need to be monitored such as improvement of nutritional status, monitoring of calcium and phosphorus levels, optimization of dialysis efficacy as well as use of biocompatible dialysis membranes [65]. Pruritus found in CKD may cause from other disorders such as liver diseases (for instance; hepatitis), endocrine disorders (for instance; Graves' disease, diabetes mellitus and hypothyroidism) and skin disorders (such as atopic dermatitis, psoriasis, contact dermatitis and urticaria). Pruritus found in these causes need specific treatments which may differ from standard treatment [53]. A step-up therapeutic approach for UP in patients with CKD is presented in Figure 1.

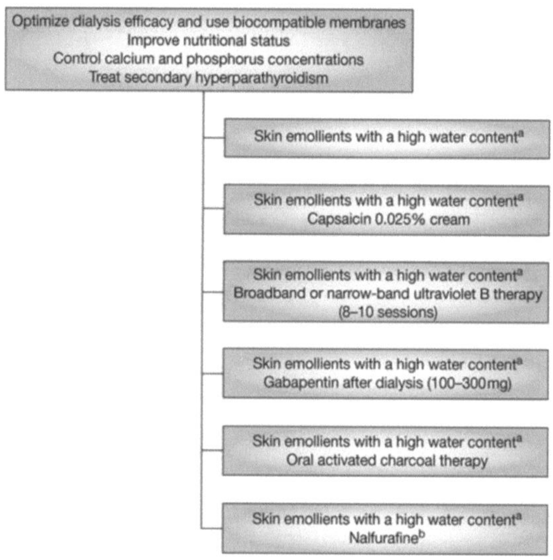

[a] Use of evening primrose oil rich in essential fatty acids (γ-linolenic acid), bath oil that contains polidocanol and cream that contains natural lipids and endocannabinoids can be attempted if simple emollients fail.

[b] For intractable UP that does not respond to nalfurafine (5 μg intravenously thrice weekly for 4 weeks), treatment with short courses of topical tacrolimus ointment (0.1% for 2-6 weeks) or oral thalidomide (100 mg daily for 2-4 weeks) can be attempted.

*Reprint with permission from publisher (Kuypers, DRJ., Skin problems in chronic kidney disease. *Nat. Clin. Pract. Nephrol.* (2009).

Figure 1. Step-up therapeutic approach for UP in a patients with CKD.

4. Physical Treatments

4.1. Modification of Dialysis Techniques and Mineral Abnormalities

The prevalence of UP declines by using biocompatible dialysis membranes [66]. Hence, the first approach to improve UP is still to optimize the dialysis efficiency, use biocompatible dialysis membranes and improve the nutrition status of patients. One study demonstrates that in a series of 30 cases, a polymethylmethacrylate (PMMA) artificial kidney may be a useful adjuvant therapy in chronic hemodialysis patients with severe UP, as it may eliminate more serum cytokines by adsorption than other types of high-flux membranes [67].

Because divalent ions, including magnesium and calcium, may possibly be involved in the pathogenesis of uremia, using a hemodialysis bath with low calcium and magnesium concentration [45,68,69] and keeping the calcium × phosphate product less than 55 mg^2/dL^2 can play a role in improving the pruritus [35]. However, drastic reduction in dialysate calcium concentration may possibly aggravate renal osteodystrophy.

4.2. Efficient Dialysis

It is a common experience that pruritus is more frequent in underdialyzed patients and improves by increasing the efficacy of dialysis. Pruritus patients tend to have higher blood urea nitrogen and lower K_t/V values [70]. Increasing the K_t/V from a mean of 1.05 to 1.24 in severely pruritic patients improved their symptoms significantly [70].

4.3. Parathyroidectomy

Patients who experience pruritus together with hypercalcemia and hyperparathyroidism should be treated by parathyroidectomy [46,71]. However, there is no relation between parathyroid hormone and UP, parathyroidectomy should not be used as a routine procedure [2]. It was found that patients with hypocalcemia or serum calcium at the normal limit can still experience pruritus. It can be concluded that the relationship between serum calcium level and pruritus is hardly found [72].

4.4. Phototherapy

The role of phototherapy in renal pruritus has been assessed by double-blind trials. Ultraviolet B (UVB) has been generally, although not uniformly, shown to be therapeutic. The mechanism of the antipruritic effect of UVB is not completely understood. Among the proposed mechanisms are inactivation of a circulating pruritogenic substance, formation of a photo-product that relieves pruritus, alteration of divalent ion content in the skin, suppression of histamine release as well as deactivation of circulating pruritogenic substances [16] and promotion of cutaneous nerve degeneration [73,74]. UVB phototherapy is well tolerated aside from occasional instances of sunburn [75]. The duration of the antipruritic effect of thrice-weekly, total body UVB phototherapy (8- 10 sessions in total) is variable but can last for several months. In

1975, Saltzer *et al.* first described successful treatment with irradiation of UVB (wavelength 280- 315 nm), [76] and the results were confirmed by several studies [32,75,77,78]. The study also showed that there was no significant difference between remission rates or length of remission between the intensive, intermediate and prolonged treatment schedule [75,79].

Later, a study by Blachley *et al.* not only showed the efficacy of UVB treatment in 17 patients clinically but also showed, by obtaining skin biopsies before and after therapy, a reduction in skin phosphorus following UVB treatment to values that were comparable with those of patients with nonpruritic uremia or healthy volunteers [77]. Further investigation has been performed using narrowband UVB phototherapy, as most of the data on UV radiation have been predominately derived from studies using broadband UVB [80]. The results showed the effectiveness of narrowband UVB, as 9 of 15 patients with UP were marked as responders; however, remission was not prolonged, as 4 of 6 responders who came back for a follow-up had a recurrence [80,81]. Due to the carcinogenic effect of UVB, ultraviolet A (UVA, wavelength 315- 400 nm), which is safer than UVB, was studied for its efficacy, however, UVA did not demonstrate any benefit [82]. Narrowband UVB, which is generally accepted to be less carcinogenic than broadband UVB, should be a better alternative treatment in both efficacy and safety aspects.

4.5. Acupuncture and Electrical Needle Therapy

Modern medicine tries to explain the efficacy of acupuncture by describing its effects on the receptors of the nervous system, its action on the endogenous endorphin enkephalin and 5-hydroxytryptamine (5-HT), or that it can increase the number of leukocytes and strengthen the defensive mechanisms of the body [83]. Some studies show the benefit of acupuncture for UP. The fundamental information indicated that pruritus was transmitted by conductive C fibers, and acupuncture generates impulses that are carried by the smaller, myelinated, and rapidly conductive beta and delta fibers, all of which reach the spinal cord. There, opiate-like substances are released that block the slower C fiber impulses [84].

Acupoint injection, at San Yin Jiao (SP6), Xuehai (SP 10), Zusanli (ST 36) and Quchi (LI 11) acupoints, has been reported to be effective in UP [85]. Using a transcutaneous electrical nerve stimulation (TENS) acupressure apparatus at those points also showed a benefit in reducing UP [86]. Duo also reported that an electric needle is effective at two similar points (Quchi and Zusanli) [87]. Che-yi *et al.* also reported that acupuncture at the Quchi (LI 11) acupoint, which is close to the hemodialysis needle puncture site but not too close for acupuncture there to interfere with hemodialysis, is also effective for relieving UP [1]. However, acupuncture does not change the level of biochemical parameters associated with the development of UP—including magnesium, iPTH, phosphate and calcium.

4.6. Thermal Therapy

Hsu *et al.* investigated the effects on UP of 40 degree Celsius thermal therapy with far-infrared rays at the Sanyinjiao acupoint for 15 minutes and found a large decrease in pruritus scores in the thermal therapy group compared with the non-thermal therapy group, even though there was no significant differences between groups [88]. The result implied that thermal therapy may have therapeutic benefits for UP.

4.7. Sauna

Stimulation of the sweat glands with a sauna has shown benefits, perhaps through augmented excretion of hypothetical pruritogen [89]. However, such treatment may cause major complications in fluid balance due to unquantifiable insensible water loss.

5. Topical Treatments

Topical treatment with skin emollient contained high water to hydrate stratum corneum is considered as a primary therapy for UP in CKD patients. In order to avoid any allergic reaction, emollients without perfumes or other additives is preferable [43,90].

5.1. Skin Emollients

Because xerosis plays at least an adjuvant role in the development of UP, emollients are a mainstay in the treatment. It has been suggested by several researchers that the use of emollients with high water content should be the first-line treatment [91,92]. The benefit of using emollients to treat dry skin in patients with UP has been reported by Morton et al. and others [9,43,93]. A pilot study on the use of urea 10% lotion with dexpanthenol, a moisturizer, showed significant improvement in skin itch [20]. The study by Balaskas *et al.* of 100 patients using glycerol and paraffin, showed a 75% improvement in UP and hence quality of life ($p<0.001$) [94]. The addition of endocannabinoids to creams containing structured physiological lipids demonstrated good efficacy and tolerance in a clinical study [61,95].

5.2. Sericin Cream

Sericin, a biopolymer with a high molecular weight, is a water-soluble protein that is obtained from the silkworm (*Bombyx mori*). Sericin is characterized by the presence of 32% serine, which is the main amino acid of the natural moisture factor (NMF) in human skin; therefore, sericin has excellent moisturizing properties that may be helpful for treating hypohidrosis. Sericin also demonstrates many biological activities and has been widely studied for potential use in medicines and biomaterials [96-100]. Moreover, sericin can significantly decrease the levels of the pro-inflammatory cytokines TNF-α and IL-1β in sericin-treated wounds in rats 7 days after an injury, compared with the levels found in normal saline-soaked wounds and cream base-treated wounds [101]. As previously mentioned, the immune-inflammatory hypothesis considers UP a dermatologic manifestation of chronic inflammation and treats the condition as a possible result of derangements in the immune system that are based on a pro-inflammatory pattern. Based on this reasoning, sericin was investigated for relieving UP. An in-subject, randomized, double-blind, placebo-controlled experimental study was designed to investigate the effects of sericin cream (concentration 8%) versus the cream base (placebo) applied twice daily for 6 weeks in reducing the symptoms of UP (itching, dryness and redness) and skin pigmentation in 47 subjects with stable maintenance hemodialysis [102]. The results showed that sericin reduces pruritus in patients with UP. The use of sericin cream significantly increased the level of skin hydration after 6 weeks of treatment compared to baseline and to the use of the cream base. The use of sericin cream also significantly reduced the level of skin irritation and pigmentation after 6 weeks of treatment compared to baseline, while use of the cream base reduced skin pigmentation slightly but not significantly. Patients' quality of life was also assessed using the Thai version of the KDQOL-SF Version 1.3, and the results showed a better quality of life in all of the measured domains, including sleep and mood/emotional distress after the treatment period. When the mean score on the enrollment day was compared with the mean score on the day after the completion of treatment, significant differences were found in some domains, including pain, the symptoms/problems list in kidney disease, the effect of kidney disease on daily life and sleep, the most relevant parameter for itching. The overall score increased from 60.00 at the time of enrollment to 61.95 after 6 weeks of treatment, although this difference was not statistically significant. The results of this study suggest that sericin cream may be a good choice for treating pruritus in hemodialysis patients. Because sericin is obtained from natural sources that have high biocompatibility, it may cause fewer allergic reactions and lower resistances compared to other chemical substances.

5.3. Capsaicin

Capsaicin (trans-8-methyl-N-vanillyl-6-nonenamide), an extract from capsicum or common pepper plant, can be used as a main ingredient in cream for the treatment of painful disorders including postherpetic neuralgia, cluster headaches, diabetic neuropathy, osteoarthritis and phantom limb [103,104]. Capsaicin blocks pain and itching by depleting and preventing the re-accumulation of substance P from local type C sensory nerve terminals [89,104]. After using 0.025% capsaicin cream for the treatment of UP in long-term dialysis patients, the results indicated that significant alleviation of pruritus was found with no serious adverse reaction [105,106]. Although topical capsaicin might be useful for the treatment of localized disease, it is impractical for large areas or generalized pruritus.

5.4. Tacrolimus

Tacrolimus is an immunomodulator targeting mainly at the T helper cells. It blocks the differentiation of Th1-type lymphocytes, and therefore, suppresses the production of IL-2. Due to these mechanisms, it was suggested that it might be beneficial in the treatment of UP. An observational study of 3 cases of severe UP in patients on peritoneal dialysis indicated a short-term efficacy of 0.03% tacrolimus ointment over 7 days. However, the use of this agent was not extended longer because of the potential carcinogenic effect of systemic tacrolimus [107], which resulted in an FDA black-box warning that was issued in 2006 against the prolonged topical use of tacrolimus creams and ointments. Nevertheless, some studies failed to demonstrate any efficacy of the topical calcineurin inhibitor in patients with UP [108,109].

6. Systemic Treatments

6.1. Opioid Antagonists

Endogenous opioids have been implicated in the genesis of the pruritus associated with cholestasis [110,111]. One study demonstrated the effect of naltrexone 50 mg/day for a week in 15 dialyzed patients with severe UP in a randomized cross-over trial, and the results indicated that short-term amelioration of UP was found and attributed to the inhibition of basophil histamine release. Only mild upper gastrointestinal tract symptoms were found to be the side effects [112]. Opioid antagonists should therefore be considered for patients with severe and persistent UP [2].

More recently, another perspective was elaborated on regarding the use of a κ-agonist, for κ-receptor stimulation inhibits μ-receptor effects both peripherally and centrally and hence might inhibit itching induced by substance P [64]. A meta-analysis approach was used to assess the efficacy of nalfurafine, which is a κ-agonist, in two randomized placebo-controlled clinical studies. Nalfurafine was administered intravenously postdialysis over 2-4 weeks, and the results were encouraging, as improvements in the worst itching, itching intensity and sleep disturbances were noted in the nalfurafine group, with significant p values [113]. In addition, the evaluation of adverse events demonstrated that nalfurafine was well tolerated.

6.2. Erythropoietin

De Marchi *et al.* studied the effect of erythropoietin in dialysis patients with elevated plasma histamine levels in a placebo-controlled, double-blind, crossover study. They found that erythropoietin improved UP and decreased plasma histamine concentrations. Further, they found that it can result in marked improvement of UP and that recurrence of pruritus occurred after discontinuation of erythropoietin [114]. However, this effect was not related to the change in hemoglobin levels [115].

6.3. Serotonin Antagonists

Serotonin has been suggested as a possible mediator of cholestasis and UP. One study indicated that ondansetron, a selective inhibitor of serotonin type 3 receptors, at 4 mg twice a day for approximately 3 months can significantly reduce the severity of UP in peritoneal dialysis patients with moderate to severe pruritus [116]. This treatment was well tolerated and showed no significant side effects. However, the study by Ashmore *et al.* failed to show any significant change in the pruritus scores in patients treated with ondansetron in comparison with the placebo group [117].

6.4. Gabapentin

Gabapentin, a γ-aminobutyric acid analog, is a potent anticonvulsant drug that was has been clearly demonstrated as effective in the treatment of neuropathic pain, especially diabetic neuropathy. Considering that neuropathic pain and pruritus share common pathogenic mechanisms, gabapentin, which is usually used to treat neuropathic pain, emerged as another possibility in the arsenal of treatment for severe UP resistant to other therapies [64]. Recent, limited data suggest that gabapentin is a promising drug in treating UP, given its efficacy and its safety [13,91,118]. In a randomized, placebo-controlled, double-blind study, 25 patients were treated with gabapentin versus a placebo for 4 weeks; the treatment was then reversed, and the mean pruritus score dropped significantly. No patient dropped out due to adverse events from gabapentin [119]. Regarding its pharmacokinetics, gabapentin is eliminated primarily through the kidney, and it is removed by hemodialysis. It has a significantly longer half-life in patients on hemodialysis than in those with normal kidney function, and thus, these patients need lower doses at less frequent intervals [64]. The recommended dose for hemodialysis patients is 200- 300 mg after each hemodialysis session, with somnolence, dizziness and fatigue being the most commonly reported side effects [120].

6.5. Antihistaminic Agents

Despite the fact that histamine might be implicated in the pathogenesis of UP and the demonstration of elevated histamine levels in patients with ESRD with pruritus [91,121], classical antihistamines showed very limited efficacy in the treatment of UP [53,54,94,121]. The response to the administration of antihistaminic agents is marginal, at best [9]. Mast cell stabilizers including ketotifen, 2-4 mg per day for 8 weeks, [55] and cromolyn sodium [55], however, were demonstrated to be effective in case series.

6.6. Long Chain Fatty Acids

Abnormalities in the plasma composition of essential fatty acids may be related to the etiology of pruritus in patients undergoing hemodialysis. After administration of 6 grams of ethyl ester of either fish oil, olive oil or safflower oil in double-blind study of 25 hemodialysis patients, the results indicated that pruritus was significantly improved due to the altered plasma fatty acid profile and increased prostaglandin E_2 (PGE_2) plasma concentration [122]. Another study indicated that the improvement in pruritus was due to an increase in PGE_1 plasma levels [123] after administration of γ-linoleic acid-rich evening primrose oil 2 grams per day for 6 weeks.

6.7. Lidocaine and Mexiletine

Parenteral administration of lidocaine, a membrane-stabilizing antiarrhythmic agent, can relieve pruritus in double-blind study however, significant side effects such as hypotension and grand mal seizures were found [124]. An oral dosage form of mexiletine, a longer half-life and less toxicity than lidocaine, was found to be ineffective for the treatment of UP [125].

6.8. Low Protein Diet

Low protein diet has been proposed for the treatment of UP due to the rational of less accumulation of renally excreted pruritogen [126]. However, low protein diet may lead to malnutrition which can be dangerous in CKD patients and detoxification showed no benefit on pruritus [2].

6.9. Oral Activated Charcoal

With the rationale of adsorbing an unidentified pruritogen, oral activated charcoal at the dose of 6 grams per day has been used for uremic pruritus. A double-blind crossover trial and a single-blind study have yielded impressive results [127,128]. This preparation is effective, inexpensive, and has a favorable side effect profile. However, this treatment has not yet been accepted and utilized in clinical practice [127,128].

6.10. Cholestyramine

The success of cholestyramine in treating PU is inconsistent. When administered at a dose of 5 grams twice a day, the gastrointestinal side effects are normally found. Moreover, the risk of acidosis must also be taken into consideration, particularly in patients who are not on dialysis [128,129].

6.11. Heparin

Patients on hemodialysis may develop pruritus when treated with porcine or bovine heparin. Pruritus is relieved promptly when another form of heparin is used, implying that these heparins act as allergens [9]. Paradoxically, administration of heparin at 75- 100 mg twice a day for 2-3 weeks can improve UP in some dialysis patients [130]. From the mechanism of action by inhibition of T-lymphocyte heparanase activity which is an important factor for T-cell migration to target tissues, low molecular weight heparin such as enoxaparin at low dose is effective in treating pruritus associated with lichen planus [2,131].

6.12. Thalidomide

Thalidomide is a relatively selective inhibitor of TNF-α production. The study indicated that thalidomide at 100 mg per day administered for 1 week can significantly reduce the intensity of pruritus by up to 80% in more than half of the subjects, suggesting a potential role for this agent in the treatment of persistent UP [132].

6.13. Nicergoline

Nicergoline is a dopamine receptor agonist and a partial α-adrenergic blocker related to ergot alkaloids. A double-blind, placebo-controlled study that investigated the effect of 30 mg per day by mouth and 5 mg per day intravenously during dialysis, indicated relief of pruritus in most patients, and the effect lasted for 24- 48 h with improvement persistent in long-term therapy (30 mg per day) in most patients who responded to the initial treatment [133].

6.14. Nicotinamide

Nicotinamide is the pyridine-3-carboxylic acid amide of niacin, a component of the vitamin B complex. Namazi *et al.* suggested 3 mechanisms through which nicotinamide can be effective in treating UP: the anti-inflammatory effect through the inhibition of the expression of major histocompatibility complex (MHC)-II and the production of IL- 12, TNF-α and IL-1; the inhibition of cyclic adenosine monophosphate (cAMP) phosphodiesterase and stabilization of mast cells and leukocytes and hence, blocking histamine release; and the increase of the biosynthesis of ceramides by keratinocytes with the resultant alleviation of xerosis [134]. For those reasons, nicotinamide could be an effective treatment for UP. However, clinical trials should be conducted to confirm its efficacy.

7. Conclusion

UP is one of the most common and disabling symptoms for patients with ESRD. It is considered to be an inflammatory systemic disease rather than a local skin disorder. Biomarkers of inflammation are increased in patients with UP, and an imbalance of the endogenous opioidergic system might be involved in the complex pathogenesis of the disease. UP affects up to 90% of patients on dialysis and is associated with a high morbidity and mortality. Given the complexity of its pathogenesis and the lack of clear evidence regarding the efficacy of more conservative therapies, the only definitive treatment is kidney transplantation.

Antihistamines, which are the most widely used antipruritic agents, are ineffective for the treatment of hemodialysis-related pruritus. Safe and effective modalities, and those that should probably be considered as first-line treatment, are topical emollients. Other physical therapies and medications should be further investigated due to the inconsistent trial results. Without definitive treatment of the underlying disease, therapy for hemodialysis-related pruritus is often palliative at best, aiming to minimize the severity of pruritus and to improve the quality of life.

The standard of care remains to optimize the dialysis dose and to use biocompatible membranes, as well as the treatment of mineral abnormalities and anemia. The reasonable course for treating hemodialysis-related pruritus should be as follows:

a. If the patients can tolerate it, dialysis should achieve a K_t/V_{urea} value greater than 1.4.

b. If the patient is sensitive to ethylene oxide or the dialysis membrane, a gamma-irradiated or noncomplement-activating membrane should be used.

c. Compliance with dietary restrictions and phosphate-binding therapy should be encouraged.

d. Epoetin alpha therapy should start at 36- 360 units/kg intravenously or subcutaneously weekly and be optimized according to hemoglobin and hematocrit values.

e. Topical emollients should be started if the symptoms persist and followed by step therapy in Figure 1.

Without definitive treatment of the underlying disease, therapy for hemodialysis-related pruritus is often palliative at best, aiming to minimize the severity of pruritus and to improve patients' quality of life.

Author details

Pornanong Aramwit[1*] and Ouppatham Supasyndh[2]

*Address all correspondence to: aramwit@gmail.com

1 Bioactive Resources for Innovative Clinical Applications Research Unit and Department of Pharmacy Practice, Faculty of Pharmaceutical Sciences, Chulalongkorn University, PhayaThai Road, Phatumwan, Bangkok, Thailand

2 Division of Nephrology, Department of Medicine, Phramongkutklao Hospital and College of Medicine, Bangkok, Thailand

References

[1] Che-Yi, C., C.Y. Wen, K. Min-Tsung, et al., Acupuncture in haemodialysis patients at the Quchi (LI11) acupoint for refractory uraemic pruritus. Nephrol Dial Transplant, 2005. 20(9): p. 1912-1915.

[2] Schwartz, I.F. and A. Iaina, Management of uremic pruritus. Semin Dial, 2000. 13(3): p. 177-180.

[3] Cho, Y.L., H.N. Liu, T.P. Huang, et al., Uremic pruritus: roles of parathyroid hormone and substance P. J Am Acad Dermatol, 1997. 36(4): p. 538-543.

[4] Pico, M.R., A. Lugo-Somolinos, J.L. Sanchez, et al., Cutaneous alterations in patients with chronic renal failure. Int J Dermatol, 1992. 31(12): p. 860-863.

[5] Szepietowski, J.C. and R.A. Schwartz, Uremic pruritus. Int J Dermatol, 1998. 37(4): p. 247-253.

[6] Stahle-Backdahl, M., Uremic pruritis. Clinical and experimental studies. Acta Dermatol Venereol (Stockh), 1989. Suppl 145: p. 1-38.

[7] Pisoni, R.L., B. Wikstrom, S.J. Elder, et al., Pruritus in haemodialysis patients: International results from the Dialysis Outcomes and Practice Patterns Study (DOPPS). Nephrol Dial Transplant, 2006. 21(12): p. 3495-3505.

[8] Khanna, D., A. Singal, and O.P. Kalra, Comparison of cutaneous manifestations in chronic kidney disease with or without dialysis. Postgrad Med J, 2010. 86(1021): p. 641-647.

[9] Gilchrest, B.A., R.S. Stern, T.I. Steinman, et al., Clinical features of pruritus among patients undergoing maintenance hemodialysis. Arch Dermatol, 1982. 118(3): p. 154-156.

[10] Szepietowski, J.C., Selected elements of the pathogenesis of pruritus in hemodialysis patients: My own study. Med Sci Monit, 1996. 2: p. 343-347.

[11] Young, A.W., Jr., E.W. Sweeney, D.S. David, et al., Dermatologic evaluation of pruritus in patients on hemodialysis. N Y State J Med, 1973. 73(22): p. 2670-2674.

[12] Stahle-Backdahl, M., O. Hagermark, and L.E. Lins, Pruritus in patients on maintenance hemodialysis. Acta Med Scand, 1988. 224(1): p. 55-60.

[13] Villa, T., J. Gommer, and A. Scates, Role of gabapentin in the treatment of uremic pruritus. Ann Pharmcother, 2008. 42(7): p. 1080-1084.

[14] Cormia, F.E., Experimental histamine pruritus. I. Influence of physical and psychological factors on threshold reactivity. J Invest Dermatol, 1952. 19(1): p. 21-34.

[15] Patel, T.S., B.I. Freedman, and G. Yosipovitch, An update on pruritus associated with CKD. Am J Kidney Dis, 2007. 50(1): p. 11-20.

[16] Markova, A., J. Lester, J. Wang, et al., Diagnosis of common dermopathies in dialysis patients: a review and update. Semin Dial, 2012. 25(4): p. 408-418.

[17] Yosipovitch, G., I. Zucker, G. Boner, et al., A questionnaire for the assessment of pruritus: validation in uremic patients. Acta Derm Venereol, 2001. 81(2): p. 108-111.

[18] Zucker, I., G. Yosipovitch, M. David, et al., Prevalence and characterization of uremic pruritus in patients undergoing hemodialysis: uremic pruritus is still a major problem for patients with end-stage renal disease. J Am Acad Dermatol, 2003. 49(5): p. 842-846.

[19] Mistik, S., S. Utas, A. Ferahbas, et al., An epidemiology study of patients with uremic pruritus. J Eur Acad Dermatol Venereol, 2006. 20(6): p. 672-678.

[20] Udayakumar, P., S. Balasubramanian, K.S. Ramalingam, et al., Cutaneous manifestations in patients with chronic renal failure on hemodialysis. Indian J Dermatol Venereol Leprol, 2006. 72(2): p. 119-125.

[21] Balaskas, E.V. and E. Grapsa, Uremic pruritus is a poor prognostic factor of outcome. Perit Dial Int, 1995. 15(2): p. 177.

[22] Dar, N.R. and A. Akhter, Clinical characteristics of uremic pruritus in patients undergoing haemodialysis. J Coll Physicians Surg Pak, 2006. 16(2): p. 94-96.

[23] Robinson-Bostom, L. and J.J. DiGiovanna, Cutaneous manifestations of end-stage renal disease. J Am Acad Dermatol, 2000. 43(6): p. 975-986;quiz 987-990.

[24] Southi, P. and C. Commens, Pruritus in dialysis patients. Med J Aust, 1987. 146(7): p. 397, 400.

[25] Balaskas, E.V., M. Chu, R.P. Uldall, et al., Pruritus in continuous ambulatory peritoneal dialysis and hemodialysis patients. Perit Dial Int, 1993. 13 Suppl 2: p. S527-532.

[26] Mettang, T., P. Fritz, J. Weber, et al., Uremic pruritus in patients on hemodialysis or continuous ambulatory peritoneal dialysis (CAPD). The role of plasma histamine and skin mast cells. Clin Nephrol, 1990. 34(3): p. 136-141.

[27] Tapia, L., Pruritus on hemodialysis. Int J Dermatol, 1979. 18(3): p. 217-218.

[28] Szepietowski, J.C., M. Sikora, M. Kusztal, et al., Uremic pruritus: a clinical study of maintenance hemodialysis patients. J Dermatol, 2002. 29(10): p. 621-627.

[29] Keithi-Reddy, S.R., T.V. Patel, A.W. Armstrong, et al., Uremic pruritus. Kidney Int, 2007. 72(3): p. 373-377.

[30] Friga, V., A. Linos, and D.A. Linos, Is aluminum toxicity responsible for uremic pruritus in chronic hemodialysis patients? Nephron, 1997. 75(1): p. 48-53.

[31] Zakrzewska-Pniewska, B. and M. Jedras, Is pruritus in chronic uremic patients related to peripheral somatic and autonomic neuropathy? Study by R-R interval variation test (RRIV) and by sympathetic skin response (SSR). Neurophysiol Clin, 2001. 31(3): p. 181-193.

[32] Kurban, M.S., A. Boueiz, and A.G. Kibbi, Cutaneous manifestations of chronic kidney disease. Clin Dermatol, 2008. 26(3): p. 255-264.

[33] Hiroshige, K. and A. Kuroiwa, Uremic pruritus. Int J Artif Organs, 1996. 19(5): p. 265-267.

[34] Akizawa, T., M. Suzuki, T. Akiba, et al., Clinical effects of maxacalcitol on secondary hyperparathyroidism of uremic patients. Am J Kidney Dis, 2001. 38(4 Suppl 1): p. S147-151.

[35] Kyriazis, J. and J. Glotsos, Dialysate calcium concentration of</=1.25 mmol/l: is it effective in suppressing uremic pruritus? Nephron, 2000. 84(1): p. 85-86.

[36] Hagermark, O. and C.F. Wahlgren, Some methods for evaluating clinical itch and their application for studying pathophysiological mechanisms. J Dermatol Sci, 1992. 4(2): p. 55-62.

[37] Gilchrest, B.A., J.W. Rowe, and M.C. Mihm, Jr., Clinical and histological skin changes in chronic renal failure: evidence for a dialysis-resistant, transplant-responsive microangiopathy. Lancet, 1980. 2(8207): p. 1271-1275.

[38] Matsumoto, M., K. Ichimaru, and A. Horie, Pruritus and mast cell proliferation of the skin in end stage renal failure. Clin Nephrol, 1985. 23(6): p. 285-288.

[39] Landing, B.H., T.R. Wells, and M.L. Williamson, Anatomy of eccrine sweat glands in children with chronic renal insufficiency and other fatal chronic diseases. Am J Clin Pathol, 1970. 54(1): p. 15-21.

[40] Rosen, T., Uremic pruritus: a review. Cutis, 1979. 23(6): p. 790-792.

[41] Yosipovitch, G., E. Tur, G. Morduchowicz, et al., Skin surface pH, moisture, and pruritus in haemodialysis patients. Nephrol Dial Transplant, 1993. 8(10): p. 1129-1132.

[42] Ostlere, L.S., C. Taylor, R. Baillod, et al., Relationship between pruritus, transepidermal water loss, and biochemical markers of renal itch in haemodialysis patients. Nephrol Dial Transplant, 1994. 9(9): p. 1302-1304.

[43] Morton, C.A., M. Lafferty, C. Hau, et al., Pruritus and skin hydration during dialysis. Nephrol Dial Transplant, 1996. 11(10): p. 2031-2036.

[44] Carmichael, A.J., M.M. McHugh, A.M. Martin, et al., Serological markers of renal itch in patients receiving long term haemodialysis. Br Med J (Clin Res Ed), 1988. 296(6636): p. 1575.

[45] Graf, H., J. Kovarik, H.K. Stummvoll, et al., Disappearance of uraemic pruritus after lowering dialysate magnesium concentration. Br Med J, 1979. 2(6203): p. 1478-1479.

[46] Massry, S.G., M.M. Popovtzer, J.W. Coburn, et al., Intractable pruritus as a manifestation of secondary hyperparathyroidism in uremia. Disappearance of itching after subtotal parathyroidectomy. N Engl J Med, 1968. 279(13): p. 697-700.

[47] Dimkovic, N., L. Djukanovic, A. Radmilovic, et al., Uremic pruritus and skin mast cells. Nephron, 1992. 61(1): p. 5-9.

[48] Dallapiccola, B., G. Tataranni, and A. Farinelli, Uraemia and mast-cell proliferation. Lancet, 1972. 1(7762): p. 1231.

[49] Tsakalos, N.D., T.C. Theoharides, S.K. Kops, et al., Induction of mast cell secretion by parathormone. Biochem Pharmacol, 1983. 32(2): p. 355-360.

[50] Leong, S.O., C.C. Tan, W.C. Lye, et al., Dermal mast cell density and pruritus in end-stage renal failure. Ann Acad Med Singapore, 1994. 23(3): p. 327-329.

[51] Szepietowski, J., T. Thepen, W.A. van Vloten, et al., Pruritus and mast cell proliferation in the skin of haemodialysis patients. Inflamm Res, 1995. 44 Suppl 1: p. S84-85.

[52] Stockenhuber, F., R.W. Kurz, K. Sertl, et al., Increased plasma histamine levels in uraemic pruritus. Clin Sci (Lond), 1990. 79(5): p. 477-482.

[53] Kuypers, D.R., Skin problems in chronic kidney disease. Nat Clin Pract Nephrol, 2009. 5(3): p. 157-170.

[54] Lugon, J.R., Uremic pruritus: a review. Hemodial Int, 2005. 9(2): p. 180-188.

[55] Francos, G.C., Y.C. Kauh, S.D. Gittlen, et al., Elevated plasma histamine in chronic uremia. Effects of ketotifen on pruritus. Int J Dermatol, 1991. 30(12): p. 884-889.

[56] De Filippi, C., R. Regazzini, V. Piazza, et al., Uraemic pruritus is not related to plasma histamine concentrations. Clin Exp Dermatol, 1995. 20(4): p. 294-296.

[57] Ponticelli, C. and P.L. Bencini, Uremic pruritus: a review. Nephron, 1992. 60(1): p. 1-5.

[58] Urbonas, A., R.A. Schwartz, and J.C. Szepietowski, Uremic pruritus--an update. Am J Nephrol, 2001. 21(5): p. 343-350.

[59] Pereira, B.J. and C.A. Dinarello, Production of cytokines and cytokine inhibitory proteins in patients on dialysis. Nephrol Dial Transplant, 1994. 9 Suppl 2: p. 60-71.

[60] Chen, Y.C., W.T. Chiu, and M.S. Wu, Therapeutic effect of topical gamma-linolenic acid on refractory uremic pruritus. Am J Kidney Dis, 2006. 48(1): p. 69-76.

[61] Szepietowski, J.C., A. Reich, and T. Szepietowski, Emollients with endocannabinoids in the treatment of uremic pruritus: discussion of the therapeutic options. Ther Apher Dial, 2005. 9(3): p. 277-279.

[62] Chodorowska, G., A. Wysokinski, and J. Chodorowski, Uremic pruritus in the chronic renal failure patients. Ann Univ Mariae Curie Sklodowska Med, 2004. 59(1): p. 174-179.

[63] Mathur, V.S., J. Lindberg, M. Germain, et al., A longitudinal study of uremic pruritus in hemodialysis patients. Clin J Am Soc Nephrol, 2010. 5(8): p. 1410-1419.

[64] Kfoury, L.W. and M.A. Jurdi, Uremic pruritus. J Nephrol, 2012. 25(5): p. 644-652.

[65] Chou, F.F., J.C. Ho, S.C. Huang, et al., A study on pruritus after parathyroidectomy for secondary hyperparathyroidism. J Am Coll Surg, 2000. 190(1): p. 65-70.

[66] Kosmadakis, G.C. and N. Zerefos, Uremic pruritus. Int J Artif Organs, 2006. 29(10): p. 938-943.

[67] Lin, H.H., Y.L. Liu, J.H. Liu, et al., Uremic pruritus, cytokines, and polymethylmethacrylate artificial kidney. Artif Organs, 2008. 32(6): p. 468-472.

[68] Duque, M.I., S. Thevarajah, Y.H. Chan, et al., Uremic pruritus is associated with higher kt/V and serum calcium concentration. Clin Nephrol, 2006. 66(3): p. 184-191.

[69] Carmichael, A.J., F. Dickinson, M.I. McHugh, et al., Magnesium free dialysis for uraemic pruritus. BMJ, 1988. 297(6663): p. 1584-1585.

[70] Hiroshige, K., N. Kabashima, M. Takasugi, et al., Optimal dialysis improves uremic pruritus. Am J Kidney Dis, 1995. 25(3): p. 413-419.

[71] Hampers, C.L., A.I. Katz, R.E. Wilson, et al., Disappearance of "uremic" itching after subtotal parathyroidectomy. N Engl J Med, 1968. 279(13): p. 695-697.

[72] Balaskas, E.V. and D.G. Oreopoulos, Uremic pruritus. Nephrol Dial Transplant, 1992. 21: p. 192-206.

[73] Fjellner, B. and O. Hagermark, Influence of ultraviolet light on itch and flare reactions in human skin induced by histamine and the histamine liberator compound 48/80. Acta Derm Venereol, 1982. 62(2): p. 137-140.

[74] Fjellner, B., Experimental and clinical pruritus. Studies on some putative peripheral mediators. The influence of ultraviolet light and transcutaneous nerve stimulation. Acta Derm Venereol Suppl (Stockh), 1981. 97: p. 1-34.

[75] Gilchrest, B.A., J.W. Rowe, R.S. Brown, et al., Ultraviolet phototherapy of uremic pruritus. Long-term results and possible mechanism of action. Ann Intern Med, 1979. 91(1): p. 17-21.

[76] Saltzer, E., Relief from uremic pruritus: A therapeutic approach. Cutis, 1975. 16: p. 298-299.

[77] Blachley, J.D., D.M. Blankenship, A. Menter, et al., Uremic pruritus: skin divalent ion content and response to ultraviolet phototherapy. Am J Kidney Dis, 1985. 5(5): p. 237-241.

[78] Gilchrest, B.A., J.W. Rowe, R.S. Brown, et al., Relief of uremic pruritus with ultraviolet phototherapy. N Engl J Med, 1977. 297(3): p. 136-138.

[79] Gilchrest, B.A., Ultraviolet phototherapy of uremic pruritus. Int J Dermatol, 1979. 18(9): p. 741-748.

[80] Seckin, D., Z. Demircay, and O. Akin, Generalized pruritus treated with narrowband UVB. Int J Dermatol, 2007. 46(4): p. 367-370.

[81] Ada, S., D. Seckin, I. Budakoglu, et al., Treatment of uremic pruritus with narrowband ultraviolet B phototherapy: an open pilot study. J Am Acad Dermatol, 2005. 53(1): p. 149-151.

[82] Spiro, J.G., S. Scott, J. MacMillan, et al., Treatment of uremic pruritus with blue light. Photodermatol, 1985. 2(5): p. 319-321.

[83] Hongmei, G., Z. Wanxiang, and W. Ying, Accupuncture treatment for 34 cases of uremic cutaneous pruritus. J Tradit Chin Med, 2002. 22: p. 29-30.

[84] Melzack, R. and P.D. Wall, Pain mechanisms: a new theory. Science, 1965. 150(3699): p. 971-979.

[85] Shapiro, R. and H. Stockard, Successful treament of uremic pruritus: The acupuncture approach revisited. Dial Transplant, 2003. 32: p. 257-265.

[86] Kilic Akca, N., S. Tasci, and N. Karatas, Effect of acupressure on patients in Turkey receiving hemodialysis treatment for uremic pruritus. Altern Ther Health Med, 2013. 19(5): p. 12-18.

[87] Duo, L.J., Electrical needle therapy of uremic pruritus. Nephron, 1987. 47(3): p. 179-183.

[88] Hsu, M.C., H.W. Chen, Y.J. Hwu, et al., Effects of thermal therapy on uremic pruritus and biochemical parameters in patients having haemodialysis. J Adv Nurs, 2009. 65(11): p. 2397-2408.

[89] Bernstein, J.E., Capsaicin in dermatologic disease. Semin Dermatol, 1988. 7(4): p. 304-309.

[90] Okada, K. and K. Matsumoto, Effect of skin care with an emollient containing a high water content on mild uremic pruritus. Ther Apher Dial, 2004. 8(5): p. 419-422.

[91] Manenti, L., A. Vaglio, and P.P. Borgatti, Gabapentin as a therapeutic option in uremic pruritus. Kidney Int, 2008. 73(4): p. 512; author reply 512-513.

[92] Fantini, F., A. Baraldi, and A. Pincelli, Neuron-specific enolase-immunoreactive fibres in uremic patients. Acta Derm Venereol, 1990. 70(4): p. 363-365.

[93] Denman, S.T., A review of pruritus. J Am Acad Dermatol, 1986. 14(3): p. 375-392.

[94] Balaskas, E., J.C. Szepietowski, D. Bessis, et al., Randomized, double-blind study with glycerol and paraffin in uremic xerosis. Clin J Am Soc Nephrol, 2011. 6(4): p. 748-752.

[95] Szepietowski, J.C., T. Szepietowski, and A. Reich, Efficacy and tolerance of the cream containing structured physiological lipids with endocannabinoids in the treatment of uremic pruritus: a preliminary study. Acta Dermatovenerol Croat, 2005. 13(2): p. 97-103.

[96] Aramwit, P. and A. Sangcakul, The effects of sericin cream on wound healing in rats. Biosci Biotechnol Biochem, 2007. 71(10): p. 2473-2477.

[97] Zhaorigetu, S., N. Yanaka, M. Sasaki, et al., Inhibitory effects of silk protein, sericin on UVB-induced acute damage and tumor promotion by reducing oxidative stress in the skin of hairless mouse. J Photochem Photobiol B, 2003. 71(1-3): p. 11-17.

[98] Zhaorigetu, S., N. Yanaka, M. Sasaki, et al., Silk protein, sericin, suppresses DMBA-TPA-induced mouse skin tumorigenesis by reducing oxidative stress, inflammatory responses and endogenous tumor promoter TNF-alpha. Oncol Rep, 2003. 10(3): p. 537-543.

[99] Aramwit, P., S. Damrongsakkul, S. Kanokpanont, et al., Properties and antityrosinase activity of sericin from various extraction methods. Biotechnol Appl Biochem, 2010. 55(2): p. 91-98.

[100] Aramwit, P., T. Siritientong, S. Kanokpanont, et al., Formulation and characterization of silk sericin-PVA scaffold crosslinked with genipin. Int J Biol Macromol, 2010. 47(5): p. 668-675.

[101] Aramwit, P., S. Kanokpanont, W. De-Eknamkul, et al., Monitoring of inflammatory mediators induced by silk sericin. J Biosci Bioeng, 2009. 107(5): p. 556-561.

[102] Aramwit, P., O. Keongamaroon, T. Siritientong, et al., Sericin cream reduces pruritus in hemodialysis patients: a randomized, double-blind, placebo-controlled experimental study. BMC Nephrol, 2012. 13: p. 119.

[103] Rumsfield, J.A. and D.P. West, Topical capsaicin in dermatologic and peripheral pain disorders. DICP, 1991. 25(4): p. 381-387.

[104] Virus, R.M. and G.F. Gebhart, Pharmacologic actions of capsaicin: apparent involvement of substance P and serotonin. Life Sci, 1979. 25(15): p. 1273-1283.

[105] Tarng, D.C., Y.L. Cho, H.N. Liu, et al., Hemodialysis-related pruritus: a double-blind, placebo-controlled, crossover study of capsaicin 0.025% cream. Nephron, 1996. 72(4): p. 617-622.

[106] Breneman, D.L., J.S. Cardone, R.F. Blumsack, et al., Topical capsaicin for treatment of hemodialysis-related pruritus. J Am Acad Dermatol, 1992. 26(1): p. 91-94.

[107] Pauli-Magnus, C., S. Klumpp, D.M. Alscher, et al., Short-term efficacy of tacrolimus ointment in severe uremic pruritus. Perit Dial Int, 2000. 20(6): p. 802-803.

[108] Ghorbani, A.R., A. Feily, A. Khalili, et al., Lack of efficacy of topical calcineurin inhibitor pimecrolimus 1% on pruritus of severely uremic patients: a randomized double-blind study in 60 patients. Dermatitis, 2011. 22(3): p. 167-168.

[109] Duque, M.I., G. Yosipovitch, A.B. Fleischer, Jr., et al., Lack of efficacy of tacrolimus ointment 0.1% for treatment of hemodialysis-related pruritus: a randomized, double-blind, vehicle-controlled study. J Am Acad Dermatol, 2005. 52(3 Pt 1): p. 519-521.

[110] Bergasa, N.V., T.L. Talbot, D.W. Alling, et al., A controlled trial of naloxone infusions for the pruritus of chronic cholestasis. Gastroenterology, 1992. 102(2): p. 544-549.

[111] Jones, E.A. and N.V. Bergasa, The pruritus of cholestasis and the opioid system. JAMA, 1992. 268(23): p. 3359-3362.

[112] Peer, G., S. Kivity, O. Agami, et al., Randomised crossover trial of naltrexone in uraemic pruritus. Lancet, 1996. 348(9041): p. 1552-1554.

[113] Wikstrom, B., R. Gellert, S.D. Ladefoged, et al., Kappa-opioid system in uremic pruritus: multicenter, randomized, double-blind, placebo-controlled clinical studies. J Am Soc Nephrol, 2005. 16(12): p. 3742-3747.

[114] Balaskas, E.V. and R.P. Uldall, Erythropoietin treatment does not improve uremic pruritus. Perit Dial Int, 1992. 12(3): p. 330-331.

[115] De Marchi, S., E. Cecchin, D. Villalta, et al., Relief of pruritus and decreases in plasma histamine concentrations during erythropoietin therapy in patients with uremia. N Engl J Med, 1992. 326(15): p. 969-974.

[116] Balaskas, E.V., G.I. Bamihas, M. Karamouzis, et al., Histamine and serotonin in uremic pruritus: effect of ondansetron in CAPD-pruritic patients. Nephron, 1998. 78(4): p. 395-402.

[117] Ashmore, S.D., C.H. Jones, C.G. Newstead, et al., Ondansetron therapy for uremic pruritus in hemodialysis patients. Am J Kidney Dis, 2000. 35(5): p. 827-831.

[118] Naini, A.E., A.A. Harandi, S. Khanbabapour, et al., Gabapentin: a promising drug for the treatment of uremic pruritus. Saudi J Kidney Dis Transpl, 2007. 18(3): p. 378-381.

[119] Gunal, A.I., G. Ozalp, T.K. Yoldas, et al., Gabapentin therapy for pruritus in haemodialysis patients: a randomized, placebo-controlled, double-blind trial. Nephrol Dial Transplant, 2004. 19(12): p. 3137-3139.

[120] Razeghi, E., D. Eskandari, M.R. Ganji, et al., Gabapentin and uremic pruritus in hemodialysis patients. Ren Fail, 2009. 31(2): p. 85-90.

[121] Legroux-Crespel, E., J. Cledes, and L. Misery, A comparative study on the effects of naltrexone and loratadine on uremic pruritus. Dermatology, 2004. 208(4): p. 326-330.

[122] Peck, L.W., E.R. Monsen, and S. Ahmad, Effect of three sources of long-chain fatty acids on the plasma fatty acid profile, plasma prostaglandin E2 concentrations, and pruritus symptoms in hemodialysis patients. Am J Clin Nutr, 1996. 64(2): p. 210-214.

[123] Yoshimoto-Furuie, K., K. Yoshimoto, T. Tanaka, et al., Effects of oral supplementation with evening primrose oil for six weeks on plasma essential fatty acids and uremic skin symptoms in hemodialysis patients. Nephron, 1999. 81(2): p. 151-159.

[124] Tapia, L., J.S. Cheigh, D.S. David, et al., Pruritus in dialysis patients treated with parenteral lidocaine. N Engl J Med, 1977. 296(5): p. 261-262.

[125] Hagermark, O., P. Anderson, and K. Nordlind, Failure of mexiletine to relieve severe pruritus. Dermatologica, 1984. 169(4): p. 188-190.

[126] Boulton-Jones, J.M., J.G. Sissons, and E.R. Harrison, Letter: Itching in renal failure. Lancet, 1974. 1(7853): p. 355.

[127] Giovannetti, S., G. Barsotti, A. Cupisti, et al., Oral activated charcoal in patients with uremic pruritus. Nephron, 1995. 70(2): p. 193-196.

[128] Pederson, J.A., B.J. Matter, A.W. Czerwinski, et al., Relief of idiopathic generalized pruritus in dialysis patients treated with activated oral charcoal. Ann Intern Med, 1980. 93(3): p. 446-448.

[129] Silverberg, D.S., A. Iaina, E. Reisin, et al., Cholestyramine in uraemic pruritus. Br Med J, 1977. 1(6063): p. 752-753.

[130] Yatzidis, H., P. Digenis, and C. Tountas, Heparin treatment of uremic itching. JAMA, 1972. 222(9): p. 1183.

[131] Hodak, E., G. Yosipovitch, M. David, et al., Low-dose low-molecular-weight heparin (enoxaparin) is beneficial in lichen planus: a preliminary report. J Am Acad Dermatol, 1998. 38(4): p. 564-568.

[132] Silva, S.R., P.C. Viana, N.V. Lugon, et al., Thalidomide for the treatment of uremic pruritus: a crossover randomized double-blind trial. Nephron, 1994. 67(3): p. 270-273.

[133] Bousquet, J., J.P. Rivory, M. Maheut, et al., Double-blind, placebo-controlled study of nicergoline in the treatment of pruritus in patients receiving maintenance hemodialysis. J Allergy Clin Immunol, 1989. 83(4): p. 825-828.

[134] Namazi, M.R., M.K. Fallahzadeh, and J. Roozbeh, Nicotinamide as a potential novel addition to the anti-uremic pruritus weaponry. Saudi J Kidney Dis Transpl, 2009. 20(2): p. 291-292.

Chapter 3

Treatment Option for Uremic Pruritus

Hiromichi Suzuki, Hiroshi Omata and Hiroo Kumagai

Additional information is available at the end of the chapter

http://dx.doi.org/10.5772/59493

1. Introduction

Uremic pruritus remains a frequent concern for hemodialysis [HD] patients with the most frustrating and disabling symptoms. Nearly 90% of patients on dialysis suffer from pruritus. Until present, there have been a lot of reviews discussing the pathophysiology and treatment of pruritus[1-14]. Previously, the word "uremic pruritus" has been used for symptoms of itching because it is a common skin derangement in patients with advanced renal failure. However, the usage of "uremic" may cause confusion because pruritus is not found in patients with acute kidney injury. In this regard Paitel et al. [9] recently proposed the term, "chronic kidney disease (CKD)-associated pruritus" instead of "uremic pruritus" as a more precise nomenclature. In this review, the words "uremic pruritus", "CKD-associated pruritus" and "pruritus" are used interchangeably because the authors would like to respect each author's contribution. The prevalence of CKD-associated pruritus was found to range from 15-90% of patients [15, 16]. Recent data from the Dialysis Outcomes and Practice Patterns Study (DOPPS) reported that the prevalence of CKD-associated pruritus was 42% [17].

2. Clinical characteristics of CKD-associated pruritus

In patients with CKD, skin lesions are usually not found. Generally, skin lesions are secondary changes such as excoriations with or without impetigo, linear crusts, papules, and ulcerations. Half of patients have generalized itching, and in the other half, pruritus is localized to the back, limbs, chest or head. Pruritus is intermittent or prolonged over hours and days, and becomes worse at night [18, 19]. Mettang & Krener [14] stated in their review that the diagnosis of uremic pruritus may be challenging because many patients with end-stage renal disease (ESRD) are suffering from other diseases, such as cardiovascular diseases, diabetes mellitus, chronic liver or hematological diseases, which may provoke itching either by itself or by medication given to treat these entities.

3. Why is pruritus problematic?

A recent longitudinal study of CKD-associated pruritus in HD patients have clearly demonstrated that significant associations were found among itching intensity, severity, and health-related quality of life [HR-QOL] measures in domains such as mood, social relations, and sleep. In Japan, Narita et al. [16] recruited a total of 1773 patients on HD and evaluated the severity of pruritus with a visual analogue scale (VAS). Four hundred and fifty-three patients had severe pruritus with a VAS score of more than or equal to 7.0. Further, 70% of these patients complained of sleep disturbances. From these data, it is clear that patients who suffer from pruritus also have a lower HR-QOL including sleep disturbances which may lead to poor prognosis.

4. Treatment for CKD-associated pruritus

4.1. Modification of dialysis techniques

The use of biocompatible dialysis membranes has been reported to reduce the prevalence of pruritus in HD patients [7]. However, it still remains uncertain whether alterations in dialysis therapy including changes in dialysis membrane can reduce pruritus [20, 21] or not [22]. Hiroshige et al. [23] analyzed data on 59 HD patients, who did not have disorders in calcium and phosphate metabolism, and found that more than 60% of them suffered from disabling pruritus possibly related to chronic uremia. Blood urea nitrogen [BUN] and plasma β_2-microglobulin, both of which are biochemical factors that are associated with the prevalence of pruritus and dialysis efficacy, were investigated and calculated by urea kinetics. After 3 months without changing the dialysis prescriptions, 16 patients had significant reductions of the pruritic score ranging from 12.6 ±5.1 to 6.3 ±3.2 ($P < 0.001$). From this study, the authors concluded that higher dialysis efficacy with good nutritional state reduces the prevalence and degree of pruritus in HD patients.

Previously, Graf et al. [24] reported that lowering the dialysate magnesium concentration can restore nerve conduction velocity towards normal in patients receiving HD, and this could be the reason for the complete disappearance of pruritus in the study by Hiroshige et al [25]. In contrast, Carmichael et al. [25] failed to demonstrate a beneficial effect of reduction in magnesium on pruritus. In their trial, although they showed that a magnesium-free dialysis fluid corrected hypermagnesaemia, it failed to improve renal itch. In addition, the fall in serum magnesium concentration was associated with an increased concentration of parathyroid hormone, as previously noted, with the potential of producing renal osteodystrophy in the long term. It is therefore difficult to generalize the findings from the study by Hiroshige and colleagues.

The role of calcium in the dialysate was discussed by Kyriazi et al. [26], who showed that reduction in dialysis calcium concentrations from 1.75 to 1.0 mmol/L was associated with a 41.421 ± 8.47% ($P < 0.05$) relief from itching in 4 HD patients, indicating that at least in some uremic individuals, ionized calcium (iCa) has a pivotal role in the neuropathophysiology of CKD-associated pruritus. It has been postulated that calcium contributes to itching by influencing the degranulation of cutaneous mast cells, thus appearing to be a modifier rather than an initiator of CKD-associated pruritus.

Polymethylmethacrylate (PMMA) artificial kidney (AK) has been reported to adsorb more serum cytokines than other high-flux AK. In 30 patients with severe uremic pruritus out of 300 chronic patients in a single center who entered this prospective study, the dialyzers were changed to PMMA AK for 4 weeks. There were no significant differences in the laboratory assay results including predialysis serum BUN, creatinine (Cr), $\beta_2$microglobulin, calcium, phosphate, calcium-phosphate product, intact parathyroid hormone (iPTH), ferritin, hematocrit, high-sensitivity C-reactive protein (hsCRP), interleukin (IL)-1β, IL-2, IL-6, IL-18, tumor necrosis factor (TNF)-α, and Kt/V. PMMA AK was effective in reducing the pruritus score from 23.46 ± 11.94 to 7.38 ± 6.42 ($P < 0.001$). The effect of uremic pruritus relief appeared after 1 week of PMMA AK use. In spite of this study, the mechanism for the beneficial effect of PMMA AK on uremic pruritus remains to be determined. However, it is proposed that PMMA AK may be a useful adjuvant therapy in chronic HD patients with severe uremic pruritus.

In line with this study, Kato et al. [27] carried out a prospective and crossover trial to investigate the effect of PMMA membrane on pruritus of HD patients with measurements of circulating levels of TNF-α and soluble TNF receptors (sTNFR-I, sTNFR-II) in 19 HD patients, who were complicated with prolonged severe pruritus for 6 months. However, there was no association between the degree of pruritus and circulating sTNFR-I and II values, although skin itching scale was significantly decreased following the use of PMMA membrane for 3 months. Combining with these finding together, it could be proposed that the PMMA dialyzer can improve renal itching.

4.2. Topical treatments

Emollients have been shown to be beneficial in patients with CKD-associated pruritus [28, 29, 30]. In general, emollients are proposed for use as first-line treatment. Among emollients, aqueous gels have been shown to reduce pruritus; previously, Okada and Matsumoto [31] demonstrated that emollients with high water content effectively reduced itch. In their report, 20 HD patients were divided into two groups; one group was treated with an aqueous gel containing 80% water (ADJUPEX Ensemble gel, ADJUPEX Co. Ltd. Tokyo, Japan) and another group did not receive any emollient treatment. The aqueous gel used in their study was composed by 80 g of water and 20 g of aloe vera extract, silk powder, naturally-derived vitamin E, squalane, and other naturally-derived ingredients. Moreover, the gel contained no synthetic and artificial substances. The emollient was applied twice daily for 2 weeks. VAS scores for itching at 2 weeks were significantly decreased compared with that at week 0. The results showed that an aqueous gel containing high water content effectively improves itching in HD patients with mild uremic pruritus. Besides, psychological discomfort also improved.

The effects of aromatherapy on mood and anxiety in HD patients had been reported by Itai et al. [32] that in HD patients, hiba oil is an effective, non-invasive treatment for depression and anxiety.

A cream with structured physiological lipids (DMS, Derma Membrane Structure) and endogenous cannabinoids was tested for 3 weeks in 21 subjects with pruritus [30]. A significant reduction in pruritus was noted during the test product application using both scales for itching intensity assessment ($P < 0.0001$). Pruritus was significantly decreased at the end of the 3-week treatment ($P = 0.02$) as compared to before treatment, and was completely eliminated in eight patients (38.1%). This is the first study to evaluate topical application of a preparation containing endocannabinoids in the treatment of uremic pruritus. Dvorak et al.[33] showed that treatment with cannabionoid receptor agonists produced reduction of histamine-induced itching and had vasodilation by these topical application.

Another naturally-derived agent that may be helpful in reducing pruritus is capsaicin, which is an alkaloid extracted from the common pepper plant and marketed as a topical analgesic. Capsaicin has a potential antipruritic property with desensitization of nociceptive nerve endings depletion of substance P and then might block the conductor of pruritus. Breneman et al. [34] carried out an open-label, uncontrolled trial and a double-blind, vehicle-controlled trial to evaluate the efficacy and safety of capsaicin 0.025% cream in the treatment of localized areas of pruritus in patients undergoing long term HD. They found marked relief of itching without serious treatment-related adverse reactions.

Further, Tarng et al. [35] reported that 19 HD patients with idiopathic, moderate (n = 5) to severe (n = 14) pruritus were examined in a double-blind, placebo-controlled, crossover study. The results showed that capsaicin was significantly more effective than placebo and a prolonged antipruritic effect was observed 8 weeks post-treatment. Moreover, no serious side effects were noted during the study and there were no significant changes in serum concentrations of albumin, calcium, phosphorus, alkaline phosphatase, or iPTH during the treatment with either capsaicin or placebo. According to their results, this study provides indirect evidence that in idiopathic pruritus in some patients on maintenance HD, substance P may be transmitted from the peripheral sensory neurons to the central nervous system because local application of capsaicin depletes the peripheral neurons of substance P and may block the conduction of pruritus. In another study, Weisshaar et al. [36] reported that 11 pruritic patients on HD and 10 controls were treated with capsaicin 0.05% liniment on the upper back three times daily for 5 days. They reported that topical capsaicin showed some antipruritic potency in HD patients, providing that topical capsaicin might be one of the choice for treatment for HD patients with pruritus.

In addition to the components described above, essential fatty acids and their derivatives are necessary for normal cutaneous function and are thus proposed as potential treatments of pruritus. Tamimi et al. [37] found that primrose oil rich in the essential fatty acid gamma-linolenic acid (GLA) may be beneficial in alleviating pruritus. Chen et al. [38] found that GLA-rich cream was better than placebo-based cream for alleviating uremic pruritus, thus it is a useful adjuvant in the management of refractory uremic pruritus.

A new topically active antipruritic medication has been derived from the Amazonian medicine Sangre de Grado [39]. The reported antipruritic effect on itch induced by insect bite was convincing, based on its role as a potent inhibitor of sensory afferent nerves. Moreover, Sangre de Grado is an effective analgesic and anti-inflammatory agent when applied topically.

Further, naturally-derived agents, chemical formulations, such as Tacrolimus, have also been studied, however there have been no convincing data reported until the present time [40, 41]. Topical steroids were also prescribed to these patients, probably based on the assumption that drugs used for itch in other conditions may also work on uremic pruritus, however, the absence of controlled studies and potential serious side effects of these agents dampen the routine prescription of such drugs to HD patients.

4.3. Ultraviolet irradiation

Ultraviolet, especially narrowband UVB, has been proposed as a potential therapeutic agent for pruritus. Although exact mechanisms of UVB therapy in CKD-associated pruritus is unknown, some possible explanations have been proposed such as inactivation of circulating pruritogenic substances [42, 43], suppression of histamine release from cutaneous mast cells [44], and reduction of cutaneous nerve fibers [45, 46]. Blachley et al. [47] reported that 17 patients presenting with severe pruritus were treated thrice weekly with total body exposure to either UVA or UVB light. UVB light resulted in resolution of pruritus in all cases. The mechanism by which UVB improves pruritus is not clear, but it has been suggested that it may in part be due to its ability to reduce cytokine production by lymphocytes.

4.4. Acupuncture

Acupuncture can be defined as the stimulation of anatomical points on the body using a variety of techniques for therapeutic purposes.

Recently, Kim et al. [48] reported a systemic review of acupuncture for treating uremic pruritus in patients with ESRD. According to their analysis, all of the included subjects reported beneficial effects of acupuncture. Che-yi et al. [49] randomized 40 HD patients with uremic pruritus into two groups and reported that; in group 1 (n = 20), acupuncture was applied unilaterally at the Quchi (LI11) acupoint thrice weekly for 1 month, and in group 2 (controls, n = 20), acupuncture was applied at a non-acupoint 2 cm lateral to Quchi (LI11) thrice weekly for 1 month. In their findings, pruritus scores before and after acupuncture, and at the 3-month follow-up were 38.3±4.3, 17.3± 5.5, and 16.5± 4.9 in group 1, and 38.3± 4.3, 37.5± 3.2, and 37.1± 5 in group 2 (controls), respectively. From these findings, the authors concluded that acupuncture at the Quchi (LI11) acupoint is an easy, safe, and effective method of relieving uremic pruritus.

In another study by Gao et al. [50], 68 cases were randomly divided by half into two groups, acupuncture or drug administration with chlor-trimenton and topical ointment for 2 weeks.

While receiving HD treatment, the acupuncture group received treatment at Quchi (LI11) with lifting-thrusting reducing method, and Zusanli (ST36) with lifting-thrusting reinforcing method for 30 min. In patients who received acupuncture therapy, after one course of treatment, 24 of 34 cases (70.6%) had complete alleviation of pruritus, 9 cases (26.5%) had obvious alleviation of pruritus, and 1 case had no improvement.

Sakurada et al. [51] reported that almost one-third of HD patients had undergone acupuncture or had a desire to try acupuncture treatment to manage common complications. Similar findings were also reported by Shapiro et al. [52] in an observational study. Further, electro-acupuncture was performed on 7 HD patients with pruritus. Surprisingly, complete relief after one session of acupuncture treatment was reported in 6 patients and effects lasted up to one year.

Our group recently demonstrated a marked improvement of symptoms related with pruritus. Acupuncture was administered in 12 HD patients 1 to 3 times a week for one year. With improvement of these symptoms, QOL as evaluated by short form 36 (SF-36) health survey showed a marked increase in physical activity and sleep quality (personal communication). Interestingly, the BUN levels were significantly decreased, and those of hemoglobin increased although it did not reach statistical significance (Figs. 1-3).

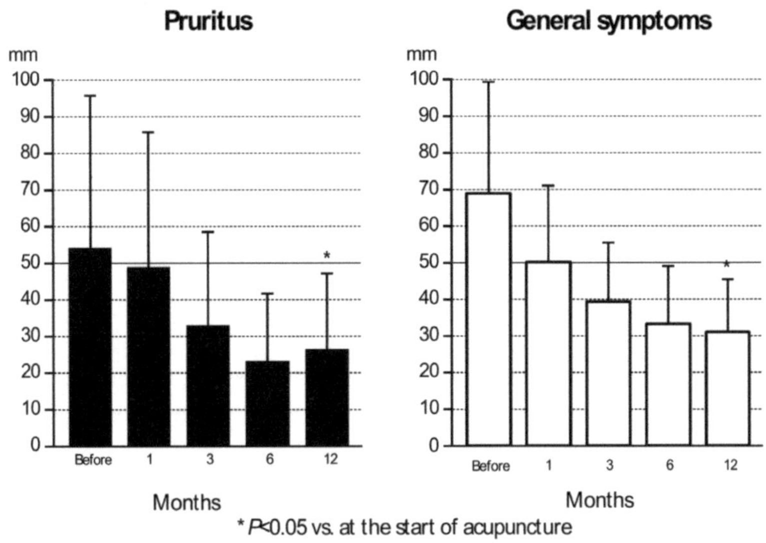

Figure 1. Changes in pruritus and general symptoms related with hemodialysis therapy by acupuncture 1 to 3 times a week for one year. Acupuncutre 1 to 3 times a week for one year produced a marked improvement in pruritus and general symptoms in patients with hemodialysis. * indicates P<0.05.

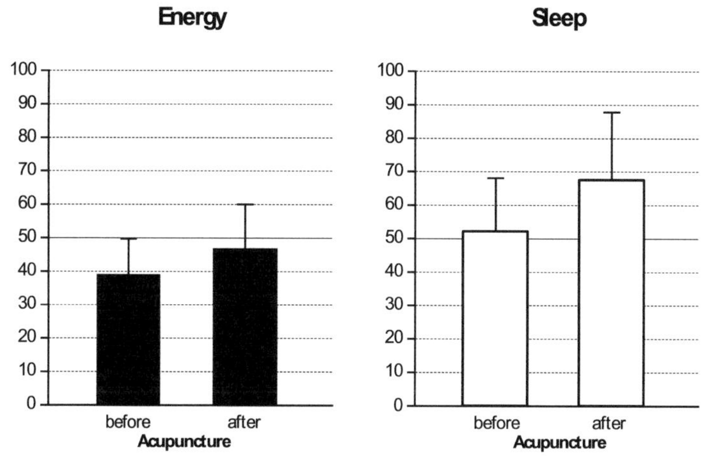

Figure 2. Changes in energy level and sleep of patients with hemodialysis by acupuncture 1 to 3 times a week for one year as evaluated by SF-36. Acupuncutre 1 to 3 times a week for one year produced a marked improvement in energy level and sleep in patients with hemodialysis.

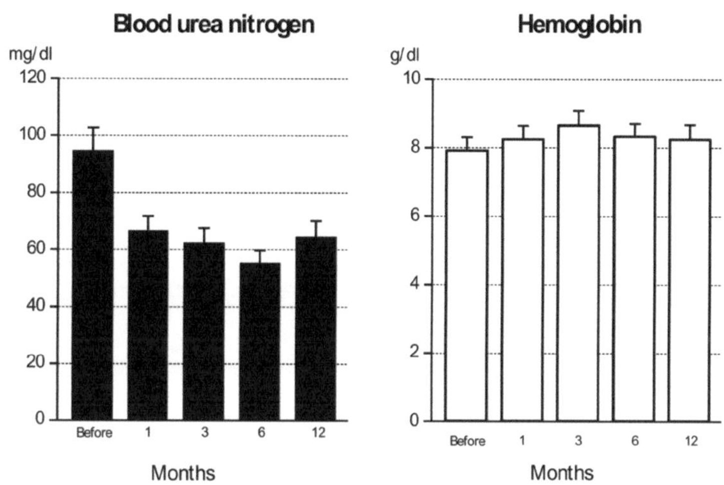

Figure 3. Changes in blood urea nitrogen and hemoglobin levels by acupuncture 1 to 3 times a week for one year. Acupuncutre 1 to 3 times a week for one year produced a marked improvement in blood urea nitrogen and hemoglobin levels in patients with hemodialysis.

4.5. Rubdown with Japanese dry towels

Our group examined the effects of "rubdown with Japanese dry towels" on CKD-associated pruritus. This method is a traditional Japanese alternative medical treatment to strengthen the barrier function of the skin. Briefly, subjects were naked or wore minimal clothing to maximally expose the skin of their body. Then, the subjects prepared three sets of Japanese dry towels made with cotton. These towels were cleansed with water and then dried under sunlight. After drying, the subjects gently rubbed their whole body with these towels, and if possible, this procedure was carried out in direct sunlight. The results are shown in Fig.4. The mechanism by which this traditional Japanese alternative medical procedure aids in symptom relief may be because skin-rubbing produces secretion of corticosteroid hormone through stimulation of the thalamus [53]. Further, skin-rubbing eliminates the bacterial flora on the surface of the skin [54]. In combination with ultraviolet rays, skin-rubbing may prevent intrusion of c-fiber from the dermis into the epidermis which is one of the causes of itch [55, 56]

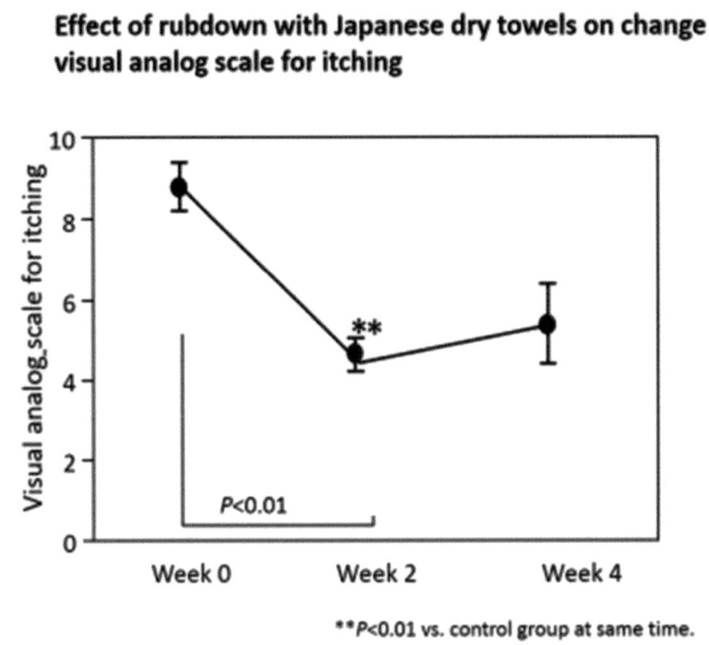

Figure 4. Effect of rubdown with Japanese dry towels on change in visual analog scale for itching. Manipulation by rubdown with Japanese dry towels produced a marked reduction in pruritus using the visual analog scale. ** indicates P<0.01.

4.6. Opioid antagonists

The use of opioid antagonists in uremic pruritus was first brought to our attention by Andersen et al. [57] when they published a case report about a terminally ill uremic patient successfully treated by naloxone for persistent itching. However, few studies were published, and these had conflicting findings. While Peer et al. [58] showed in a small placebo-controlled clinical trial that naltrexone, which is a μ-receptor antagonist, is effective, Pauli-Magnus et al. [40] failed to demonstrate any efficacy of naltrexone in the treatment of uremic pruritus. Later, Legroux-Crespel et al. [59] conducted a comparative study between naltrexone and loratadine, and concluded that naltrexone is not effective and not well-tolerated because of frequent side effects, except in a small subset of patients. More recently, another perspective was elaborated regarding the use of a κ-agonist, for κ -receptor stimulation inhibits μ-receptor effects both peripherally and centrally, and hence might inhibit itching induced by substance P. In line with this concept, Wikstrom et al. [60] conducted two multicenter, randomized, double-blind, placebo-controlled studies that enrolled 144 patients with uremic pruritus to receive post-dialysis intravenous treatment with either nalfurafine, a novel κ -receptor agonist, or placebo for 2 to 4 weeks. Statistically significant reductions in itching, itching intensity, excoriations, and sleep disturbances were noted in the nalfurafine group as compared to the placebo group.

In light of all these findings, Toray Industries, Inc., Japan, recently developed nalfurafine, with refined opioid receptor affinity and selectivity, as an agent for relief of pruritus [61, 62]. In studies using animal models, nalfurafine exerted antipruritic activity not only for antihistamine-sensitive itch, but also for antihistamine-resistant itch [63, 64].

Kumagai et al. [65] carried out a prospective, randomized, double-blind comparative study for 2 weeks to compare the antipruritic effect of oral nalfurafine (2.5 and 5.0 μg) with a placebo in 337 patients. The mean pruritus value as assessed by VAS was 75.2 mm during the pre-observation period, which decreased significantly to 50.9 in weeks 2. The mean decrease in VAS from baseline was significantly larger in the 2 μg (n=112, P = 0.0001) and 5 μg (n=114, P = 0.0002) nalfurafine groups than in the placebo group (n=111). However, adverse drug reactions (ADRs) occurred in 103 patients, and the incidence was 25.0% in the 2.5 μg group, 35.1% in the 5 μg group, and 16.2% in the placebo group. The most common ADR was insomnia, observed in 24 of the 226 nalfurafine patients (22.3%). It is interesting to note that the group that received placebo also had a similar decrease in itching. It is well known that placebo-induced expectancies have been shown to decrease pain in a manner reversible by opioid antagonists. This phenomenon is corroborated by the findings of Wager et al. [66], who demonstrated using functional magnetic resonance image that placebo analgesia was related to decreased brain activity in pain-sensitive brain regions, including the thalamus, insula, and anterior cingulate cortex.

Further, Kumagai et al. [67] carried out an open-label study examining the effects and ADRs of 52-week oral administration of nalfurafine hydrochloride in 211 HD patients with treatment-resistant itch. They found that the mean pruritus values as assessed by the VAS was 75.2 mm during the pre-observation period, which decreased significantly to 50.9 and 30.9 mm in weeks 52, indicating a long-lasting efficacy. ADRs occurred in 103 patients. Frequent ADRs were insomnia (19.4%), constipation (7.1%), and increased blood prolactin (3.3%).

5. Future perspectives

As stated in this review, recent advances in pathophysiology of itch and treatment for CKD-associated pruritus have improved this condition remarkably, however, there are still a lot of obstacles to overcome in order to achieve satisfactory comfort and relief from unpleasant symptoms stemming from pruritus. It is therefore of the utmost importance for investigators and physicians to study and research in this area.

Author details

Hiromichi Suzuki[1*], Hiroshi Omata [2] and Hiroo Kumagai[3]

*Address all correspondence to: iromichi@saitama-med.ac.jp

1 Department of Nephrology, Saitama Medical University, Japan

2 Department of Oriental Medicine, Saitama Medical University, Japan

3 Department of Nephrology and Endocrinology National Defense Medical College, Japan

References

[1] Stahle-Backdahl M. Uremic pruritus. Clinical and experimental studies. Acta Derm Venereol Suppl [Stockh]. 1989;145:1-38.

[2] Stahle-Backdahl M. Pruritus in hemodialysis patients. Skin Pharmacol. 1992;5:14-20.

[3] Stahle-Backdahl M. Uremic pruritus. Semin Dermatol. 1995;14:297-301.

[4] Manenti L, Tansinda P, Vaglio A. Uraemic pruritus: clinical characteristics, pathophysiology and treatment. Drugs. 2009;69:251-63.

[5] Yosipovitch G, Greaves MW, Schmelz M. Itch. The Lancet. 2003;361:690-4.

[6] Lugon JR. Uremic pruritus: a review. Hemodial Int. 2005;9:180-8.

[7] Kosmadakis GC, Zerefos N. Uremic pruritus. Int J Artif Organs. 2006;29:938-43.

[8] Greaves MW. Recent advances in pathophysiology and current management of itch. Ann Acad Med Singapore. 2007;36:788-92.

[9] Patel TS, Freedman BI, Yosipovitch G. An update on pruritus associated with CKD. Am J Kidney Dis. 2007;50:11-20.

[10] Narita I, Iguchi S, Omori K, Gejyo F. Uremic pruritus in chronic hemodialysis patients. J Nephrol. 2008;21:161-5.

[11] Berger TG, Steinhoff M. Pruritus and renal failure. Semin Cutan Med Surg. 2011;30:99-100.

[12] Greaves MW. Pathogenesis and treatment of pruritus. Curr Allergy Asthma Rep. 2010;10:236-42.

[13] Kfoury LW, Jurdi MA. Uremic pruritus. J Nephrol. 2012;25:644-52.

[14] Mettang T, Kremer AE. Uremic pruritus. Kidney Int. advance online publication, 8 January 2014;doi:10.1038

http://dx.doi.org/10.5772/59493

[15] Pontremoli R, Sofia A, Ravera M, Nicolella C, Viazzi F, Tirotta A, et al. Prevalence and clinical correlates of microalbuminuria in essential hypertension The MAGIC Study. Hypertension. 1997;30:1135-43.

[16] Narita I, Alchi B, Omori K, Sato F, Ajiro J, Saga D, et al. Etiology and prognostic significance of severe uremic pruritus in chronic hemodialysis patients. Kidney Int. 2006;69:1626-32.

[17] Pisoni RL, Wikstrom B, Elder SJ, Akizawa T, Asano Y, Keen ML, et al. Pruritus in haemodialysis patients: International results from the Dialysis Outcomes and Practice Patterns Study (DOPPS). Nephrol Dial Transplant. 2006;21(12):3495-505.

[18] Gilchrest BA, Stern RS, Steinman TI, Brown RS, Arndt KA, Anderson WW. Clinical features of pruritus among patients undergoing maintenance hemodialysis. Arch Dermatol. 1982;118:154-6.

[19] Dar NR, Akhter A. Clinical characteristics of uremic pruritus in patients undergoing haemodialysis. J Coll Physicians Surg Pak. 2006;16:94-6.

[20] Liakopoulos V, Krishnan M, Stefanidis I, Savaj S, Ghareeb S, Musso C, et al. Improvement in uremic symptoms after increasing daily dialysate volume in patients on chronic peritoneal dialysis with declining renal function. Int Urol Nephrol. 2004;36:437-43.

[21] Szepietowski JC, Reich A, Szepietowski T. Emollients with endocannabinoids in the treatment of uremic pruritus: discussion of the therapeutic options. Ther Apher Dial. 2005;9:277-9.

[22] Novak MJ, Sheth H, Bender FH, Fried L, Piraino B. Improvement in Pittsburgh Symptom Score index after initiation of peritoneal dialysis. Adv Perit Dial. 2008;24:46-50.

[23] Hiroshige K, Kabashima N, Takasugi M, Kuroiwa A. Optimal dialysis improves uremic pruritus. Am J Kidney Dis. 1995;25:413-9.

[24] Graf H, Kovarik J, Stummvoll HK, Wolf A. Disappearance of uraemic pruritus after lowering dialysate magnesium concentration. Br Med J. 1979;2(6203):1478-9.

[25] Carmichael AJ, Dickinson F, McHugh MI, Martin AM, Farrow M. Magnesium free dialysis for uraemic pruritus. BMJ. 1988;297(6663):1584-5.

[26] Kyriazis J, Glotsos J. Dialysate calcium concentration of</=1.25 mmol/l: is it effective in suppressing uremic pruritus? Nephron. 2000;84:85-6.

[27] Kato A, Takita T, Furuhashi M, Takahashi T, Watanabe T, Maruyama Y, et al. Polymethylmethacrylate efficacy in reduction of renal itching in hemodialysis patients: crossover study and role of tumor necrosis factor-alpha. Artif Organs. 2001;25:441-7.

[28] Morton CA, Lafferty M, Hau C, Henderson I, Jones M, Lowe JG. Pruritus and skin hydration during dialysis. Nephrol Dial Transplant. 1996;11:2031-6.

[29] Twycross R, Greaves MW, Handwerker H, Jones EA, Libretto SE, Szepietowski JC, et al. Itch: scratching more than the surface. QJM. 2003;96:7-26.

[30] Szepietowski JC, Szepietowski T, Reich A. Efficacy and tolerance of the cream containing structured physiological lipids with endocannabinoids in the treatment of uremic pruritus: a preliminary study. Acta Dermatovenerol Croat. 2005;13:97-103.

[31] Okada K, Matsumoto K. Effect of skin care with an emollient containing a high water content on mild uremic pruritus. Ther Apher Dial. 2004;8:419-22.

[32] Itai T, Amayasu H, Kuribayashi M, Kawamura N, Okada M, Momose A, et al. Psychological effects of aromatherapy on chronic hemodialysis patients. Psychiatry Clin Neurosci. 2000;54:393-7.

[33] Dvorak M, Watkinson A, McGlone F, Rukwied R. Histamine induced responses are attenuated by a cannabinoid receptor agonist in human skin. Inflamm Res. 2003;52:238-45.

[34] Breneman DL, Cardone JS, Blumsack RF, Lather RM, Searle EA, Pollack VE. Topical capsaicin for treatment of hemodialysis-related pruritus. J Am Acad Dermatol. 1992;26:91-4.

[35] Tarng DC, Cho YL, Liu HN, Huang TP. Hemodialysis-related pruritus: a double-blind, placebo-controlled, crossover study of capsaicin 0.025% cream. Nephron. 1996;72:617-22.

[36] Weisshaar E, Dunker N, Gollnick H. Topical capsaicin therapy in humans with hemodialysis-related pruritus. Neurosci Lett. 2003;345:192-4.

[37] Tamimi NA, Mikhail AI, Stevens PE. Role of gamma-linolenic acid in uraemic pruritus. Nephron. 1999;83:170-1.

[38] Chen YC, Chiu WT, Wu MS. Therapeutic effect of topical gamma-linolenic acid on refractory uremic pruritus. Am J Kidney Dis. 2006;48:69-76.

[39] Miller MJS, Vergnolle N, McKnight W, Musah RA, Davison CA, Trentacosti AM, et al. Inhibition of Neurogenic Inflammation by the Amazonian Herbal Medicine Sangre de Grado. 2001;117:725-30.

[40] Pauli-Magnus C, Mikus G, Alscher DM, Kirschner T, Nagel W, Gugeler N, et al. Naltrexone does not relieve uremic pruritus: results of a randomized, double-blind, placebo-controlled crossover study. J Am Soc Nephrol. 2000;11:514-9.

[41] Duque MI, Thevarajah S, Chan YH, Tuttle AB, Freedman BI, Yosipovitch G. Uremic pruritus is associated with higher kt/V and serum calcium concentration. Clin Nephrol. 2006;66:184-91.

[42] Gilchrest BA, Rowe JW, Brown RS, Steinman TI, Arndt KA. Ultraviolet phototherapy of uremic pruritus. Long-term results and possible mechanism of action. Ann Intern Med. 1979;91:17-21.

[43] Shultz B, Roenigk H. Uremic pruritus treated with ultraviolet light. JAMA. 1980;243:1836-7.

[44] Imazu LE, Tachibana T, Danno K, Tanaka M, Imamura S. Histamine-releasing factor[s] in sera of uraemic pruritus patients in a possible mechanism of UVB therapy. Arch Dermatol Res. 1993;285:423-7.

[45] Fjellner B, Hagermark O. Influence of ultraviolet light on itch and flare reactions in human skin induced by histamine and the histamine liberator compound 48/80. Acta Derm Venereol. 1982;62:137-40.

[46] Wallengren J, Sundler F. Phototherapy reduces the number of epidermal and CGRP-positive dermal nerve fibres. Acta Derm Venereol. 2004;84:111-5.

[47] Blachley JD, Blankenship DM, Menter A, Parker TF, 3rd, Knochel JP. Uremic pruritus: skin divalent ion content and response to ultraviolet phototherapy. Am J Kidney Dis. 1985;5:237-41.

[48] Kim KH, Lee MS, Choi SM. Acupuncture for treating uremic pruritus in patients with end-stage renal disease: a systematic review. J Pain Symptom Manage. 2010;40:117-25.

[49] Che-Yi C, Wen CY, Min-Tsung K, Chiu-Ching H. Acupuncture in haemodialysis patients at the Quchi (LI11) acupoint for refractory uraemic pruritus. Nephrol Dial Transplant. 2005;20:1912-5.

[50] Gao H, Zhang W, Wang Y. Acupuncture treatment for 34 cases of uremic cutaneous pruritus. J Tradit Chin Med. 2002;22[1]:29-30.

[51] Sakuraba H, Takeuchi H, Takeuchi M, Syoji M, Moriyama T. Questionnaire survey of complaints and accupuncutre treatment in maintenance hemodialysis patients. Nihon Toseki Igakkai Zasshi 2007;40:513-6.

[52] Shapiro R, Stockard H, Schank A. Successful treatment of uremic pruritus with acupuncutre.. Am J Acupunct. 1986;14:235-42.

[53] Antoni F. Hypothalamic control of adrenocorticotropin secretion : advnaces ince the discovery of 41-redue corticotropin-releasing factor. Endocr Rev. 1986;7:351-78.

[54] Percival SL, Emanuel C, Cutting KF, Williams DW. Microbiology of the skin and the role of biofilms in infection. Int Wound J. 2012;9:14-32.

[55] Tominaga M, Takamori K. An update on peripheral mechanisms and treatments of itch. Biol Pharm Bull. 2013;36:1241-7.

[56] Tominaga M, Takamori K. Sensitization of Itch Signaling: Itch Sensitization-Nerve Growth Factor, Semaphorins. 2014.

[57] Andersen LW, Friedberg M, Lokkegaard N. Naloxone in the treatment of uremic pruritus: a case history. Clin Nephrol. 1984;21:355-6.

[58] Peer G, Kivity S, Agami O, Fireman E, Silverberg D, Blum M, et al. Randomised crossover trial of naltrexone in uraemic pruritus. Lancet. 1996;348:1552-4.

[59] Legroux-Crespel E, Cledes J, Misery L. A comparative study on the effects of naltrexone and loratadine on uremic pruritus. Dermatology. 2004;208:326-30.

[60] Wikstrom B, Gellert R, Ladefoged SD, Danda Y, Akai M, Ide K, et al. Kappa-opioid system in uremic pruritus: multicenter, randomized, double-blind, placebo-controlled clinical studies. J Am Soc Nephrol. 2005;16:3742-7.

[61] Seki T, Awamura S, Kimura C, Ide S, Sakano K, Minami M, et al. Pharmacological properties of TRK-820 on cloned mu-, delta- and kappa-opioid receptors and nociceptin receptor. Eur J Pharmacol. 1999;376:159-67.

[62] Nagase H, Hayakawa J, Kawamura K, Kawai K, Takezawa Y, Matsuura H, et al. Discovery of a structurally novel opioid kappa-agonist derived from 4,5-epoxymorphinan. Chem Pharm Bull (Tokyo). 1998;46:366-9.

[63] Wakasa Y, Fujiwara A, Umeuchi H, Endoh T, Okano K, Tanaka T, et al. Inhibitory effects of TRK-820 on systemic skin scratching induced by morphine in rhesus monkeys. Life Sci. 2004;75:2947-57.

[64] Togashi Y, Umeuchi H, Okano K, Ando N, Yoshizawa Y, Honda T, et al. Antipruritic activity of the kappa-opioid receptor agonist, TRK-820. Eur J Pharmacol. 2002;435:259-64.

[65] Kumagai H, Ebata T, Takamori K, Muramatsu T, Nakamoto H, Suzuki H. Effect of a novel kappa-receptor agonist, nalfurafine hydrochloride, on severe itch in 337 haemodialysis patients: a Phase III, randomized, double-blind, placebo-controlled study. Nephrol Dial Transplant. 2010;25:1251-7.

[66] Wager TD, Rilling JK, Smith EE, Sokolik A, Casey KL, Davidson RJ, et al. Placebo-induced changes in FMRI in the anticipation and experience of pain. Science. 2004;303:1162-7.

[67] Kumagai H, Ebata T, Takamori K, Miyasato K, Muramatsu T, Nakamoto H, et al. Efficacy and safety of a novel k-agonist for managing intractable pruritus in dialysis patients. Am J Nephrol. 2012;36:175-83.

Chapter 4

Iatrogenic Iron Overload in Dialysis Patients

Guy Rostoker, Mireille Griuncelli,
Christelle Loridon and Yves Cohen

Additional information is available at the end of the chapter

http://dx.doi.org/10.5772/59316

1. Introduction

During the past two decades, routine use of recombinant erythropoeisis-stimulating agents (ESA) has enabled anemia to be corrected in most patients with end-stage renal disease, permitting better outcomes and improving quality of life [1]. The use of ESA is frequently associated with iron deficiency, resulting primarily from massive transfer of stored iron to erythroid progenitor cells [2]. Mobilization of iron from repleted storage sites may also be inadequate, resulting in functional iron deficiency [3]. Moreover, blood loss related to hemodialysis itself and to occult intestinal bleeding due to uremic enteropathy can markedly aggravate iron deficiency in this setting [1]. As successful use of ESA requires sufficient available iron before and during therapy, almost all dialysis patients on ESA currently receive parenteral iron therapy [3]. The dual risk of iron deficiency and iron overload must therefore be closely monitored in dialysis patients. Interestingly, most relevant studies published in the last two decades have focused chiefly on the detection and treatment of iron deficiency in dialysis patients, while very few have examined iron overload [3-4].

Until recently it was widely considered that iron overload among dialysis patients was more prevalent during the pre-ESA era, when blood transfusion was frequently used to treat anemia and when intravenous iron therapy was given without concomitant ESA administration; iron overload was therefore considered rare, or even exceptional, among dialysis patients in the ESA era but is now an increasingly recognized clinical situation [3-7].

The only laboratory parameter available to screen for iron overload in dialysis patients is serum ferritin, but confirmation necessitates liver or bone biopsy, and few data were available on patients with end-stage renal disease until now, owing to the aggressiveness of these histological examinations [4]. Moreover, serum ferritin is an acute-phase reactant, and these patients' frequent systemic inflammation may inhibit both iron mobilization from reticuloendothelial stores and intestinal iron absorption via hepcidin modulation; the relationship between ferritin and iron stores may therefore be blunted or skewed [4, 8].

American and European clinical practice guidelines (KDOQI-2006 and European Best Practice Guideline-2009) warned against regular iron administration when the ferritin concentration exceeds 500 μg/L, although the former guideline allowed clinicians to make a decision on IV iron administration above this level after carefully weighing up ESA responsiveness, hemoglobin and transferrin saturation, and the patient's clinical status [1, 9]. It is also worthy of note that the recent KDIGO-2012 guideline proposed a trial of IV iron in dialysis patients prior to ESA use, with the aims of sparing these expensive drugs and of reaching high TSAT (30%) and ferritin (500 μg/L) target values [10]; however, these new KDIGO target values for iron biomarkers were not fully endorsed by EDTA-ERA because of the potential risk of iron overload [11]. Likewise, the Japanese Society for Dialysis recently proposed that a minimal amount of IV iron (up to 650 mg in the induction phase) should be given to dialysis patients, and only in case of true iron deficiency (ferritin <100 μg/L), while also warning against maintenance intravenous iron therapy because of the risk of iron toxicity [12].

2. Normal iron metabolism

Iron stores in healthy humans average 3 to 4 g in men and 2.2 to 3.5 g in women [13, 14]. About 60% of iron is located within the hemoglobin protein of circulating erythrocytes and, to a lesser degree, in medullary erythrocytes; 20% of iron stores are located in the liver (hepatocytes and Kupffer cells) and in the reticulo-endothelial system (mainly in spleen macrophages), in the form of the iron-storage protein ferritin (marginally in haemosiderin) whereas muscle myoglobin accounts for about 10% of body iron [8, 13, 14]. Iron-containing enzymes represent only 1% of iron stores, while plasma transferrin-bound iron represents only a small fraction (0.2%=3 mg) of total body iron [13, 14]. Each day, macrophages of the reticulo-endothelial system recycle about 30 mg of iron from senescent erythrocytes, thus providing the 20-30 mg of iron required for normal erythropoïesis [8, 13, 14]. Physiological iron losses are estimated at about 1 mg/day (urinary loss: 0.1 mg/day; gut loss secondary to enterocyte desquamation: 0.6 mg/day; skin loss: 0.3 mg/day) but are increased in women by menstruation (the main cause of iron-deficiency anemia worldwide), pregnancy and breast-feeding [14]. Therefore, recommended daily dietary iron intake to compensate for iron losses is 10 mg/day generally (because of an absorption rate of only 10%) and 30 mg/day in pregnant women and nursing mothers [14]. Hepcidin-25, a hormone synthesized in the liver, is the master regulator of iron metabolism, acting negatively on both intestinal iron absorption and iron release from reticulo-endothelial macrophages and liver cells by decreasing the expression of ferroportin, a protein that regulates iron export from these cells [8]. Hepcidin-25 synthesis is increased by iron itself and by inflammation (via IL6), and decreased by anemia, hypoxia, iron deficiency, haemorrhage, erythropoïetin, and increased medullary erythropoïesis [8]. The mechanism by which this latter situation down-regulates hepcidin synthesis was recently linked to a new peptide hormone, erythroferrone, secreted by erythroblasts and acting directly on the liver [15]. Defective hepcidin-25 synthesis plays a paramount pathophysiological role in genetic hemo-

http://dx.doi.org/10.5772/59316

chromatoses, whereas excessive, unregulated hepcidin synthesis is the mainstay of a newly discovered genetic (autosomal recessive) form of iron-deficiency anemia called IRIDA (iron refractory iron deficiency anemia) related to mutation of the *TMPRSS6* gene (encoding matriptase-2); IRIDA is refractory to oral iron but partially responsive to IV iron products [16].

3. Blood loss in hemodialysis patients

With the ready availability of ESA and IV iron, iatrogenic blood losses, which are major contributors to iron deficiency in dialysis patients, have often been neglected. There are three distinct and cumulative sources of blood loss in this setting: 1) the dialytic technique itself; 2) regular blood sampling for patient monitoring, and 3) occult intestinal blood loss. Traditionally estimated to be between 4 and 12 liters/year, these blood losses classically represent 2 to 6 g of iron lost per year (1 L of blood contains about 500 mg of iron, although the value may be lower in dialysis patients because of a lower hematocrit) [17]. These classical approximations clearly overestimate dialysis-related blood loss. In addition, the type of vascular access and comorbidities may strongly influence both the type and magnitude of blood loss.

Two recent publications have quantified blood loss associated with modern dialysis membranes at respectively 0.3 ml/session [18] and 0.9 ml/session [19], while blood-line losses have been calculated to be about 0.2 ml/session [18]. Thus, taking a value of 1.1 ml/session, annual blood losses due to conventional hemodialysis *per se* (3 sessions/week, 150 sessions/year) would be about 165 ml/year. But the major source of blood loss in dialysis units stems from the care of tunnelized double-lumen catheters, when nurses apply the universal protocol of purging 7 to 10 ml of blood in each branch at the outset of the hemodialysis session, leading to a yearly blood loss of 2.4 L, to which should be added 288 ml for routine monthly bacterial cultures of the anticoagulant locks. Thus, the total annual blood loss related to catheter care is about 2.68 L [20]. Use of a recent protocol proposed by Prof. Bernard Canaud, based on the purge of only 2 ml of blood instead of 7-10 ml/branch, would lessen catheter-related blood loss to only 888 ml/year, representing a net 77% reduction [20].

In a recent survey in France, blood samples for regular patient monitoring were quantified in 10 dialysis centers run by the healthcare provider Générale de Santé at between 350 ml and 450 ml/year [20], a volume close to the 368 ml found by Sargent and Acchiardo in patients dialysed at the University of Tennessee in Memphis in 2004 [17]. Note that blood sampling may be far more abundant in academic hospitals conducting clinical trials or pathophysiological studies.

The third source of blood losses in hemodialysis patients is the gut. These losses are occult, being below the detection limit of stool tests. They are favoured by uremic enteropathy and thrombopathy, anticoagulation of the extracorporeal circuit during dialysis sessions, and also antiplatelet and antivitamin K drugs [21, 22]. Rosenblatt and coworkers, in a study performed in the 1980s using chromium 51-labelled erythrocytes, quantified faecal blood loss at 0.83 ml/day in healthy controls, 3.15 ml/day in non dialysis chronic kidney disease (CKD) patients and 6.27 ml/day (2.2 L/year) in hemodialysis patients [21]. These occult faecal blood losses are increased by antiplatelet and antivitamin K drugs: dialysis patients thus treated require higher IV iron dosages to replenish their iron stores (e.g 703 to 961 mg/year) [22, 23]. Thus, total blood losses in a hemodialysis patient with a native arteriovenous fistulae treated in a non academic center and not receiving antiplatelet or antivitamin K drugs can be estimated at 2.85 L/year (1.425 g of iron/year), whereas a patient with the same clinical profile but a double-lumen tunnelized catheter will lose 5.5 L/year (2.765 g of iron); note that both values are far lower than the classical estimates of 2 to 6 g/year [20].

4. Evolving concept of iron as an adjuvant of erythropoiesis —Stimulating agent therapy over the last two decades

With the advent of erythropoietin replacement therapy in the eighties, the goal of iron therapy was to maintain iron stores and thereby prevent true iron deficiency, mainly with oral iron supplements when the serum ferritin level was less than 50 µg/L; IV iron was advocated at that time as a second-line option in case of severe iron deficiency, poor tolerance or inefficacy of oral iron salts [24, 25]. Parenteral iron therapy has gained popularity in the nephrology community in the last fifteen years because of its convenience (infusion during dialysis sessions), its superiority over oral preparations for treating true iron deficiency, and its ability to overcome functional iron deficiency, a very common clinical situation in hemodialysis patients; in addition, this treatment enabled cost savings of about 20%-30% on expensive ESA drugs [1, 9].

Based solely on bone marrow studies and the lack of known long-term adverse effects, recent guidelines have redefined iron deficiency and adjusted iron-store repletion criteria to even higher levels (the KDIGO 2012 target for "upper normal" ferritin in hemodialysis patients is now 500 µg/L), underlining the risk of functional iron deficiency during ESA treatment and the ability of IV iron to spare ESA use, and even going so far as to advocate a trial of IV iron prior to ESA initiation. All these changes have amplified the use of parenteral iron products [7, 10, 26].

5. Increased use of IV iron in dialysis patients worldwide in the last two decades

A recent epidemiological analysis of the management of anemia in hemodialysis patients in the USA, based on USRDS data, showed an increase in the use of IV iron from 64% of patients in 2002 to 76% in 2008, together with an increase in the infused dose from 166 mg/month to 216 mg/month [27]. In addition, during the first year of hemodialysis, the usual monthly infused dose of iron was shown to be far higher, ranging from 270 mg to 305 mg [27]. The change made to the ESA label by the Food and Drug Administration in June 2010 also led to an increase in the percentage of US patients receiving IV iron, from 57% (August 2010) to 71% (August 2011), together with a significant decline in the ESA dosage and an increase in the median ferritin level from 556 to 650 μg/L, with values exceeding 800 μg/L in 34% of patients [28]. While the median dose of IV iron remained largely stable at 190 mg/month, it is noteworthy that 18% of patients received more than 500 mg/month during this period [28].

Very similar trends in the use of IV iron were recently observed in other industrialised countries, with the exception of Japan: the percentage of patients treated with IV iron rose between 1999 and 2010 from 50% to 71% overall, from 65% to 80% in Canada, from 55% to 70% in France, from 65% to 80% in Germany, and from 60% to 80% in the UK; during the same period (1999-2010), the mean ferritin level rose from 380 to 450 μg/L in Canada, from 420 to 580 μg/L in Germany and from 400 to 500 μg/L in the UK, while it remained stable in France at around 400 μg/L [29]. In Japan, the percentage of patients receiving IV iron rose only from 25% to 36% and the mean ferritin level rose only from 280 to 320 μg/L [29]. The overall mean monthly iron dose administered in industrialized countries other than the U.S. rose by 21%, from 232 mg/month in 1992 to 281 mg/month in 2010 [29].

6. Hemodialysis-associated hemosiderosis in the pre-ESA era

Post-mortem studies performed at the end of the 1970s and early 1980s showed that iron deposits were abundant in the adrenal glands, lymph nodes and lungs of dialysis patients with severe hepatosplenic siderosis, and generally sparser in the heart, kidney and pancreas [30-32]. In the liver, the earliest detectable iron deposits were observed within cells lining the sinusoids and in Kupffer cells; as hepatic siderosis progressed, iron appeared within hepatocytes, first in the peripheral zones of the hepatic lobules in the vicinity of portal triads and subsequently throughout the lobules [30]. In the spleen, the principal site of iron storage was also the cells lining the splenic sinusoids, while the white pulp was generally spared [30]. Even in case of massive hepatic siderosis there was no cytological evidence of cell damage, but reticulin and trichrome stains showed an increase in the hepatic fibroconjunctive network, together with loss of liver cells [30-32]. Similarly, most patients who had marked hemosiderosis and underwent liver biopsy had focal portal fibrosis [33]. These post-mortem studies also showed a strong link between iron overload and both blood transfusions and intravenous high-molecular-weight iron dextran (IMFERON®); interestingly, the closest relationship was between hepatic siderosis and IV iron [5][31-32]. Iron overload was usually absent in patients who had received little or no IV iron [31], whereas massive hepatosplenic siderosis was only seen in patients with a dialysis vintage of more than 3 years [5][32]. Adrenal involvement was observed in 11/24 unselected patients in the work of Pitts and coworkers [32] but in 17/18 patients with severe hepatosplenic siderosis studied by Ali [30]. Pancreatic involvement was less frequent, affecting 7/24 patients studied by Pitts and coworkers and 5/18 patients with severe hepatoplenic siderosis studied by Ali [30]. Interestingly, significant cardiac iron deposits were found in respectively 16.6% (4/24) and 22% (5/22) of unselected patients in the autopsy studies of Pitts [31] and Gokal [32], whereas cardiac involvement was found in 44% (8/18) of the patients with severe hepatosplenic siderosis studied post-mortem by Ali [30].

In the pre-ESA era, one strategy to avoid blood transfusion-related iron overload in dialysis patients with transfusion-dependent anemia was to use young instead of mature erythrocytes for transfusions [33]. Tissue iron depletion with the chelator desferrioxamine was advocated to prevent hemosiderosis or to cure organ dysfunction due to iron overload [33].

At the beginning of the 1990s, the advent of recombinant human erythropoïetin allowed simultaneous treatment of anemia and iron overload by allowing massive mobilization of iron stores and effective phlebotomy (by partial letting of the extracorporeal circuit) at the end of dialysis sessions in patients rendered non anemic [34], together with the first successful use of non invasive radiological tools (liver quantitative computer tomography) to diagnose hemodialysis-associated hemosiderosis and to monitor iron stores [35].

7. Liver iron content and modern non invasive imaging of iron stores

The liver is the main iron storage site in humans, and the liver iron concentration (LIC) correlates closely with total body iron stores in patients with secondary hemosideroses such as thalassemia major, sickle cell disease and genetic hemochromatosis [36, 37]. In order to avoid liver biopsy, a number of non invasive techniques have been developed to estimate liver iron stores, including the superconducting quantum interference device (SQUID), liver quantitative computer tomography (qCT), and magnetic resonance imaging (MRI) [38-39]. MRI has became the dominant technique, because of its sensitivity, reproducibility, availability and ability to image multiple organs in a single session [39]. Hepatic MRI is now considered the gold standard method for estimating and monitoring iron stores in secondary hemosideroses and genetic hemochromatoses ("iterative radiological biopsy"), and has been a major contributor to knowledge and care in this field during the last decade [37, 40].

As one specific feature of hemodialysis patients receiving intravenous iron in the pre-ESA era was that their bone marrow iron content was paradoxically low in up to one-third of cases despite severe hepatosplenic siderosis; thus LIC seems to be the best indicator of iron overload in hemodialysis patients, given that bone marrow analysis may be misleading even in the ESA era [5].

SQUID (also called magnetic susceptometry) is based on the determination of the magnetic volume susceptibility of paramagnetic ferritin/haemosiderin iron in the liver and has been validated by comparison with percutaneous biopsy; it does not distinguish ferritin from haemosiderin iron [38-39]. The limitations of this method relate to its scarcity (only 5 devices worldwide), its very high cost (about 1000 euros/exam) and the lack of calibration homogeneity (risk of underestimating LIC) [38-39].

Liver quantitative computer tomography (qCT) was superseded by MRI at the beginning of the 21st century [38-39]. Quantitative MRI for LIC estimation is based on the paramagnetic properties of iron, leading to a reduction in the magnetic resonance signal as the liver iron concentration increases; it does not distinguish ferritin from haemosiderin iron [39]. It is a low-cost (about 300 euros/exam), non irradiating technique that does not require gadolinium (therefore safe in CKD patients) and is available everywhere [39].

http://dx.doi.org/10.5772/59316

There are three valuable hepatic MRI methods for determining LIC: the signal-intensitity ratio, R2 relaxometry, and R2* relaxometry [39]. The signal-intensity ratio is the reference method. It was established at Rennes University in France on a 1.5 Tesla apparatus in 2004, and is predominantly used in Europe [41]. It was validated in a cohort of 191 patients with secondary hemosiderosis, genetic hemochromatosis and hepatic diseases who underwent liver biopsy for biochemical iron assay [41]; the results were successfully replicated in 3 prospective cohorts studied by independent teams in France, the Netherlands and Spain [42-44]. Two of these studies were performed by comparison with liver biopsy [42-44]. This approach is based on a comparison between liver and muscle intensity on various sequences (T1, PD, T2, T2+, T2++) and requires a specific algorithm to analyse the results (free software available on the website of Rennes University) (figure 1)[41]. It has a sensitivity of 89% and a specificity of 80% for the diagnosis of iron overload disease, and values are linear up to 350 μmol/g of dry liver [41]; a complementary algorithm established by a Spanish team is required for higher values [39].

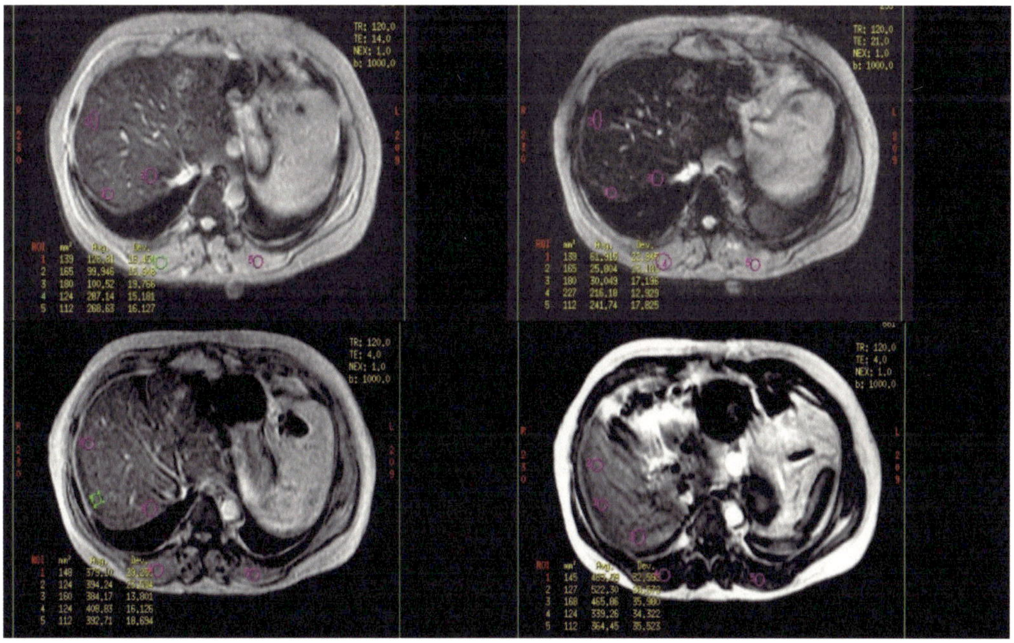

Figure 1. Magnetic resonance imaging quantification of hepatic iron stores according to the method of Rennes University

The second MRI technique for iron store quantification was established in Australia in 2005 on a 1.5 Tesla apparatus and is based on R2 relaxometry; it was validated in a cohort of 105 patients with thalassemia, genetic hemochromatosis and hepatic diseases who underwent liver biopsy for biochemical iron assay, and was also compared to SQUID in 23 patients [45]. It is based on R2/T2 sequences. It has a sensitivity of 86% and a specificity of 88% for the diagnosis of iron overload disease, and is linear up to 700 μmol/g of dry liver; however, it requires calibration of the apparatus with phantoms and also a specific configuration of the machine [45]. It is mainly used (and called Ferriscan) in Australia, New Zealand and North America.

The third MRI technique for iron store quantification is based on R2* relaxometry: it is the most promising tool and can be used on a 1.5 Tesla apparatus with specific software; it not only quantifies iron in liver but also detects (in the same session lasting about 20 minutes) iron overload in heart, spleen and pancreas [46]. Its main limitation for LIC determination is its validation on only a small number of liver biopsies [38-39, 46].

Normal hepatic iron stores on MRI have been established on the basis of liver biopsy findings, together with categories of gradually increasing iron overload reflecting the risk of complications; moreover, as the upper 95% of LIC in healthy adults is 32 µmol/g of dry liver and hepatic MRI accurately detects liver iron overload exceeding 50 µmol/g of dry liver, the upper limit of normal was set at 50 µmol/g in many studies [6][41][45]. According to Rennes University, LIC values between 51 and 100 µmol/g represent mild iron overload, values between 101 and 200 µmol/g moderate iron overload, and values ≥ 201 µmol/g severe iron overload [41]. Management modalities for different clinically relevant thresholds of MRI-determined LIC have been forwarded by hepatologists and haematologists (e.g chelation in hemosiderosis, phlebotomy in genetic hemochromatosis, and specific follow-up of target organs)(Table 1) [37-41][45].

Liver Iron content (µmol/g)	Clinical thresholds of LIC in secondary hemosiderosis and genetic hemochromatosis
125 µmol/g (7 mg/g)	threshold for increased risk of iron induced complications and level of decision for chelation therapy or phlebotomy
143 µmol/g (8 mg/g)	threshold of saturation of reticulo-endothelial system in sickle-cell disease
160 µmol/g (9 mg/g)	threshold of hepatic fibrosis in sickle cell disease
269 µmol/g (15 mg/g)	threshold of risk of hepatic fibrosis and cardiac disease in thalassemia major
331 µmol/g (18 mg/g)	threshold of risk of hepatic fibrosis or cirrhosis in patients with genetic hemochromatosis

Table 1. Clinicaly relevant LIC thresholds in secondary hemosiderosis and genetic hemochromatosis

It is very likely that radiologists will be heavily solicited in the near future by nephrology teams requesting quantitative hepatic MRI for dialysis patients, both for research purposes and for diagnosis and follow-up of iron overload. Radiologists and nephrologists should also be aware of the marked differences in the pharmacological properties of available intravenous iron products, and their potential interference with MRI (summarized in table 2) [47].

Trade Name	Carbohydrate composition	Molecular weight (Dalton)	Half Life in the plasma (hours)	Time for complete elimination of the plasma	Informations in the Label about MRI	Scientific publications on biological clearance and MRI interference	Advised time between last iron infusion and MRI
VENOFER®	iron sucrose	34 000 to 60 000	5.3-6	30 hours	No	Yes (PETSCAN)	One week
COSMOFER® (Europe) INFeD® (USA)	iron dextran of low molecular weight	165 000	20	4 days	No	No	One month
FERRLECIT®	iron gluconate	289 000 to 444 000	1.42	1 day	No	No	One week
DEXFERRUM®	iron dextran of high molecular weight	265 000	9.4 to 87.4	2 to 18 days	No	No	3 months
MONOFER®	iron isomaltoside	150 000	23.2	5 days	No	No	One month
FERINJECT® (Europe) INJECTAFER® (USA)	iron carboxy-maltose	150 000	7 to 12	1 day and half to 2 days and half	**Yes** **no influence** of Ferinject/Injectafer on MRI	Yes (PETSCAN)	One week
RIENSO® (Europe) FERAHEME®(Europe)	ferumoxytol (polyglucose sorbitol carboxy methyl ether iron)	750 000	14.7	3 days	**Yes** **Inference with MRI** Respect a delay of 3 months between infusion and MRI	Yes (Interference with MRI)	6 months

(according to Rostoker G and Cohen Y. *Magnetic resonance imaging repercussions of intravenous iron products used for iron-deficiency anemia and dialysis associated anemia.* J Comp Assist Tomogr 2014: Sept 16)

Table 2. IV iron preparations: Physicochemical and pharmacokinetic parameters and influence on MRI

8. Hemodialysis-associated hemosiderosis in the era of erythropoiesis-stimulating agents

Recent studies using SQUID and quantitative MRI to estimate liver iron stores in hemodialysis patients suggest a strong link between the infused iron dose and the risk of iron overload. They also strongly challenge the assumed safety of IV iron products, the reliability of current iron biomarker cutoffs, and current monitoring of iron stores in dialysis patients.

Two recent studies have focused on iron overload in hemodialysis patients with serum ferritin levels well above 500 µg/L: Ferrari et al measured hepatic iron content by magnetic resonance relaxometry R2 in 15 Australian patients with a median ferritin of 782 µg/L and found iron overload in 60% of them [48], whereas Ghoti et al [49] more recently analyzed LIC by T2*MRI, along with spleen, pancreas and heart iron deposits, in 21 iron-overloaded hemodialysis patients with serum ferritin levels above 1000 µg/L; they found hepatic siderosis in 19 patients (90%)(mild in 8, moderate in 5 and severe in 6), and spleen involvement in every case (21/21); pancreas involvement was sought in only 8 patients (because of poor compliance with the exam) and was found in 3 patients (37%); none of the patients had an abnormal cardiac R2*[49].

Two modern studies have analyzed hepatic iron stores by SQUID, one in 2004 [50] and the other in 2012 with quantitative MRI based on the Rennes University protocol [6], in cohorts of hemodialysis patients treated according to KDOQI and EDTA-ERBP guidelines with ferritin levels within the target range. Canavese et al used the SQUID technique to study 40 Italian patients and found normal LIC in 30% of them (median ferritin 245 µg/L), mild iron overload in 32.5% (median ferritin 329 µg/L) and moderate iron overload in 37.5% (median ferritin 482 µg/L) [50]. It was subsequently claimed that these findings could not be extrapolated to the general hemodialysis population, owing to possible biased selection of an iron-overloaded population [51].

We recently showed that 84% of a cohort of 119 fit hemodialysis patients treated according to contemporary guidelines had hepatic iron overload on MRI (≥ 51 µmol/g dry weight); mild iron overload was seen in 42 patients (35.3%) and moderate iron overload in 22 patients (18.5%), while 36 of these 119 patients (30%) had severe iron overload (≥ 201 µmol/g dry weight) at levels usually seen in genetic hemochromatosis; MRI also revealed spleen anomalies (a sign of secondary hemosiderosis) in several patients [6].

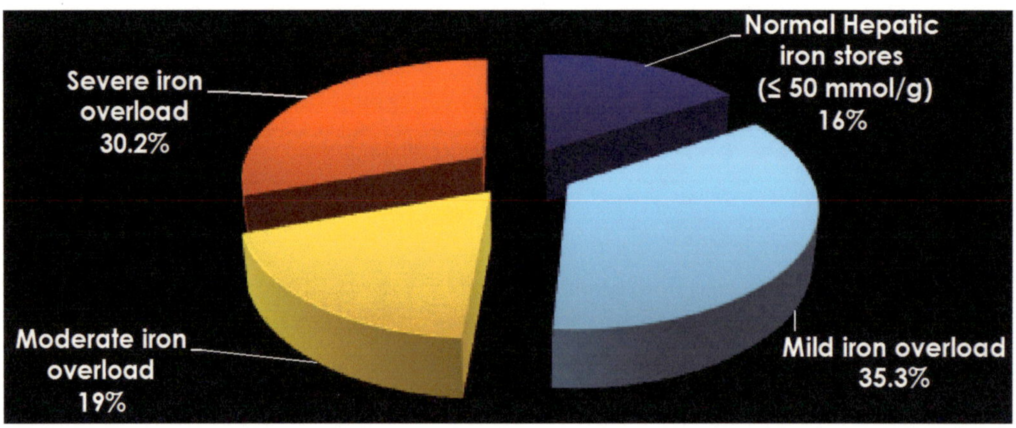

(according Rostoker G, Griuncelli M, Loridon C et al. Hemodialysis-associated hemosiderosis in the era of erythropoiesis-stimulating agents: a MRI study. Am J Med 2012; 125: 991-999)

Figure 2. Results of a cross-sectional study of 119 hemodialysis patients

In our cross-sectional study, infused iron, hepcidin and C-reactive protein values correlated with hepatic iron stores in both univariate analysis ($p<0.05$, Spearman test) and binary logistic regression ($p<0.05$). We found no relationship between the LIC of hemodialysis patients and alcohol consumption (assessed by the AUDIT score) or the major HFE mutation C282Y [6]. Like Canavese et al [50], we found an increased relative risk of iron overload in female patients (relative risk for females: 3.36 (95% CI: 1.03-10.9))[6]. In 11 patients who were monitored closely during parenteral iron therapy, the iron dose infused per month correlated strongly with both the overall increase and the monthly increase in the liver iron concentration (respectively rho=0.66, p=0.0306 and rho=0.85, p=0.0015, Spearman test)(figures 3 and 4)[6].

http://dx.doi.org/10.5772/59316

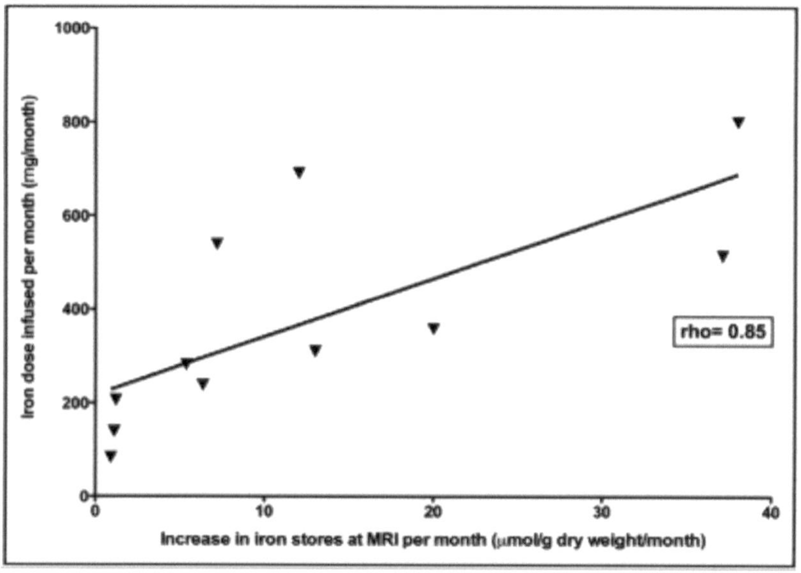

Figure 3. Correlation between the infused iron dose and iron stores in 11 hemodialysis patients. Relationship between the monthly infused dose of iron and the monthly increase in iron stores evaluated by magnetic resonance imaging (MRI) in 11 hemodialysis patients. The relationship was studied with the Spearman test, which showed a very strong correlation (rho=0.854; *P*=0.0015).

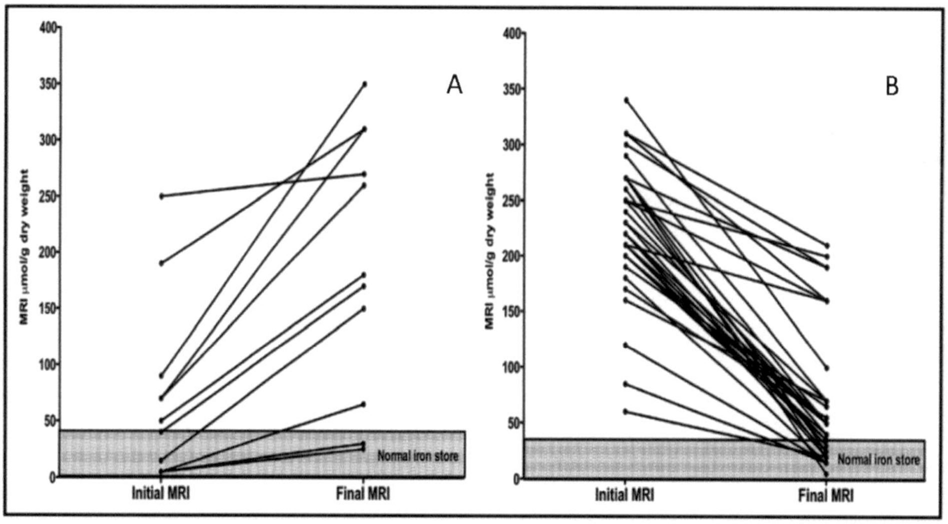

Figure 4. Time course of hepatic iron stores studied by magnetic resonance imaging in hemodialysis patients. (A) Initial and final hepatic iron concentrations on MRI in 11 patients during iron therapy. (B) Initial and final hepatic iron concentrations on MRI in 33 patients with hepatic iron overload after iron withdrawal (n=19) or after a major iron dose reduction (n=14) (according Rostoker G, Griuncelli M, Loridon C et al. Hemodialysis-associated hemosiderosis in the era of erythropoiesis-stimulating agents: a MRI study. Am J Med 2012; 125: 991-999).

In the 33 patients with iron overload, iron stores fell significantly after iron withdrawal or after a major reduction in the iron dose (first MRI: 220 µmol/g (CI: 60-340); last MRI: 50 µmol/g (CI: 5-210); p< 0.0001, Wilcoxon's paired test)(figure 4)[6]. The slope of the decline in hepatic iron was not significantly different after iron withdrawal (17.9 µmol/g dry weight/month), iron dose reduction (12.8 µmol/g dry weight/month), and renal transplantation (11.9 µmol/g dry weight/month)(p>0.05, Kruskal-Wallis test) [6]. Thus, the frequency of iron overload appears to be markedly underestimated in hemodialysis patients receiving both erythropoeisis-stimulating agents and parenteral iron [6,7]. We concluded that most hemodialysis patients receiving ESA and intravenous iron supplementation likely have hepatic iron overload on MRI and called for a revision of guidelines on iron therapy in this setting, especially regarding the amount of iron infused and the use of non invasive methods for monitoring iron stores [6,7].

9. Detrimental effects of iron overload in dialysis patients

The classical (although rare) clinical picture of hemodialysis-associated hemosiderosis in the pre-ESA era (pigmented skin, cirrhosis and cardiac failure associated with multiple endocrine disorders) has totally disappeared from dialysis centers for at least 3 decades [5]. It is also noteworthy that genetic hemochromatosis and secondary hemosiderosis related to hematological disorders are now diagnosed very early, long before any organ dysfunction is detected [37,40]. Therefore, iron overload in dialysis patients in the ESA era is more likely to silently increase the burden of complications of dialysed CKD than to have obvious clinical effects.

Three recent epidemiological studies convergently show that excessive IV iron administration can adversely affect the prognosis of hemodialysis patients by increasing mortality and cardiovascular events [52-54]. In a prospective cohort study conducted in Taiwan, 1239 hemodialysis patients were followed for one year: 583 patients not receiving iron therapy were compared to 656 patients treated with IV ferric chloride hexahydrate, the latter patients being divided into 3 subgroups according the cumulative dose of IV iron: 40-800 mg/6 months, 840-1600 mg/6 months and 1640-2400 mg/6 month [52]. Patients in the 2 subgroups with the largest cumulative iron dose had higher adjusted mortality (Hazard ratio (HR) 3.1 and 3.7) and more cardiovascular events (HR 3.5 and 5.1) than those not receiving IV iron and those having received less than 820 mg/6 months (136 mg/month) [52]. Similarly, Kuragano and coworkers prospectively followed 1086 Japanese hemodialysis patients during 2 years and compared 4 subgroups of patients: an oral iron group, an oral iron+very low IV iron group, a low IV iron group (< 200 mg/month), and a high IV iron group (> 200 mg/month) [53]. They observed more acute cardiocerebral vascular disease (hazard ratio 6.02) and hospitalizations (hazard ratio 2.77) in the high IV iron group, whereas both low (hazard ratio 1.78) and high (hazard ratio 5.22) IV iron regimens increased the frequency of infections but at different rates [53]. High ferritin levels (consistently above 100 µg/L) were associated with an increase risk of acute cardiocerebral vascular disease (hazard ratio 2.22), infections (hazard ratio 1.76) and death (hazard ratio 2.28) [53]. Similarly, a jump in the ferritin level from low to high (from less to more than 100 µg/L) was associated with an increased risk of acute cardiocerebral vascular disease (hazard ratio 1.59) and death (hazard ratio 6.18) [53]. More recently, the DOPPS study, using Cox regression models with multiple adjustments, analyzed associations between IV iron and outcomes in 32 435 hemodialysis patients followed in 12 countries from 2002 to 2011 and found an increased adjusted mortality rate among patients receiving 300-399 mg/month (HR: 1.13) and 400 mg/month or more (HR: 1.18) as compared with those receiving no iron and those receiving 1-99, 100-199 and 200-299 mg of IV iron per month [54]. Similarly, the risk of hospitalization was elevated (HR: 1.12) in patients receiving 300 mg/month or more of IV iron as compared to those receiving 100-199 mg/month [54]. The results of the Japanese study on the risk of infection are convergent with recent results fom an American study showing that iron maintenance therapy at 200 mg/month is not associated with an increased short-term risk of infections, as encountered with bolus characterized by monthly iron exposure of 700 mg [55].

Three mechanisms may act synergystically to increase mortality and cardiovascular events in iron-overloaded dialysis patients, namely increased levels of hepcidin and oxidative stress, and arterial structural changes.

Some authors recently advocated critical re-evaluation of hepcidin levels in renal failure patients, postulating that hepcidin is not intrinsically elevated in hemodialysis patients but rather reflects poor matching with healthy subjects and frequently excessive iron stores in these patients [56]. It thus seems that hepcidin elevation in fact represents a physiologic defense mechanism against iron overload that is preserved in CKD, even during dialysis [56]. Moreover, increased levels of hepcidin-25 in patients with severe iron overload on MRI have been shown to normalize in parallel with LIC normalization [6]. As high levels of hepcidin-25 in dialysis patients have recently been linked to fatal and nonfatal cardiovascular events, it is tempting to postulate that the main pathophysiological pathway between iron overload and these events involves pleiotropic effects of hepcidin-25 [57]. The worsening of oxidative stress usually encountered in end-stage renal disease by IV iron infusions and iron overload (mediated by the release of labile, non transferrin-bound iron) may also adversely affect the vascular bed and act as a "second hit" [58, 59]. Finally, in the hemodialysis population, excess iron may also play a direct role in the high burden of cardiovascular complications by impairing endothelial function, as shown in patients with hereditary hemochromatosis [60], and also by favoring atherosclerosis [61, 62].

Given data on heterozygotous genetic hemochromatosis and secondary hemosideroses, the risk/benefit ratio of iron therapy may remain favorable in hemodialysis patients with mild iron overload (LIC $<$ 100 μmol/g), whereas the risk in patients with moderate iron overload (LIC $>$ 100 μmol/g and $<$ LIC $<$ 200 μmol/g) needs to be ascertained [6,7]. It is also tempting to postulate that hemodialysis patients with severe hepatic iron overload (e.g. $>$ 200 μmol/g) are at risk of silent and gradual multiple organ dysfunctions due to hemosiderosis, together with a higher burden of cardiovascular complications [6,7].

10. Future directions

Iron overload in hemodialysis patients may be favored by reimbursement policies in the USA and many other developed countries, which have led to a dramatic increase in the use of intravenous iron preparations in order to offset the cost of ESA therapy; the situation may also be aggravated by excessive advocated doses of intravenous iron and erroneous iron biomarker targets aimed at "repleting exaggerately" iron stores [6,7]. A new pharmacometric and economic approach to iron therapy has recently been advocated [6,7,26,58]. Moreover, the KDIGO Controversies Conference on Iron Management in Chronic Kidney Disease, which took place in San Francisco on March 27-30, 2014 and was attended by nephrologists, hematologists, hepatologists and specialists in iron metabolism, recognized the entity of iron overload in hemodialysis patients and called for an agenda of research on this topic, especially by means of MRI [63]. Analysis of liver iron content in dialysis patients by means of quantitative MRI, a new research tool that overcomes a major hypothetical limitation in hemodialysis patients, namely bone marrow iron depletion despite severe hepatosplenic siderosis, and allows safe non aggressive iterative "radiological liver biopsy" might, in combination with data-mining statistical methods and classical statistical methods such as AUC determination and logistic regression, allow nephrologists to determine both a non toxic dose of infused iron and relevant target values for biological markers of iron metabolism, thereby improving the safety of parenteral iron products in dialysis patients [6,7,26,58, 63]. Finally, specific MRI protocols need to be established in radiology and nephrology divisions for each pharmaceutical iron product, in order to avoid spurious results [47].

Permissions

Parts of the chapter are reproduced from the authors' previous publication "Maximal Standard Dose of Parenteral Iron for Hemodialysis Patients: An MRI-Based Decision Tree Learning Analysis" Guy Rostoker, Mireille Griuncelli, Christelle Loridon, Théophile Magna, Philippe Janklewicz, Gilles Drahi, Hervé Dahan, Yves Cohen.

PLoS One. 2014 Dec 15; 9(12):e115096. doi: 10.1371/journal.pone.0115096. eCollection 2014.

Parts of the chapter are reproduced from the authors' previous publication "Hemodialysis-associated hemosiderosis in the era of erythropoiesis-stimulating agents: a MRI study." Rostoker G1, Griuncelli M, Loridon C, Couprie R, Benmaadi A, Bounhiol C, Roy M, Machado G, Janklewicz P, Drahi G, Dahan H, Cohen Y. Am J Med. 2012 Oct; 125(10):991-999.e1. doi: 10.1016/j.amjmed.2012.01.015.

Author details

Guy Rostoker[1*], Mireille Griuncelli[1], Christelle Loridon[1] and Yves Cohen[2]

*Address all correspondence to: rostotom@orange.fr

1 Division of Nephrology and Dialysis, HP Claude Galien, Ramsay Générale de Santé, Quincy sous Sénart, France

2 Division of Radiology, HP Claude Galien, Ramsay Générale de Santé, Quincy sous Sénart, France

References

[1] KDOQI National Kidney Foundation. ll. Clinical practice guidelines and clinical practice recommendations for anemia in chronic kidney disease in adults. Am J Kidney Dis 2006; 47(5 Suppl. 3): Sl6-S85

[2] Eschbach JW, Egrie JC, Downing MR et al. Correction of the anemia of end-stage renal disease with recombinant human erythropoietin. Results of a combined phase I and II clinical trial. N Engl J Med 1987; 316(2): 73-78

[3] Hörl WH. Clinical aspects of iron use in the anemia of kidney disease. J Am Soc Nephrol 2007; 18(2): 382-393

[4] Kalantar-Zadeh K, Kalantar-Zadeh K, Lee GH. The fascinating but deceptive ferritin: to measure it or not to measure it in chronic kidney disease? Clin J Am Soc Nephrol 2006; 1 Suppl 1: S9-S18

[5] Ali M, Fayemi AO, Frascino J, et al. Failure of serum ferritin levels to predict bone-marrow iron content after intravenous iron-dextran therapy. Lancet 1982 Mar 20; 1(8273): 652-655

[6] Rostoker G, Griuncelli M, Loridon C et al. Hemodialysis-associated hemosiderosis in the era of erythropoiesis-stimulating agents: a MRI study. Am J Med 2012; 125(10): 991-999

[7] Vaziri ND. Epidemic of iron overload in dialysis population caused by intravenous iron products: a plea for moderation. Am J Med 2012; 125(10): 951-952

[8] Himmelfarb J. Iron regulation. J Am Soc Nephrol 2007; 18(2): 379-381

[9] Locatelli F, Covic A, Eckardt KU et al. Anaemia management in patients with chronic kidney disease: a position statement by the Anaemia Working Group of European Renal Best Practice (ERBP). Nephrol Dial Transplant 2009; 24(2): 348-354

[10] KDIGO Clinical practice Guideline for anemia in chronic kidney disease. Kidney Int Suppl 2012; 2: 279-335

[11] Locatelli F, Bárány P, Covic A et al on behalf of the ERA-EDTA ERBP advisory board. Kidney disease: Improving global outcomes guidelines on anaemia management in chronic kidney disease: an European Renal Best Practice position statement; Nephrol Dial Transplant; 2013; 28(6): 1346-1359

[12] Yamamoto H, Tsubakihara Y. Limiting iron supplementation for anemia in dialysis patients--the Basis for Japan's conservative guidelines. Semin Dial 2011; 24(3): 269-271

[13] Kohgo Y, Ikuta K, Ohtake T, et al. Body iron metabolism and pathophysiology of iron overload. Int J Hematol. 2008; 88(1):7-15.

[14] Scientific advisory committee on nutrition. Iron and health. 2010, London, TSO.

[15] Kautz L, Jung G, Valore EV et al. Identification of erythroferrone as an erythroid regulator of iron metabolism. Nature Genet 2014; 46(7): 678-684

[16] De Falco L, Sanchez M, Silvestri L et al. Iron refractory deficiency anemia. Haematologica 2013; 98 (6): 845-853

[17] Sargent JA and Acchiardo SR. Iron requirements in hemodialysis. Blood Purif 2004; 22(1): 112-123

[18] Otti T, Khajehdehi P, Fawzy A et al. Comparison of blood loss with different high-flux and high-efficiency hemodialysis membranes. Am J Nephrol 2001; 21(1): 16-19

[19] Kalocheretis P, Vlamis I, Belesi C et al. Residual blood loss in single use dialyzers: effect of different membranes and flux. Int J Artif Organs 2006; 29(3): 286-292

[20] Rottembourg J and Rostoker G. Use of intravenous iron products in chronic kidney disease. Submitted for publication

[21] Rosenblatt SG, Drake S, Fadem S et al. Gastrointestinal blood loss in patients with chronic renal failure. Am J Kidney Dis 1982; 1(4): 232-236

[22] Flint S, Taylor E, Beavis J et al. Increased iron requirement in hemodialysis patients on antiplatelet agents or warfarin. Nephron Clin Pract 2009; 113(1): c38-c45

[23] Goicoechea M, Caramelo C, Ochando A, et al. Antiplatelet therapy alters iron requirements in hemodialysis patients. Am J Kidney Dis 2000; 36(1): 80-87

[24] Anastassiades EG, Howarth D, Howarth J et al. Monitoring of iron requirements in renal patients on erythropoietin. Nephrol Dial transplant 1993; 8(9): 846-853

[25] Van Wyck DB. Iron deficiency in patients with dialysis–associated anemia during erythropoietin replacement therapy: strategies for assessment and management. Semin Nephrol 1989; 9 (1 Suppl 2): 21-24

[26] Gaweda AE, Ginzburg YZ, Chait Y et al. Iron dosing in kidney disease: inconsistency of evidence and clinical practice. Nephrol Dial Transplant 2014; doi 10.1093/ndt/gfu 104. First published online: May 12, 2014.

[27] Freburger JK, Ng LJ, Bradbury B et al. Changing patterns of anemia management in US hemodialysis patients. Am J Med 2012; 125(9): 906-914

[28] Pisoni RL, Fuller DS, Bieber BA et al. The DOPPS practice monitor for US dialysis care: trends through August 2011. Am J Kidney Diseases 2012; 60(1): 160-165

[29] Bailie GR, Larkina M, Goodkin DA et al. Variation in intravenous iron use internationally and over time: the Dialysis Outcomes and Practice Patterns Study (DOPPS). Nephrol Dial Transplant 2013; 28(10): 2570-2579

[30] Ali M, Fayemi AO, Rigolosi R et al. Hemosiderosis in hemodialysis patients. An autopsy study of 50 cases. JAMA 1980; 244(4): 343-345

[31] Pitts TO, Barbour GL. Hemosiderosis secondary to chronic parenteral iron therapy in maintenance hemodialysis patients. Nephron 1978; 22(4-6): 316-321

[32] Gokal R, Millard PR, Weatherall DJ et al. Iron metabolism in haemodialysis patients. A study of the management of iron therapy and overload. Q J Med 1979; 48(191): 369-391

[33] Simon P. Detoxification in hemosiderosis. Blood Purif 1985; 3(1-3): 75-88

[34] Agroyannis B, Koutsicos D, Tzanatou-Exarchou H et al. Combined recombinant human erythropoetin-blood letting stategy for treating anemia and iron overload in hemodialysis patients. Int J Artificial Organs 1991; 14(7): 403-406

[35] Cecchin E, De Marchi S, Querin F et al. Efficacy of hepatic computed tomography to detect iron overload in chronic hemodialysis. Kidney Int 1990; 37(3): 943-950.

[36] Angelucci E, Brittenham GM, McLaren CE, et al. Hepatic iron concentration and total body iron stores in thalassemia major. N Engl J Med 2000; 343(5): 327–331.

[37] Brissot P, Troadec MB, Bardou-Jacquet E et al. Current approach to hemochromatosis. Blood Rev 2008; 22(4): 195-210

[38] Fischer R, Harmatz PR. Non-invasive assessment of tissue iron overload. Hematology Am Soc Hematol Educ Program 2009: 215-221

[39] Alústiza JM, Castiella A, De Juan MD et al. Iron overload in the liver diagnostic and quantification. Eur J Radiol 2007; 61(3): 499-506

[40] Angelucci E, Barosi G, Camaschella C et al. Italian Society of Hematology practice guidelines for the management of iron overload in thalassemia major and related disorders. Haematologica 2008; 93(5): 741-752

[41] Gandon Y, Olivié D, Guyader D et al. Non-invasive assessment of hepatic iron stores by MRI. Lancet 2004; 363(9406): 357-362

[42] Rose C, Vandevenne P, Bourgeois E et Al. Liver iron content assessment by routine and simple magnetic resonance imaging procedure in highly transfused patients. Eur J Haematol 2006; 77(2): 14-149

[43] lthof AW, Sijens PE, Kreeftenberg HG et al. Non-invasive liver iron concentration measurement by MRI: comparison of two validated protocols. Eur J Radiol 2009; 71: 116-121

[44] Castiella A, Alustiza JM, Emparanza JI et al. Liver iron quantification by MRI : are recommended protocols accurate enough for clinical practice. Eur J Radiol 2011; 21(1): 137-141

[45] St Pierre TG, Clark PR, Chua-Anusom W et al. Noninvasive measurement and imaging of liver iron concentrations using proton magnetic resonance. Blood 2005; 105(2): 855-861

[46] Wood JC, Enriquez C, Ghugre N et al. MRI R2 and R2*mapping accurately estimates hepatic iron concentration in transfusion-dependent thalassemia and sickle cell disease patients. Blood 2005; 106(4): 1460-1465

[47] Rostoker G and Cohen Y. Magnetic resonance imaging repercussions of intravenous iron products used for iron-deficiency anemia and dialysis-associated anemia. J Comp Assist Tomogr 2014, Sept 16

[48] Ferrari P, Kulkarni H, Dheda S et al. Serum iron markers are inadequate for guiding iron repletion in chronic kidney disease. Clin J Am Soc Nephrol 2011; 6(1): 77-83

[49] Ghoti H, Rachmilewitz EA, Simon-Lopez R et al. Evidence for tissue iron overload in long-term hemodialysis patients and the impact of withdrawing parenteral iron. Eur J Haematol 2012; 89(1): 87-93

[50] Canavese C, Bergamo D, Ciccone G et al. Validation of serum ferritin values by magnetic susceptometry in predicting iron overload in dialysis patients. Kidney Int 2004; 65(3): 1091-1098

[51] Fishbane S, Miyawaki N, Masani N. Hepatic iron in hemodialysis patients. Kidney Int 2004; 66(4): 1714-1715

[52] Kuo KL, Hung SC, Lin YP et al. Intravenous ferric chloride hexahydrate supplementation induced endothelial dysfunction and increased cardiovascular risk among hemodialysis patients. PloS One 2012; 7(12): e50295

[53] Kuragano T, Matsumura O, Matsuda A et al. Association between hemoglobin variability, serum ferritin levels, and adverse events/mortality in maintenance hemodialysis patients. Kidney International, 23 april 2014; doi: 10.1038/ki.2014.114

[54] Bailie GR, Larkina M, Goodkin DA et al. Data from the Dialysis Outcomes and Practice Patterns Study validate an association between high intravenous iron doses and mortality. Kidney Int 30 july 2014 /doi: 10.1038 /ki.2014.275

[55] Brookhart MA, Freburger JK, Ellis AR et al. Infection risk with bolus versus maintenance iron supplementation in hemodialysis patients. JASN 2013; 24(7): 1151-1158

[56] Valenti L, Messa P, Pelusi S et al. Hepcidin levels in chronic hemodialysis patients: a critical evaluation. Clin Chem and Lab Med 2014; 52(5): 613-619

[57] Van der Weerd NC, Grooteman MP, Bots ML et al. Hepcidin-25 is related to cardiovascular events in chronic haemodialysis patients. Nephrol Dial Transplant 2013; 28(12): 3062-3071

[58] Fishbane S, Mathew A, Vaziri ND. Iron toxicity: relevance for dialysis patients. Nephrol Dial Transplant 2014; 29(2): 255-259.

[59] Morena M, Delbosc S, Dupuy AM, Canaud B, Cristol JP. Overproduction of reactive oxygen species in end-stage renal disease patients: a potential component of hemodialysis-associated inflammation. Hemodial Int 2005; 9(1): 37-46

[60] Gaenzer H, Marschang P, Sturm W et al. Association between increased iron stores and impaired endothelial function in patients with hereditary hemochromatosis. J Am Coll Cardiol 2002; 40(12): 2189-2194

[61] Drüeke T, Witko-Sarsat V, Massy Z et al. Iron therapy, advanced oxidation protein products and carotid artery intima-media thickness in end-stage renal disease. Circulation 2002; 106(17): 2212-2217

[62] Reis KA, Guz G, Ozdemir H et al. Intravenous iron therapy as a possible risk factor for atherosclerosis in end-stage renal disease. Int Heart J 2005; 46(2): 255-264

[63] KDIGO Controversies Conference on iron management in chronic kidney disease, March 27-30, 2014, San-Francisco, USA.

Chapter 5

Bone Fragility in Hemodialysis Patients

Shozo Yano

Additional information is available at the end of the chapter

http://dx.doi.org/10.5772/59408

1. Introduction

According to WHO technical report in 1994, osteoporosis is a disease characterized by low bone mass and microarchitectural deterioration of bone tissue leading to enhanced bone fragility, and consequently increases the fracture risk. Since fracture does not solely depend on bone mass, osteoporosis was defined by NIH as a skeletal disorder, characterized by compromised bone strength predisposing to an increased risk of fracture. Although aging is a major risk for fracture, it is a strong risk for chronic kidney disease (CKD) as well. Thus, patients having comorbidity of CKD and osteoporosis are sometimes found. According to a study NHANES III (the Third National Health and Nutrition Examination Survey, 1988-1994) in the US, in women with osteoporosis, 85% (95%CI: 79-91%) showed Creatinine clearance (Ccr)≤60mL/min and 24% (95%CI: 19-29%) were of Ccr<35mL/min [1]. Another study demonstrated that Ccr≤60mL/min is an independent risk factor for fracture at vertebra, femur and radius [2].

In addition to aging, a female sex, low bone mineral density (BMD), prevalent fracture, family history of fracture and lower body weight, life style such as drinking, smoking and excise and common diseases would affect risk for fracture [3, 4]. Recent studies demonstrate that measurement of BMD by Dual-energy X-ray absorptiometry (DXA), which is a gold standard for diagnosis of osteoporosis, is less useful for the fracture prediction in the patients with diabetes mellitus and the patients under glucocorticoid therapy [5-8]. Among these population, BMD-independent bone fragility and falls may be involved in an elevation of the risk for fracture. Therefore, much interest is focused on the link between kidney dysfunction /CKD and fracture /osteoporosis [9].

2. Elevated risk for fracture in end-stage kidney disease

Compared with general population, the risk for fracture is reported to be much higher in end-stage kidney disease (ESKD) (Table 1) [10-14]. A multicenter cohort study in the US having more than 320,000 dialysis patients, 13.6 in women and 7.5 in men had an incident hip fracture among 1,000 person-years [10].The incidence ratio standardized with age was about 4.4 times higher than that of healthy subjects. Another study in a single institution in the US having 1,272 dialysis patients, 13.9 (24.1 in women and 11.7 in men) had an incident hip fracture among 1,000 person-years, which was 17.4 times higher than that of general population [11]. Increased risk of hip fracture was shown among Japanese hemodialysis (HD) patients, in which the risk was about 5 times higher than that of general population [12]. Facture risk of HD patients was increased in the west part of Japan, which showed similar results to the general population [12, 15]. A multicenter prospective study (DOPPS II) in 12,782 patients from 12 countries showed that 8.9/1,000 person-years had a hip fracture [13]. In addition, risk for fracture may even be higher for 3 years after kidney transplantation [16].

Study design	Subjects	Fracture type	Fracture incidence of 1,000 person-years and RR (95%CI) for general population			Reference
Retrospective cohort study	326,464 dialysis patients in the US	hip	men	7.45	4.44 (4.16-4.75)	[10]
			women	13.63	4.40 (4.17-4.64)	
Retrospective cohort study	1,272 dialysis patients in the US	hip	men	11.7	14.2 (9.3-28.6)	[11]
			women	24.1	17.2 (7.1-19.4)	
			all	13.9	17.4 (12.4-34.0)	
Prospective cohort study	12,782 HD patients in 320 HD facilities from 12 countries	hip	men, 15-54		1.00 (Ref)	[13]
			men, 55-64		2.15 (1.06-4.57)	
			men, 65-74		2.38 (1.07-5.26)	
			men, 75-		5.05 (2.36-10.82)	
			women, 15-54		0.85 (0.30-2.35)	
			women, 55-64		1.85 (0.75-4.59)	
			women, 65-74		4.67 (2.22-9.83)	
			women, 75-		7.79 (3.69-16.43)	
			all	8.9 (8.4-9.4)		
		any	men, 15-54		1.00 (Ref)	
			men, 55-64		1.25 (0.84-1.85)	
			men, 65-74		1.65 (1.10-2.48)	
			men, 75-		1.86 (1.24-2.77)	
			women, 15-54		1.07 (0.67-1.69)	
			women, 55-64		2.36 (1.56-3.54)	
			women, 65-74		2.58 (1.79-3.63)	
			women, 75-		3.43 (2.33-5.06)	
			all	25.6 (24.4-27.0)		
Retrospective cohort study	128,141 HD patients in Japan	hip	men	7.57	6.2 (5.7-6.8)	[12]
			women	17.43	4.9 (4.6-5.3)	

Table 1. Elevated fracture risk in ESKD

Mean age of incident fracture in dialysis patients is reported to be 61.4 in women and 64.4 in men, which are much younger than those of general population (74 and 80, respectively), indicating that dialysis patients apt to suffer from bone fractures at younger age [11]. The incidence of hip fracture in dialysis patients of 60 and 70 years old is comparable to those of 75 and 80 years, respectively [13, 14].

CKD is not only at risk for fracture but also at mortality risk after fracture [11, 17, 18]. Coco et al. reported the mortality rate was 64% a year after hip fracture in HD patients, whereas it was about 20% in the healthy subjects [11]. Among HD patients, mortality rate was showed to be 2.7 times greater in patients with incident fracture, compared to those without fracture [17]. Moreover, significant elevation of fracture-associated mortality risk was found in patients even before the initiation of HD therapy [18].Although bisphosphonates may not be recommended in ESKD patients, they are useful in osteoporotic patients with great risk reduction for fracture [19]. PTH agent such as teriparatide, and selective estrogen receptor modulator (SERM) are also established therapies with 50% or more of relative risk reduction [20, 21].Thus, early starts of therapy for osteoporosis will prevent fracture. These findings suggest that clinicians need to evaluate bone status and initiate osteoporosis therapy in patients with CKD in early stages.

3. Elevated risk for fracture in early stages of CKD

Although considerably high risk for fracture has been shown in ESKD patients, recent epidemiological studies indicate that the risk for fracture is elevated in CKD patients, even in early stages (Table 2). Nickolas et al. reported that CKD was an independent predictor of prevalent hip fracture [22]. When categorized 6,270 participants by estimated glomerular filtration rate (eGFR) using MDRD formula, prevalent hip fracture was found in 5.2% and 2.0% of those with eGFR 15-60mL/min/1.73m^{2}and eGFR>60mL/min/1.73m^2, respectively. Odds ratio of prevalent hip fracture in those with CKD was 2.12 (95%CI: 1.18-3.80), compared with those with eGFR>100mL/min/1.73m^2. Multiple logistic analysis for prevalent hip fracture showed that osteoporosis (OR=2.52, 95%CI: 1.08-5.91), low activity (OR=2.10, 95%CI: 1.03-4.27) and CKD (OR=2.32, 95%CI: 1.13-4.74) were the risk factors independent of age, sex, body weight, race, BMD, history of hip fracture in mother, dietary calcium intake, and 25(OH)D blood level and propensity score to CKD. In ≥75 years subjects with and without prevalent fracture, the ratio of CKD suffered was 32.1% and 32.2%, respectively, whereas in < 75 years subjects, the ratio was 19.2% and 6.2%, respectively. This finding suggests that the younger patients with prevalent fractures suffer from CKD almost 3 times more frequently, compared to those without fractures. Thus, CKD (eGFR: 15-60mL/min/1.73m^2) is an independent risk of hip fracture, especially in subjects with <75 years old.

Ensrud et al. conducted a prospective study to examine risk for fracture in 9,704 women with >65 years, stratified by CCr (Cockcroft-Gault formula) corrected with body surface area [23]. During 6 years observational period, hazard ratios of hip fracture were 2.32 (95%CI: 1.15-4.68) in CCr<45 mL/min/1.73m^2 and 1.57 (95%CI: 0.89-2.76) in CCr45-59 mL/min/1.73m^2, compared to CCr≥60 mL/min/1.73m^2. These results suggest that decreased kidney function is a risk for incident hip fracture independent of age, body weight and calcaneal BMD. However, significant difference disappeared after adjustment by healthy status, smoking, walking excise,

Study design	Subjects	Kidney function	Odds ratio of fracture risk (95%CI)		Reference
Cross-sectional study	5313 osteoporotic patients aged >65 in Germany	CCr <65mL/min	hip radius vertebra	1.57 (1.18–2.09) 1.79 (1.39–2.31) 1.31 (1.19–1.55)	[2]
Cross-sectional study	6270 subjects aged >50 in the US	eGFR <60mL/min/1.73m²	hip	2.32 (1.13–4.74)	[22]
Cohort study	9704 women aged >65 in the US	CCr 45~59mL/min CCr <45mL/min CCr 45~59mL/min CCr <45mL/min CCr 45~59mL/min CCr <45mL/min	femoral neck femoral neck trochanter trochanter vertebra vertebra	1.24 (0.60–2.56) 1.41(0.59–3.36) 3.69(1.21–11.24) 5.04(1.38–18.45) 1.08(0.61–1.92) 1.33(0.63–2.80)	[23]
Case-control study	6458 postmenopausal osteoporotic women in Canada	CCr <45mL/min	all vertebra	1.3(1.0–1.6) 2.5(1.6–3.9)	[66]
Cohort study	4699 subjects aged >65 in the US	eGFR<60mL/min/1.73m² Cystatin C 1SD above	hip hip	1.38(0.99–1.94) 1.16(1.01–1.33)	[25]
Case-control study	397 incident hip fracture cases and 397 matched controls in the US	eGFR<60mL/min/1.73m²	hip	2.50(1.32–4.72)	[67]
Case-control study	659 postmenopausal women in Japan	CCr 60~89mL/min	vertebra	2.79(1.31–5.95)	[26]

Table 2. Elevated fracture risk in CKD

diabetes mellitus (DM), and history of fracture occurred after 50 years old. On the other hand, only a tendency was observed using eGFR by MDRD formula instead of CCr. Moreover, the analysis of fracture sites shows that the risk for fracture was elevated at the trochanter not at the femoral neck, indicating that hip fracture in CKD patients could be associated with the frailty [24].

Since sarcopenia or protein-energy wasting (PEW) is commonly seen in CKD patients, eGFR derived from creatinine often underestimates actual kidney function. Cystatin C is more accurate estimate for kidney function than eGFR calculated from creatinine, especially in elderly people whose muscle mass is reduced. Fried et al. demonstrated a significant association between cystatin C blood level and hip fracture risk in 4,699 subjects in their prospective study. Women with eGFR<60 mL/min/1.73m² have an increased risk for fracture even after adjusting the covariates [25].

So far, few studies are performed to evaluate the relationship between kidney function and vertebral fractures. In a case-control study of 659 postmenopausal osteoporotic women with an average age of 64.5 years, 45.3% of those with eGFR<60 mL/min/1.73m² had prevalent vertebral fractures and the ratio was significantly higher than those with eGFR 60-89 mL/min/1.73m² (25.3%) and eGFR≥90 mL/min/1.73m² (23.8%) [26]. Multiple logistic regression analysis showed that CCr was selected as a significant predictor of prevalent vertebral fracture after adjustment for years after menopause, smoking, drinking, and BMD at vertebrae (OR=0.359, 95%CI: 0.168-0.765, p=0.01). There were significant positive correlations between eGFR and BMD at the femoral neck and the radius. These findings suggest that the reduction of BMD and the elevation of risk for fracture may start during early CKD (eGFR<90 mL/min/1.73m^2).

However, Ensrud et al. could not find a significant association of incident vertebral fractures with kidney function calculated by C-G as well as MDRD formulas [23]. The discrepancies of these two reports could be derived from the differences of participants' background such as race, age, and kidney function, and the methodology. In the latter study, 150 patients, who had incident vertebral fractures, were relatively older (mean age: 73.1 years) than those of the former study. In addition, the second X-ray was not performed in 22% of women possibly due to bed rest or death. Thus, such limitation should be taken into account when the results of prospective study are assessed.

Previous studies suggest that the risk for fracture is elevated in parallel with a decrease in kidney function. We estimated the risk for fracture with the assessment tool FRAX® (http://www.shef.ac.uk/FRAX/) in 1,935 community-dwelling healthy Japanese people (1,123 women and 812 men, mean age: 68.9) [27]. Estimated risk of hip fracture for 10 years was 2.1% in men and 4.6% in women, respectively (Figure 1), and the risk was inversely proportionate to eGFR. Significant increase of the risk for fracture was observed in men with eGFR<60 ml/min/1.73m^2 and women with eGFR<75 ml/min/1.73m^2. Major risk of osteoporotic fracture (vertebrae, hip, radius and humerus) for 10 years was estimated as 6.8% in men and 14.0% in women, which was also elevated as a loss of kidney function. As we have shown the elevated risk for fracture in CKD population using FRAX®, this tool has originally been developed for the screening of patients with high risk for fracture. Indeed, Jamal et al. have recently reported the utility of FRAX® in CKD patients [28].

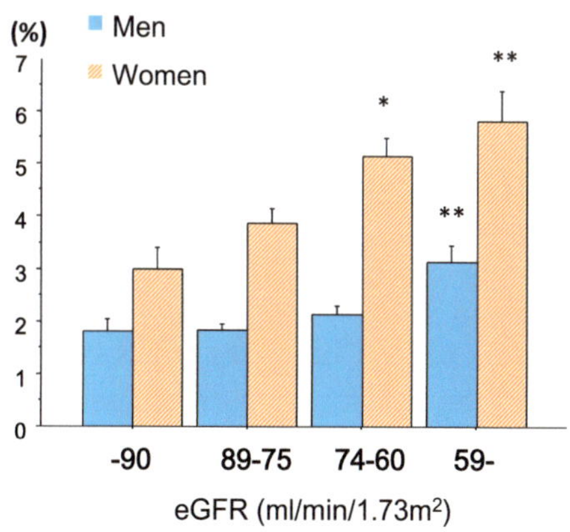

Figure 1. Association between eGFR and 10 year-hip fracture incidence calculated by FRAX® In 1,935 community-dwelling healthy Japanese people (1,123 women and 812 men, mean age: 68.9), association between eGFR (MDRD formula) and 10 year-hip fracture incidence calculated by FRAX® was shown. *; p<0.001and **; p<0.005 (vs eGFR 90-ml/min/1.73m^2), Post-hoc test (Fisher's PLSD) (modified by ref. [27])

In this part, terms such as eGFR and CCr were used followed by the original reports. Moreover, CCr was corrected with body surface in some reports and not in others. Kidney function is prone to be underestimated in C-G formula and overestimated in MDRD, which may lead confusion and the discrepancy among study results as described by Ensrud et al. [23].

4. Pathophysiology of elevated risk for fracture in CKD

Low BMD is a risk for fracture in the general population, and this is also true for CKD patients [29-32]. Recent longitudinal studies using high resolution peripheral quantitative computed tomography (HR-pQCT) have demonstrated that loss of kidney function is associated with a decrease in BMD, independent of age and body mass [29-32]. HR-pQCT is developed to measure volumetric bone mass, and to discriminate between cortical bone and trabecular bone. Volumetric BMD measured by HR-pQCT is more accurate than areal BMD by DXA, because areal BMD depends on body size and cannot exclude aortic calcification [33]. Cejka et al. reported the characteristics of bone microarchitecture of 74 HD patients, where cortical and trabecular microarchitecture was significantly impaired in patients with fracture [34]. Trabecular BMD at the tibia was the strongest determinant of fracture in these patients. In 70 patients aged ≥50 with CKD stage 2-4, trabecular BMD at the tibia and radius, trabecular number and cortical thickness were significantly decreased and trabecular separation was increased [35]. Another study by Nickolas demonstrated a significant loss of cortical BMD at the distal radius, and marked increase in cortical porosity without any changes in trabecular indices in CKD patients [36]. There was a significant association between kidney dysfunction and cortical bone loss as well as increased porosity [35]. Although DXA has a lower discriminatory power than HR-pQCT measured volumetric density, a recent report suggests a benefit of BMD measurement even with DXA to identify HD patients with high risk of fracture [32].

Although bone histological analysis is the most accurate method, a few studies have been reported because of its invasiveness and difficulty. Tomiyama et al. conducted bone biopsy at the iliac crest of 50 CKD patients after tetracycline labelling [37]. Interestingly, histomorphometry showed low turnover of bone in most patients; 100% in stage 2, 88% in stage 3, and 78% in stage 4. This finding suggests that the bone formation rate is markedly depressed in CKD at early stages.

Bone strength depends not only on BMD but also on the other factors, which have been called as a bone quality. In primary osteoporosis, bone strength is explained about 70% by BMD and the rest by bone quality. Since the risk for fracture is dissociated with BMD especially in patients with DM and with glucocorticoid-induced osteoporosis, areal BMD cannot effectively predict fracture [5-8]. This might be the case in CKD, and the factors other than BMD, such as bone quality would play a part in bone fragility, especially in later stages of CKD. Especially in patients with type 2 DM, bone strength is significantly decreased, while BMD tends to be increased due to obesity. Because DM is a leading cause of ESKD, at least to some extent DM affects risk for fracture in CKD population. Actually, previous reports demonstrated the significant elevation of risk for fracture in ESKD patients with DM, compared to those without

DM [38]. Pathogenesis of elevated risk for fracture in DM is explained by deteriorated bone quality as well as increased incidence of falls. DM patients treated by insulin have 2.78 times higher risk for falls than non-DM subjects [39]. In addition, DM is an independent risk for falls in HD patients with OR of 2.75 [40]. Increased risk of falls in DM may be caused by impaired neuromuscular function, increased instability, loss of vision, hypoglycemia, arthritis, cardiovascular disorders, depression and medication such as hypnotics or tranquilizers. Thus, these factors including DM should be the risks for falls and fracture in CKD patients.

Many factors are known as a risk for fracture including low BMD, factors independent of BMD such as older age, female sex, prevalent fracture, smoking, drinking, steroid use, family history for fracture, excise, and factors dependent of BMD such as low body weight [3, 4]. On the other hand, in CKD patients, there may be additional factors including history of kidney transplant, decreased $1,25(OH)_2D$, increased parathyroid hormone (PTH), other hormonal changes, metabolic acidosis, uremic toxins, inflammatory cytokines, and homocysteine play a role [41-48]. Although each occurs at different stages of CKD, all can affect the bone at the end-stage. Bone changes can be associated with PTH and bone metabolic markers. However, increase in serum PTH level generally starts at GFR <45mL/min. Actually, recent studies using cystatin C demonstrated that PTH, inflammation, and bone turnover did not affect the risk for fracture at least in early CKD [49, 50]. On the contrary, increasing evidences suggest that fibroblast growth factor 23 (FGF23) level is elevated to suppress bone formation at CKD stage 2, which occurs at an earlier time than the increase in PTH or decrease in $1,25(OH)_2D$ [51-53]. In addition, FGF23 may be an independent risk of vertebral fracture [54].

Bone quality is classified by material and structural properties, both of which are considered to be altered in CKD. As for structural properties, cortical thinning, porosity, and irregular thickness and loss of connectivity in trabecular bone have been reported [36]. On the other hand, material properties are not well understood. Animal study shows the changes in chemical composition of cortical bone and the deterioration in the quality of bone matrix proteins, such as type I collagen and collagen crosslinking [55], although there is a controversy [56]. These changes are thought to be resulted from an increase in advanced glycation end products (AGEs) including pentosidine that causes loss of normal crosslinking; which are mediated by high glucose, homocysteine, reactive oxygen species and low vitamin B_6 [57, 58]. Therefore, both loss of bone volume and deterioration of bone quality (altered material and structural properties at micro and macro levels) may be involved in the progression of bone fragility in CKD. Future study is needed to elucidate the deteriorated bone quality in CKD including functional changes in osteocytes and involvement of sclerostin, which regulates osteoblastic activity.

At present, however, most conceivable reason for increased risk for fracture in CKD patients is that CKD and osteoporosis have a lot of common risk factors for the pathogenesis and disease progression (Figure 2). This fact is supported by clinical findings [20, 46]. The factors including aging, inflammation, renin-angiotensin axis, oxidative stress, insulin resistance, hyperglycemia, AGEs, smoking, menopause, lack of exercise, homocysteine, uremic toxins, ADMA, and FGF23 are possible common candidates. At the same time, these factors are thought to be involved in the development of vascular calcification [46, 59-63]. In addition to the relationship between vascular calcification/ atherosclerosis and osteoporosis, so called bone-vascular relationship, hypertension and chronic obstructive pulmonary disease (COPD) also become aware of fracture risks. On the other hand, cortical bone thickness measured by HR-pQCT was reported to be the best predictor for hip fracture in CKD patients [64]. Since bone turnover markers such as P1NP and TRACP5b are risk factors for fracture independent of BMD in CKD patients, combination of BMD and bone turnover markers makes it possible to discriminate subjects with bone fragility [64]. Further studies are necessary to identify noninvasive assessment tools for fracture risk.

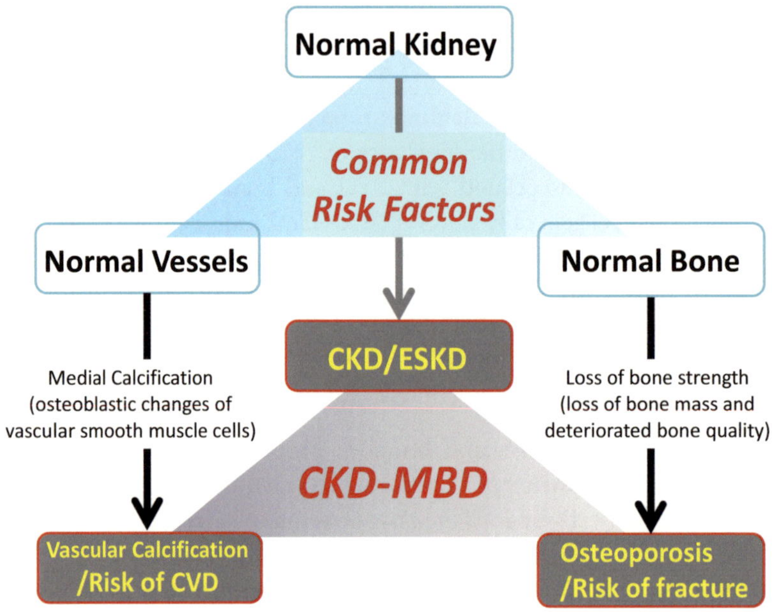

Figure 2. Mechanisms of elevated risk for fracture in CKD patients. Although precise mechanisms remain uncertain, CKD and osteoporosis have many common risk factors, and in addition, CKD progression is associated with increased risk for fracture probably due to bone loss as well as deterioration of bone quality. Aging, inflammation, renin-angiotensin axis, oxidative stress, insulin resistance, hyperglycemia, AGEs, smoking, menopause, lack of exercise, homocysteine, uremic toxins, ADMA, and FGF23 are possible candidates for the common factors, and at the same time, these are thought to be involved in the development of vascular calcification.

5. Conclusion

CKD is not a single disease but a kind of syndrome. Thus, hypertension, obesity, atherosclerosis, gout, nephrolithiasis and life style are highly linked to the pathogenesis and the development of CKD. Diabetic nephropathy and hypertensive nephropathy are commonly observed in CKD, and these are probably at high risk for fracture. Because prevalence of CKD and osteoporosis increases in parallel with age, aged people often suffer from both disorders. Nowadays, CKD has been established as a risk factor for fragility fracture independent of age and BMD. Not only CKD progression but also bone loss is associated with mortality [61-63]. Thus, bone should be cared in early stages of CKD, at least followed by guidelines [42, 65]. Since bisphosphonates are not recommended in ESKD patients, future work is necessary to establish treatment of osteoporosis or osteopenia complicated with ESKD.

Acknowledgements

This work is partly supported by Grant-In-Aids for Scientific research, Kakenhi (C) (24591230).

Author details

Shozo Yano*

Address all correspondence to: syano@med.shimane-u.ac.jp

Department of Laboratory Medicine, Shimane University Faculty of Medicine, Izumo city, Shimane, Japan

References

[1] Klawansky S, Komaroff E, Cavanaugh PF Jr, Mitchell DY, Gordon MJ, Connelly JE, Ross SD. Relationship between age, renal function and bone mineral density in the US population. Osteoporos Int 2003; 14: 570-576.

[2] Dukas L, Schacht E, Stähelin HB: In elderly men and women treated for osteoporosis a low creatinine clearance of<65 ml/min is a risk factor for falls and fractures. Osteoporos Int 2005; 16: 1683–1690.

[3] NIH Consensus Development Panel on Osteoporosis Prevention, Diagnosis, and Therapy. Osteoporosis Prevention, Diagnosis, and Therapy. JAMA 2001; 285: 785-795.

[4] Kanis JA, Johnell O, Oden A, Johansson H, McCloskey E. FRAX™ and the assessment of fracture probability in men and women from the UK. Osteoporos Int 2008; 19: 385-397.

[5] Kanis JA, Johansson H, Oden A, Johnell O, de Laet C, Melton III LJ, Tenenhouse A, Reeve J, Silman AJ, Pols HA, Eisman JA, McCloskey EV, Mellstrom D. A meta-analysis of prior corticosteroid use and fracture risk. J Bone Miner Res 2004; 19: 893-899.

[6] Vestergaard P. Discrepancies in bone and mineral density and fracture risk in patients with type1 and type2 diabetes – a meta-analysis. Osteoporos Int 2007; 18: 427-444.

[7] Janghorbani M, Van Dam RM, Willett WC, Hu FB: Systematic review of type 1 and type 2 diabetes mellitus and risk of fracture. Am J Epidemiol 2007; 166: 495-505.

[8] Yamamoto M, Yamaguchi T, Yamauchi M, Kaji H, Sugimoto T. Diabetic patients have an increased risk of vertebral fractures independent of BMD or diabetic complications. J Bone Miner Res 2009; 24: 702-709.

[9] Nickolas TL, Leonard MB, Shane E: Chronic kidney disease and bone fracture: a growing concern. Kidney Int 2008; 74: 721-731.

[10] Alem AM, Sherrard DJ, Gillen DL, Weiss NS, Beresford SA, Heckbert SR, Wong C, Stehman-Breen C. Increased risk of hip fracture among patients with end-stage renal disease. Kidney Int 2000; 58: 396-399.

[11] Coco M, Rush H: Increased incidence of hip fractures in dialysis patients with low serum parathyroid hormone. Am J Kidney Dis 2000; 36: 1115-1121.

[12] Wakasugi M, Kazama JJ, Taniguchi M, Wada A, Iseki K, Tsubakihara Y, Narita I. Increased risk of hip fracture among Japanese hemodialysis patients.J Bone Miner Metab 2013; 31: 315-321.

[13] Jadoul M, Albert JM, Akiba T, Akizawa T, Arab L, Bragg-Gresham JL, Mason N, Prutz KG, Young EW, Pisoni RL. Incidence and risk factors for hip or other bone fractures among hemodialysis patients in the Dialysis Outcomes and Practice Patterns Study. Kidney Int 2006; 70: 1358-1366.

[14] Sherrard DJ: Renal osteodystrophy and aging. Semin Nephrol 2009; 29: 636-642.

[15] Wakasugi M, Kazama JJ, Wada A, Taniguchi M, Tsubakihara Y, Iseki K, Narita I. Regional variation in hip fracture incidence among Japanese hemodialysis patients. Ther Apher Dial. 2014; 18: 162-166.

[16] Ball AM, Gillen DL, Sherrard D, Weiss NS, Emerson SS, Seliger SL, Kestenbaum BR, Stehman-Breen C: Risk of hip fracture among dialysis and renal transplant recipients. JAMA 2002; 288(23):3014-3018.

[17] Danese MD, Kim J, Doan QV, Dylan M, Griffiths R, Chertow GM: PTH and the risks for hip, vertebral, and pelvic fractures among patients on dialysis. Am J kidney Dis 2006; 47: 149-156.

[18] Nitsch D, Mylne A, Roderick PJ, Smeeth L, Hubbard R, Fletcher A. Chronic kidney disease and hip fracture-related mortality in older people in the UK. Nephrol Dial Transplant 2009; 24: 1539-1544.

[19] Wells GA, Cranney A, Peterson J, Boucher M, Shea B, Robinson V, Coyle D, Tugwell P. Alendronate for the primary and secondary prevention of osteoporotic fractures in postmenopausal women. Cochrane Database Syst Rev 2008; CD001155.

[20] Seeman E, Crans GG, Diez-Perez A, Pinette KV, Delmas PD. Anti-vertebral fracture efficacy of raloxifene: a meta-analysis. Osteoporos Int 2006; 17: 313-316.

[21] Neer RM, Arnaud CD, Zanchetta JR, Prince R, Gaich GA, Reginster JY, Hodsman AB, Eriksen EF, Ish-Shalom S, Genant HK, Wang O, Mitlak BH. Effect of parathyroid hormone (1-34) on fractures and bone mineral density in postmenopausal women with osteoporosis. N Engl J Med 2001; 344: 1434-1441.

[22] Nickolas TL, McMahon DJ, Shane E. Relationship between moderate to severe kidney disease and hip fracture in the United States. J Am Soc Nephrol 2006; 17: 3223–3232.

[23] Ensrud KE, Lui LY, Taylor BC,Ishani A, Shlipak MG, Stone KL, Cauley JA, Jamal SA, Antoniucci DM, Cummings SR; Osteoporotic Fractures Research Group. Renal function and risk of hip and vertebral fractures in older women. Arch Intern Med 2007; 167: 133-139.

[24] Shlipak MG, Stehman-Breen C, Fried LF, Song X, Siscovick D, Fried LP, Psaty BM, Newman AB. The presence of frailty in elderly persons with chronic renal insufficiency. Am J Kidney Dis 2004; 43: 861-867.

[25] Fried LF, Biggs ML, Shlipak MG, Seliger S, Kestenbaum B, Stehman-Breen C, Sarnak M, Siscovick D, Harris T, Cauley J, Newman AB, Robbins J. Association of kidney function with incident hip fracture in older adults. J Am Soc Nephrol 2007; 18: 282–286.

[26] Kaji H, Yamauchi M, Yamaguchi T, Shigematsu T, Sugimoto T. Mild renal dysfunction is a risk factor for a decrease in bone mineral density and vertebral fractures in Japanese postmenopausal women. J Clin Endocrinol Metab 2010; 95: 4635-4642.

[27] Yano S, Nabika T, Shiwaku K, Yamaguchi S, Sugimoto T. Relationship between fracture risk and kidney function in the community-dwelling population: a cross-sectional study using FRAX® (Shimane CoHRE study). Osteoporosis Japan (in Japanese) 2012; 20: 98-101.

[28] Jamal SA, West SL, Nickolas TL. The clinical utility of FRAX to discriminate fracture status in men and women with chronic kidney disease. Osteoporos Int 2014; 25: 71-76.

[29] Jassal SK, von Muhlen D, Barrett-Connor E. Measures of Renal Function, BMD, Bone Loss, and Osteoporotic Fracture in Older Adults: The Rancho Bernardo Study. J Bone Miner Res 2007; 22: 203-210.

[30] Fried L, Shlipak M, Stehman-Breen C, Mittalhenkle A, Seliger S, Sarnak M, Robbins R, Siscovick D, Harris T, Newman A, Cauley J: Cystatin C as a predictor of loss of bone mineral density. J Gerontol Med Sci 2006;61: 743-748.

[31] Ishani A, Paudel M, Taylor BC, Barrett-Connor E, Jamal S, Canales M, Steffes M, Fink HA, Orwoll E, Cummings SR, Ensrud KE; Osteoporotic Fractures in Men (MrOS) Study Group. Renal function and rate of hip bone loss in older men: the Osteoporotic Fractures in Men Study. Osteoporos Int 2008; 19: 1549-1556.

[32] Iimori S, Mori Y, Akita W, Kuyama T, Takada S, Asai T, Kuwahara M, Sasaki S, Tsukamoto Y. Diagnostic usefulness of bone mineral density and biochemical markers of bone turnover in predicting fracture in CKD stage 5D patients — a single-center cohort study. Nephrol Dial Transplant 2012; 27: 345-351.

[33] Leonard MB: A structural approach to skeletal fragility in chronic kidney disease. Semin Nephrol 2009; 29: 133-143.

[34] Cejka D, Patsch JM, Weber M,Diarra D, Riegersperger M, Kikic Z, Krestan C, Schueller-Weidekamm C, Kainberger F, Haas M. Bone microarchitecture in hemodialysis patients assessed by HR-pQCT. Clin J Am Soc Nephrol 2011; 6: 2264-2271.

[35] Bacchetta J, Boutroy S, Vilayphiou N, Juillard L, Guebre-Egziabher F, Rognant N, Sornay-Rendu E, Szulc P, Laville M, Delmas PD, Fouque D, Chapurlat R: Early impairment of trabecular microarchitecture assessed with HR-pQCT in patients with stage II-IV chronic kidney disease. J Bone Miner Res 2010; 25:849-857.

[36] Nickolas TL, Stein EM, Dworakowski E, Nishiyama KK, Komandah-Kosseh M, Zhang CA, McMahon DJ, Liu XS, Boutroy S, Cremers S, Shane E. Rapid cortical bone loss in patients with chronic kidney disease. J Bone Miner Res 2013; 28: 1811-1820.

[37] Tomiyama C, Carvalho AB, Higa A,Jorgetti V, Draibe SA, Canziani ME.Coronary calcification is associated with lower bone formation rate in CKD patients not yet in dialysis treatment. J Bone Miner Res 2010; 25: 499-504.

[38] Inaba M, Okuno S, Kumeda T, Yamakawa T, Ishimura E, Nishizawa Y. Increased incidence of vertebral fracture in older female hemodialyzed patients with type2 diabetes mellitus. Calcif Tissue Int 2005; 76: 256-260.

[39] Schwartz AV, Sellmeyer DE, Strotmeyer ES, Tylavsky FA, Feingold KR, Resnick HE, Shorr RI, Nevitt MC, Black DM, Cauley JA, Cummings SR,Harris TB; Health ABC Study. Diabetes and bone loss at the hip in older black and white adults. J Bone Miner Res 2005; 20: 596-603.

[40] Desmet C, Beguin C, Swine C, Jadoul M; Université Catholique de Louvain Collaborative Group. Falls in hemodialysis patients: prospective study of incidence, risk factors, and complications. Am J Kidney Dis 2005; 45: 148-153.

[41] Pitts TO, Piraino BH, Mitro R, Chen TC, Segre GV, Greenberg A, Puschett JB. Hyperparathyroidism and 1,25-dihydroxyvitamin D deficiency in mild, moderate, and severe renal failure. J Clin Endocrinol Metab 1988; 67: 876-881.

[42] National Kidney Foundation: K/DOQI clinical practice guidelines for bone metabolism, disease in chronic kidney disease. Am J Kidney Dis 2003; 42: S1-201.

[43] van Meurs JBJ, Dhonukshe-Rutten RAM, Pluijm SMF, van der Klift M, de Jonge R, Lindemans J, de Groot LCPGM, Hofman A, Witteman JCM, van Leeuwen JPTM, Breteler MMB, Lips P, Pols HAP, Uitterlinden AG: Homocysteine levels and the risk of osteoporotic fracture. N Engl J Med 2004; 350: 2033-2041.

[44] McLean RR, Jaques PF, Selhub J, Tucker KL, Samelson EJ, Broe KE, Hannah MT, Cupples LA, Kiel DP: Homocysteine as a predictive factor for hip fractures in older persons. N Engl J Med 2004; 350: 2042-2049.

[45] Keller CR, Odden MC, Fried LF, Newman AB, Angleman S, Green CA, Cummings SR, Harris TB, Shlipak MG. Kidney function and markers of inflammation in elderly persons without chronic kidney disease: the health, aging, and body composition study. Kidney Int 2007; 71: 239-244.

[46] Jamal SA, Leiter RE, Bauer DC. Hyperhomocysteinaemia and aortic calcification are associated with fractures in patients on haemodialysis. QJM 98: 575-579, 2005

[47] Nii-Kono T, Iwasaki Y, Uchida M, Fujieda A, Hosokawa A, Motojima M, Yamato H, Kurokawa K, Fukagawa M.Indoxyl sulfate induces skeletal resistance to parathyroid hormone in cultured osteoblastic cells. Kidney Int 2007; 71: 738-743.

[48] Yano S, Yamaguchi T, Kanazawa I, Ogawa N, Hayashi K, Yamauchi M, Sugimoto T.Uraemic toxin, phenylacetic acid, inhibits osteoblastic proliferation and differentiation: an implication for the pathogenesis of low turnover bone in chronic renal failure. Nephrol Dial Transplant 2007; 22: 3160-3165.

[49] Ensrud KE, Parimi N, Fink HA, Ishani A, Taylor BC, Steffes M, Cauley JA, Lewis CE, Orwoll ES; Osteoporotic Fractures in Men Study Group. Estimated GFR and risk of hip fracture in older men: comparison of associations using cystatin C and creatinine. Am J Kidney Dis 2014: 63; 31-39.

[50] Fujita Y, Iki M, Tamaki J, Kouda K, Yura A, Kadowaki E, Sato Y, Moon JS, Tomioka K, Okamoto N, Kurumatani N. Renal function and bone mineral density in community-dwelling elderly Japanese men: the Fujiwara-kyo Osteoporosis Risk in Men (FORMEN) Study. Bone. 2013; 56: 61-66.

[51] Fliser D, Kollerits B, Neyer U, Ankerst DP, Lhotta K, Lingenhel A, Rits E, Kronenberg F, Kuen E, König P, Kraatz G, Mann JF, Müller GA, Köhler H, Riegler P, the MMKD Study Group. Fibroblast growth factor 23 (FGF23) predicts progression of chronic kidney disease: the mild to moderate kidney disease (MMKD) study. J Am SocNephrol 2007; 18: 2600-2608.

[52] Manghat P, Fraser WD, Wierzbicki AS, Fogelman I, Goldsmith DJ, Hampson G. Fibroblast growth factor-23 is associated with C-reactive protein, serum phosphate and bone mineral density in chronic kidney disease. Osteoporos Int 2010; 21: 1853-1861.

[53] Ix JH, Shlipak MG, Wassel CL, Whooley MA: Fibroblast growth factor-23 and early decrements in kidney function: the Heart and Soul Study. Nephrol Dial Transplant 2010; 25: 993-997.

[54] Kanda E, Yoshida M, Sasaki S. Applicability of fibroblast growth factor 23 for evaluation of risk of vertebral fracture and chronic kidney disease-mineral bone disease in elderly chronic kidney disease patients. BMC Nephrol. 2012; 13: 122.

[55] Iwasaki Y, Kazama JJ, Yamato H, Fukagawa M. Changes in chemical composition of cortical bone associated with bone fragility in rat model with chronic kidney disease. Bone 2011; 48: 1260-1267.

[56] Newman CL, Moe SM, Chen NX, Hammond MA, Wallace JM, Nyman JS, Allen MR. Cortical bone mechanical properties are altered in an animal model of progressive chronic kidney disease. PLoS One 2014; 9: e99262.

[57] Saito M, Marumo K. Collagen cross-links as a determinant of bone quality: a possible explanation for bone fragility in aging, osteoporosis, and diabetes mellitus. Osteoporos Int 2010; 21: 195-214.

[58] Mitome J, Yamamoto H, Saito M, Yokoyama K, Marumo K, Hosoya T. Nonenzymatic cross-linking pentosidine increase in bone collage and are associated with disorders of bone mineralization in dialysis patients. Calcif Tissue Int 2011; 88: 521-529.

[59] Schulz E, Arfai K, Liu X, Sayre J, Gilsanz V. Aortic calcification and the risk of osteoporosis and fractures. J Clin Endocrinol Metab 2004; 89: 4246-4253.

[60] Fang Y, Ginsberg C, Sugatani T, Monier-Faugere MC, Malluche H, Hruska KA. Early chronic kidney disease-mineral bone disorder stimulates vascular calcification. Kidney Int 2014; 85: 142-150.

[61] Rodríguez-García M, Gómez-Alonso C, Naves-Díaz M, Diaz-Lopez JB, Diaz-Corte C, Cannata-Andía JB; Asturias Study Group. Vascular calcifications, vertebral fractures and mortality in haemodialysis patients. Nephrol Dial Transplant 2009; 24: 239-246.

[62] Taal MW, Roe S, Masud T, Green D, Porter C, Cassidy MJ. Total hip bone mass predicts survival in chronic hemodialysis patients. Kidney Int 2003; 63:1116-1120.

[63] Kohno K, Inaba M, Okuno S, Maeno Y, Maekawa K, Yamakawa T, Ishimura E, Nishizawa Y. Association of reduction in bone mineral density with mortality in male hemodialysis patients. Calcif Tissue Int 2009; 84: 180-185.

[64] Nickolas TL, Cremers S, Zhang A, Thomas V, Stein E, Cohen A, Chauncey R, Nikkel L, Yin MT, Liu XS, Boutroy S, Staron RB, Leonard MB, McMahon DJ, Dworakowski

E, Shane E. Discriminants of prevalent fractures in chronic kidney disease. J Am Soc Nephrol 2011; 22: 1560-1572.

[65] KDIGO Clinical Practice Guideline for the Diagnosis, Evaluation, Prevention, and Treatment of Chronic Kidney Disease-Mineral and Bone Disorder (CKDMBD). Kidney Int 2009; 76 (Suppl 113) : S1-S130.

[66] Jamal SA, Bauer DC, Ensrud KE, Cauley JA, Hochberg M, Ishani A, Cummings SR. Alendronate treatment in women with normal to severely impaired renal function: an analysis of the Fracture Intervention Trial. J Bone Miner Res 2007; 22: 503-508.

[67] LaCroix AZ, Lee JS, Wu L, Cauley JA, Shlipak MG, Ott SM, Robbins J, Curb JD, Leboff M, Bauer DC, Jackson RD, Kooperberg CL, Cummings SR; Women's Health Initiative Observational.Cystatin-C, renal function, and incidence of hip fracture in postmenopausal women. J Am Geriatr Soc 2008; 56: 1434-1441.

Chapter 6

Dyspepsia — An Underestimated Problem among End-stage Renal Disease Patients

Paulo Roberto Santos

Additional information is available at the end of the chapter

http://dx.doi.org/10.5772/59426

1. Introduction

Dyspepsia is the most common gastrointestinal disorder in primary medical assistance. In the general population, 40% of people will suffer from dyspepsia during their lifetime [1]. The most frequent category of dyspepsia is functional dyspepsia (FD). Among categories of dyspepsia, FD accounts for roughly 50% of the cases and is defined as dyspeptic symptoms not explained by structural or organic upper gastrointestinal disease [2]. The categories associated with organic alterations of the upper gastrointestinal tract are: reflux disease with normal endoscopy (20%); reflux esophagitis (20%); peptic ulcer disease (10%); and more rarely, Barret's esophagus and malignancy [2].

Dyspeptic symptoms comprise a heterogeneous group of symptoms that have in common their location. The symptoms must be located in the epigastrium and can be included in two syndromes: postprandial distress syndrome (PDS) and epigastric discomfort syndrome (EDS). PDS comprises bothersome postprandial fullness and early satiation; EDS includes epigastric pain or burning. In practice, it is common for symptoms to overlap, and as a rule patients are defined as dyspeptic when suffering symptoms of both syndromes [3]. Heartburn is not considered a dyspeptic symptom, as established in the latest definition by the Rome III consensus in 2006 [4].

The current definition of FD according to the Rome III consensus is the presence of one or more symptoms, with onset at least six months beforehand, being present during the last three months, in the absence of structural disease of the upper gastrointestinal tract (in clinical practice, ruled out by endoscopy and testing for *Helicobacter pylori*). The Rome III consensus gives the definitions of each of the four dyspeptic symptoms (Table 1). Nonetheless, even judicious criteria like these are not totally accurate to diagnose FD. There are reports showing only modest performance of the Rome III criteria, reaching only 60.7% sensitivity and 68.7% specificity for diagnosis of FD [5].

Symptom	Definition
Postprandial fullness	Unpleasant sensation of prolonged persistence of food in the stomach after a meal
Early satiation	Feeling that the stomach is overfilled soon after starting to eat, out of proportion to the size of the meal being eaten, so that the meal cannot be finished
Epigastric pain	Subjective, intense and unpleasant sensation in the epigastrium, which can lead patients to believe that some tissue damage is occurring
Epigastric burning	Unpleasant subjective sensation of heat in the epigastrium

Table 1. Definition of dyspeptic symptoms as proposed by the Rome III consensus

Why do I classify FD as underestimated among end-stage renal disease (ESRD) patients? In my view, dyspepsia really deserves special attention among ESRD patients on hemodialysis (HD) for many reasons:

1. The most common non-renal complaints in HD patients are gastrointestinal symptoms, mainly dyspeptic symptoms [6].
2. The negative effect of dyspepsia on quality of life (QOL) is well known [7]. From the perspective of ESRD, the association between dyspepsia and impaired quality of life has greater implications due to central role of QOL among HD patients [8-13].
3. Dyspepsia is also associated with another important condition: nutritional status [14].
4. ESRD allows several lines of investigations about the pathophysiology of FD. The clinical research about the interactions between typical features of ESRD (like neuropathy, uremic toxins, abnormal gut motility and excess of extracellular volume) and FD need to advance [15-23]. Meanwhile, the pathophysiology of FD in ESRD is still not completely understood and the clinical therapy of dyspeptic symptoms typically fails.
5. Treatment challenge of FD is specific in HD patients due to the polypharmacy imposed on these patients, the high prevalence of depressive feelings, which can modulate dyspeptic symptoms, and the multi-factorial mechanisms of uremia acting on the gastrointestinal tract.

Despite the above, from my observations dyspepsia is not routinely screened in dialysis units as is done for cardiovascular disease, osteodystrophy and nutritional status. There is also a lack of randomized, placebo-controlled studies about treatment of FD among HD patients, and a clear explanation of the physiopathological mechanisms regarding FD in ESRD is missing.

In my institution, Federal University of Ceará in Brazil, data have been collected since the 1980s on the relationships between volemic status and gastric motility, especially in animal models, but also among healthy subjects [18-23]. As an attending physician, I have under my care at the dialysis unit of Santa Casa de Sobral Hospital ESRD patients who form an ideal sample for studying FD, gastric dismotility and hypervolemia. Thus, currently I am trying to find clinical evidence of the link between the results coming from bench research about the relationships of volemia and gastric emptying with gastroparesis, hypervolemia and FD, which are highly prevalent among HD patients. Therefore, I propose in this chapter to organize bench and clinical data on gastric motility, volume expansion and FD in ESRD patients, to provide insight to help the daily approach to FD among HD patients.

2. How to assess dyspeptic symptoms

Dyspeptic symptoms can be easily assessed by interview. This can be done by applying the Functional Dyspepsia Module [24], one of several diagnostic questionnaires based on the Rome III Consensus [25]. The Functional Dyspepsia Module allows quantitative analysis of dyspeptic symptoms. It contains 18 items. Responses are given according to 4-item and 6-item Likert scales. If a symptom is absent, the respondent skips the questions, so opening the possibility of completing the test without answering all the 18 items. Diagnostic criteria include: one of the symptoms (bothersome postprandial fullness or early satiation or epigastric pain or epigastric burning) with a minimum intensity as assessed by the Likert scale plus a normal endoscopy and a "yes" answer to the "yes-no-questions" about the persistence of a symptom for the past three months, with symptoms' onset at least six months ago.

The Functional Dyspepsia Module is an important and validated diagnostic tool of FD. However, a validated instrument is lacking to specifically detect changes of dyspeptic symptoms over time. This gap could be filled by a kind of patient-reported outcomes questionnaire in line with the Rome III consensus aiming to evaluate the evolution of symptoms. Such a questionnaire would encourage clinicians to routinely check the effects of therapies, and would allow increased studies on treatment of FD. In this sense, it is important to mention a recent pilot study designed to develop a questionnaire to evaluate the outcomes of PDS [26].

3. Impact of dyspepsia on quality of life and nutritional condition

It is well-known that dyspepsia can lower QOL in the general population [7]. In the context of ESRD, quality of life deserves special attention. Compared to the most frequent chronic diseases, like heart failure, angina, diabetes, chronic lung disease, arthritis and cancer, ESRD impairs quality of life the most [27]. Furthermore, high mortality among ESRD patients is stationary despite the recent technical advances in dialysis therapy and the availability of several updated guidelines and recommendations for ESRD treatment. Indeed, in recent years, QOL has become the main outcome of dialysis treatment, either as a self-perceived outcome by the patient or as an objective quality parameter of the dialysis procedure. Unfortunately, many factors associated with low QOL in HD patients are non-modifiable. Consequently, both physical and mental aspects of QOL among HD patients have not been improving during the last decade [12].

My main research line is self-perceived outcomes among HD patients. Since 2006 my research group has been producing studies in this area [8-10, 28-36]. Our sample consists of ESRD patients treated in the only two dialysis units in an area of 34.560 km^2 (37.3 inhabitants/ km^2) in the northern region of Ceará state, northeast Brazil. There we found, as others, a very low level of QOL in HD patients, mainly related to physical aspects. Recently, we presented our results about QOL in dyspeptic patients at the Paulista Congress of Nephrology, in Atibaia, São Paulo, Brazil [37]. We used the SF-36 instrument to evaluate QOL. SF-36 gives results on a scale from 0 (worst result) to 100 (best result) related to eight dimensions of QOL: physical functioning, role-physical, bodily pain, general health, vitality, social functioning, role-emotional and mental health. We used the Functional Dyspepsia Module of Rome III Diagnostic Questionnaires to search for dyspeptic symptoms. Our results showed that physical (bodily pain, general health and vitality) and also mental (role-emotional and mental health) aspects are lower in dyspeptic compared to non-dyspeptic HD patients. Notably, general health and role-emotional are the two dimensions rated below 50 according to the SF-36 scale among dyspeptics. It is exciting to think about FD as a modifiable factor associated with QOL. We urgently need randomized, controlled studies to test the effect of FD treatment on QOL among HD patients.

Another crucial impact of dyspepsia is related to nutritional condition. In the general population, weight loss is taken as an alarm symptom that raises suspicion of organic disease. However, weight loss also occurs in FD [38]. In nephrology, there are many studies on nutrition among HD patients. The most well-known factors associated with malnutrition in ESRD are anorexia and chronic inflammation [39]. FD is not well studied as a factor linked to malnutrition among ESRD patients. We exposed our preliminary data on this question at the Third Conference on Nephrology, held in Valencia, Spain [40]. In our experience, dyspeptic HD patients have a lower calorie and protein intake compared to non-dyspeptics. Like in the case of QOL, it is encouraging to think about FD as a modifiable factor associated with malnutrition, particularly because to same extent FD is easier to treat than anorexia and chronic inflammation. Again, as happens in the context of FD and QOL, clinical trials about the beneficial effects of treating FD on caloric and protein intake are necessary.

4. Hypervolemia and gastroparesis in ESRD: Associated pathways explaining dyspepsia?

As commented above, two groups of dyspeptic symptoms can be distinguished: PDS and EDS. However, in clinical practice there is an overlap between these two groups. Most of the time patients classified as having PDS also present EPS and vice versa [3]. Thus, more than a classification of the symptoms, we need to understand the physiopathological mechanisms involved in order to establish more effective treatment for FD. Gut dismotility can have a central role in the genesis of dyspeptic symptoms among ESRD patients. Moreover, volemic status may be a modulator of gastric emptying.

The first reports of gastric emptying delay in ESRD appeared at the end of the 1970s [41]. Nonetheless, currently the pathogenesis of gastroparesis in ESRD patients is still unknown. Several features of ESRD have at least a partial role in gastric delay, like anemia, metabolic acidosis and uremic neuropathy [16,17]. However, none of these is considered the main cause of FD, and the treatment of each one of these features is not effective in decreasing the prevalence of FD among HD patients.

In theory, among diabetics on HD features of ESRD act together with alterations of diabetes to cause gastroparesis. Hyperglycemia and decreased action of insulin provoke slow gastric emptying by compromising cellular elements of the stomach (loss or damage of the interstitial cells of Cajal and enteric glial cells), altering motor gastric functions (autonomic neuropathy of the vagal innervations of the stomach), and triggering disturbances of enteral hormones (especially, glucagon-like polypeptide-1) [42]. Despite all this, two facts should be highlighted. First, in primary medical assistance the prevalence of gastroparesis among diabetics is as low as 5% for type 1 diabetes and 1% for type 2 diabetes [43]. Indeed, it is likely that reports of high prevalence of gastroparesis in patients with diabetes are due to a bias caused by reports covering diabetics treated in tertiary medical care. Second, specifically among ESRD patients undergoing HD, the prevalence of FD is the same among diabetics and non-diabetics [15,44,45]. In the future perhaps a specific therapy for gastroparesis among diabetics could be developed, targeting alterations of gastric motility provoked by diabetes. However, as things now stand except for glycemic control, treatment of FD and gastroparesis does not differ between diabetics and non-diabetics on HD.

One attractive hypothesis is that volemia is the main modulator of gastric motility, and that hypervolemia elicits gastroparesis. Since ESRD is typically a condition of excessive extracellular volume, this hypothesis could explain the high prevalence of FD among patients on HD (the prevalence is nearly 70%) [15]. It also opens a field for therapeutic strategies to control extracellular volume among HD patients, aiming to relieve dyspeptic symptoms. At the Federal University of Ceará, researchers from the Department of Physiology and Pharmacology of the Faculty of Medicine have been performing experiments to understand the relationships between extracellular volume and gastrointestinal motility during the past 35 years. Data have been accumulated suggesting a negative correlation between extracellular volume and gastric emptying time, especially in animal models (see Table 2 for details about the method of evaluating gastric emptying in rats), but also in humans. Results converge to clearly show that hypervolemia decreases gastric and intestinal motility [18-23]. Neural and humoral pathways have been suggested to explain this correlation [21]. Also, gastric motility and permeability are closely related, and hypervolemia increases secretion of fluids and electrolytes while dehydration decreases secretion [46-48]. Healthy blood donors make good subjects for *in vivo* experiments to test the relationship between volemic status and gastric emptying [23]. Among them, it was found that gastric compliance (measured by barostat) increases after donating 450 ml of blood (functioning as acute hypovolemia). Conversely, compliance returns to physiologic levels after infusion of the same volume of saline.

No doubt ESRD patients compose an ideal model to study the effects of hypervolemia on gastric motility *in vivo*. The drawback is the lack of simple and accurate methods for assessing volemia in clinical studies. Table 3 shows the available clinical tools for detecting hypervolemia.

• 1.5 ml of the test meal (0.5 mg mL^{-1} phenol red in 5% glucose solution) given orally through a stainless steel tube
• Animals killed by i.v. thiopental overdose at 0 (standard) or 10 min after the test meal
• Stomach exposed by laparotomy, clamped at the pylorus and cardia ends, and excised
• Removed stomach placed in 100 ml of 0.1 $_N$ NaOH, cut into small pieces and homogenized for 30 seconds
• Settling for 30 min
• 10 ml of the resulting supernatant centrifuged for 10 min (2800 r.p.m.)
• Proteins in 5 ml of this supernatant precipitated with 0.5 ml of trichloroaetic acid, centrifuged for 20 min and 3 mL of the supernatant added to 4 mL of 0.5 $_N$ NaOH
• Absorbance of the sample read at a wavelength of 560 nm by spectrophotometry
The formula for calculating gastric emptying:
• % Gastric emptying = 1 – [(amount of phenol red covered from test stomach)/ (average amount of phenol red covered from standard stomachs] x 100
Standard stomachs:
• Rats killed immediately after gavage

Table 2. Step-by-step description of the method for measuring gastric emptying of liquid in rats

Atrial natriuretic peptic
Cyclic guanidine monophosphate (post dialysis level higher than 20 pmol/L indicates fluid overload)
Bioimpendane analysis
Blood volume monitoring (change in hematocrit or protein during hemodialysis procedure)
Inferior vena cava diameter (by echocardiography)

Table 3. Tools for clinical estimation of fluid overload

Based on results of bioimpedance analysis, we have shown that among HD patients, relative fluid overload higher than 15% is associated with higher prevalence of FD compared to patients with lower fluid overload (66% *versus* 34%) [49]. Figure 1 shows the bioimpedance device used by us: a body composition monitor specifically designed to assess extracellular water in patients with kidney failure. In addition, we found that dyspeptic patients on HD present longer gastric emptying time compared to non-dyspeptics (238 minutes *versus* 185 minutes) [15]. Since gastric dismotility seems to be crucial to trigger FD, and due to the complexity of measuring gastric emptying time *in vivo*, I summarize this study below.

The simplicity of assessing FD by interview contrasts with the complexity of assessing gastric emptying time *in vivo*. The tools available for clinical estimation of gastric emptying time are: technetium-99m scintigraphy (gold standard) [50]; time of appearance of acetaminophen in blood after its ingestion [51]; imaging studies using 3D ultrasonography and nuclear resonance [52, 53]; the smart pill (which seems to be a practical and promising method) [54]; and octanoic

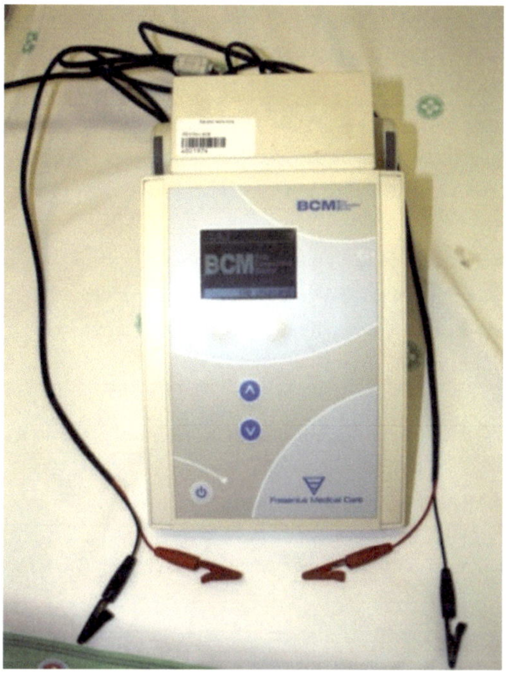

Figure 1. Body Composition Monitor® by Fresenius

acid breath test using ^{13}carbon (a very attractive method with 89% sensitivity compared to the gold standard technetium-99m scintigraphy) [55]. We used the last method in our study to assess gastric emptying time in a sample of HD patients from our clinic [15]. See Table 4 for details about the method of evaluating gastric emptying time in humans. Patients ate a scrambled egg with carbon linked to octanoic acid. Octanoic acid remains firmly attached to the egg in its passage through the stomach, but after that it is absorbed in the duodenum and eliminated in the breath. Patients breathe into bags before the test meal (baseline), every 15 minutes during 2 hours and then every 30 minutes for a further 2 hours. The gastric emptying time was defined by half-emptying time (the so-called T ½). T ½ is the time in minutes for the first half of the carbon dose in the test meal to be eliminated. Dyspeptic symptoms were assessed by a validated Brazilian version of a standardized questionnaire named the Porto Alegre Dyspeptic Symptoms Questionnaire (PADYQ). We found longer T ½ (longer gastric emptying time) among dyspeptics compared to non-dyspeptics. Moreover, we found a positive linear correlation between T ½ and dyspepsia score, in other words, the longer the gastric emptying time, the more severe the dyspeptic symptoms [15].

In short, the series of studies at our university demonstrate two findings to support clinical approaches to FD among ESRD patients: first, hypervolemia elicits gastric emptying delay [18-23]; second, dyspeptic patients on HD have longer gastric emptying time and higher fluid overload than non-dyspeptics [15, 49]. Table 5 summarizes the body of evidence on the relationships between volemia, gastric motility and dyspepsia produced in my Institution.

• Patients are instructed to avoid smoking and eating foods rich in C-4 plants, like corn (including baked goods made with cornmeal) and pineapples, in the week before the study • For the test: a minimum of 10 hours of fasting • The test meal consists of a scrambled egg with the yolk labeled with 100 μg of ^{13}carbon octanoic acid (after homogenizing the yolk, the egg white is added, beaten and baked) • The test meal is ingested with 60 g of white bread and 5 g of margarine during 1 to 5 min and followed immediately by 150 mL of water • To collect the breath samples, the patient exhales into closed aluminized plastic bags, before the test meal (baseline), and then at 15-minute intervals during 2 hours and then every 30 min for a further 2 hours • Patients are advised to remain seated and refrain from physical activity during the test • The gastric emptying time is defined by half-emptying time (T ½)
The formula for calculating T ½: • T ½ = time in minutes for the first half of the ^{13}carbon dose in the test meal to be metabolized
The cut-off: • T ½ of more than 200 minutes identifies gastric emptying delay

Table 4. Step-by-step description of the method for measuring gastric emptying time in humans

Evidence	Sample	Year [Reference]
Gastric compliance is modulated by blood volume	Anesthetized dogs	1983 [18]
Blood volume expansion decreases gastrointestinal flow while blood volume retraction increases it	Rats	1990 [19]
Expansion of blood volume delays gastrointestinal transit	Awake rats	1998 [20]
Vagal pathway is involved in the delay of gastric emptying elicited by acute blood volume expansion	Awake rats	1999 [21]
Stomach is an adjustable reservoir according to blood volume level	Anesthetized rats	2002 [22]
Acute blood shedding increases gastric compliance	Humans (healthy subjects)	2005 [23]
Gastric emptying delay is associated to functional dyspepsia	Patients on hemodialysis	2013 [15]
Fluid overload is associated to higher prevalence of functional dyspepsia	Patients on hemodialysis	2013 [49]

Table 5. Studies of volemia, gastric motility and dyspepsia produced at Federal University of Ceará, Brazil

5. Treatment

Confirming our finding that dyspepsia is underestimated despite the well-known impacts of FD on QOL and nutritional condition, there is a lack of randomized, placebo-controlled studies of treatment strategies for FD in ESRD patients. Most data on treatment of FD come from studies in the general population. This fact is worrying due to many peculiarities of uremia and its effects on gastrointestinal tract. Nevertheless, a common finding in the general population and among dialysis patients is the inefficiency of drug therapy. Only half of the dyspeptic patients become asymptomatic in population samples [56]. This is similar to our finding of 60% symptomatic HD patients under treatment for FD [15].

Initial treatment of FD in HD patients is usually empirical after performing an endoscopy to exclude ulcer (and other sorts of organic lesions) and a test for absence of *Helicobacter pylori*. The first step for treating FD can be to try acid-suppression therapy, either by an H2-receptor antagonist (H2-RA) or proton pump inhibitor (PPI) [57,58]. Favoring the initial use of PPI instead of H2-RA is the consensus of the superior acid secretion suppression of PPIs over H2-RAs. Favoring acid suppression therapy is the recent evidence coming from studies in healthy subjects that acid secretion can impair gastric motility [59,60]. Thus, theoretically PPIs can ameliorate FD by acting on both pain and dysmotility-like symptoms. Even though widely used clinically, the double-dose of PPIs in case of persistence of dyspeptic symptoms is not supported. There are reports that standard and double doses have the same results [61].

Effective	Ineffective	Under investigation
Metoclopramide (not tolerated in some) [64,71] Domperidone (not used in USA) [57] Levosulpiride [63]	Mosapiride [65] Tegaserod [66] Itopride [67] ABT-229 [68]	Acotiamide [69]
References in square brackets		

Table 6. Prokinetics for relief of dyspeptic symptoms

Prokinetics can be a second drug to add to PPI in case of treatment failure, or the first option if PDS is the main clinical presentation, or in most cases of overlap of PDS and EDS. At least, two drugs are individually superior over placebo in the treatment of FD: domperidone and cisapride [57]. Unfortunately, the accumulated data on the effects of cisapride (one of the most studied prokinetics) is of no value since the use of cisapride has been withdrawn due to risk of arrhythmia [62]. Domperidone is used in Brazil, but it is not available in many countries including the United States. A newer drug named levosulpiride shows the same positive results found with the use of cisapride [63]. In our daily practice, we prefer an old drug in use since 1960, metoclopramide. Metoclopramide is traditionally used for gastroparesis in diabetics before each meal and at bedtime, and has proven to improve the nutritional status in non-diabetics on dialysis [64]. However, metoclopramide has a limitation on its use, because it can provoke dyskinesia. New prokinetics, like mosapride, tegaserod, itopride and ABT-229, seem to be no better than the former drugs [65-68]. Currently, acotiamed is under investigation [69]. In comparison to PPIs, prokinetics have no advantage in the treatment of dyspepsia, based on studies performed in the general population [70]. However, in light of the extensive evidence of the close relationship between gastric delay and FD in ESRD discussed previously, it is my opinion that prokinetics should have a leading role in the treatment of FD in patients undergoing HD. Furthermore, there are reports favoring prokinetics regarding improvement of nutritional condition in ESRD patients [64,71]. Table 6 shows a list of effective, ineffective and under-investigation prokinetics.

Among the peculiarities of FD in ESRD patients, there is the extensive list of stressors associated with HD: illness effects, dietary constraints, time restriction, functional limitations, changes in employment, sexual dysfunction, and high mortality [13]. This explains why depression and anxiety are highly prevalent among HD patients [9,11]. Anxiety and depression can be manifested by dyspepsia (somatization). This fact forces the inclusion of depression in the differential diagnosis of FD alongside gallbladder, pancreatitis, medications, and hepatobiliary causes. On the other hand, dyspeptic symptoms of FD are more likely to be severe in depressive patients. There are several studies showing benefits of anxiolytics and antidepressants, especially tricyclic antidepressants, in the relief of dyspeptic symptoms, although their results are not superior to those of PPIs or prokinetics in the general population [72]. Once again, we have to be careful to extrapolate these population data to specific samples of ESRD patients. Due to the previously reported list of associated stressors and high prevalence of depression among HD patients, it is plausible that the effects of antidepressants can be more pronounced among HD patients than in the general population. Taking two specific drugs: amitriptyline (tricyclic antidepressant) and sertroline (selective serotonin reuptake inhibitor antidepressant) can be effective. Amitriptyline ameliorates dyspeptic symptoms in subjects who did not obtain relief with antacids and prokinetics [73]. Sertroline is a very attractive drug to test for FD in HD patients because of its additional effect of decreasing the serum level of interleukin-6 in HD patients on HD [74]. However, treatment of depression among HD patients is not simple. Drug therapy alone for depression has proven to be ineffective among HD patients. One of the reasons is that drug therapy by itself cannot eliminate the powerful stressors associated with HD therapy. For instance, among women undergoing HD, the sole use of drugs for depression will fail if there is not a concurrent approach to sexual dysfunction [75]. To my thinking, it is clear that treatment of FD in HD patients should include screening for depressive symptoms, and if depression exists, psychotherapy is necessary along with the use of drugs. Supporting this opinion, psychotherapy was proved to be beneficial for FD in controlled random trials [76].

6. Alternative medications and emerging therapies

Due to high therapy failure and risk of drug side effects from FD treatment, alternative medicine is attractive. Alternative medicine includes herbal medicine, traditional Chinese medicine and the emerging therapies, especially invasive procedures for gastroparesis.

STW 5 (also known as Iberogast) is one of the most studied mixtures of herbs proven to be effective in relieving dyspeptic symptoms. The main and active ingredient of STW 5 is *Iberis amara,* which acts both to reduce acid secretion and accelerate gastric emptying [77]. The last action is a result of its different effects on gastric portions, inhibiting the proximal portion of the stomach while exciting the tonus of the distal stomach [78]. Its prokinetic action is similar to cisapride [79]. Usual dosage of STW 5 is 20 drops three times a day. Data on other alternative medications are limited, such as artichoke leaf extract, blend of peppermint oil and caraway oil, banana powder capsules, and antioxidant astaxanthin [80].

Less available in other cultures, Xiaoban Xiatang and Zhizhu Tang are the two herbal infusions most used by traditional Chinese physicians to treat dyspeptic symptoms [81]. However, regarding traditional Chinese medicine, acupuncture is undoubtedly the procedure that deserves most attention. It has been shown that acupuncture accelerates gastric emptying time and reduces postprandial fullness, early satiety and bloating [82].

Among emerging therapies for gastroparesis, there are invasive procedures like gastric electrical stimulation and pyloric botulinum toxin injection. Gastric electrical stimulation consists of surgical implantation of electrodes into the muscle layer of the gastric antrum. A pulse generator in the abdominal wall delivers low-energy electrical pulses at high frequency to the electrodes. Meta-analyses have shown benefits of this technique, and isolated studies have demonstrated improvement of dyspeptic symptoms, quality of life, weight, body mass index and albumin level [83-86]. Gastric electrical stimulation seems to work less because of its motor effects on gastric motility, and more because of its effects in altering the sensory function of afferent nerves of the stomach. Surgical complications occur in 10% of cases, indicating that this method should be prescribed only for refractory cases and not as routine therapy. Another invasive procedure for gastroparesis is the injection of the botulinum toxin (botox) in a circumferential manner into the pyloris. Due to its effect of inhibiting acetylcholine release, botox accelerates gastric emptying and improves dyspeptic symptoms in open-label trials [87-89]. The procedure consists of intrapyloric injection of 100-200 units of botox during endoscopy and has been proven to be safe. However, botox injection cannot be currently recommended since at least two double-blind placebo controlled studies showed the same effects of botox and placebo [90,91]. Table 7 summarizes the treatment options for FD.

Established interventions
Antacids
Prokinetics
Antidepressants
Psychotherapy
Alternative medicine
Acupuncture
STW 5 (Iberogast)
Xiaoban Xiatang
Zhizhu Tang
Artichoke leaf extract
Peppermint oil + caraway oil
Banana powder capsules
Antioxidant astaxanthin
Emerging therapies for gastroparesis
Gastric electrical stimulation
Pyloric botulinum toxin injection

Table 7. Treatment options for functional dyspepsia

7. How to treat: My opinion

It is clear that the traditional algorithm indicating use of anti-secretory agents for ulcer-like FD and prokinetics for dysmotility-like FD does not meet the complexity of FD in the context of ESRD. The ordinary exclusion of patients with inadequate dialysis clearance from studies about FD implies that hypervolemia can be involved in the high prevalence of FD in the cases of more typical patients on HD (those excluded from the studies). In these cases, hypervolemia could trigger gastric emptying delay. I think that patients on HD with FD should first have their dry-weight re-evaluated. Indeed, FD can be an extra tool to help estimate real dry-weight of our HD patients. Second, metoclopramide can be used before each meal and at bedtime. Its beneficial effects on nutritional status are widely documented [62,69]. Third, screening for depressive symptoms and psychotherapy are essential in the treatment of FD among HD patients. Concerning anti-depressant drugs, sertraline is a good option because of its anti-inflammatory effects. Finally, acupuncture can be tried to ameliorate dyspeptic symptoms. Acupuncture's action in accelerating gastric emptying is particularly attractive.

8. Conclusion

Dyspepsia is highly prevalent among ESRD patients undergoing HD. It can affect central aspects, like QOL and nutritional status. The division of FD into PDS and EDS is didactic but not reasonable in clinical practice. The fact is that most dyspeptic patients present symptoms of both syndromes. Treatment is known to be ineffective. Therapy directed toward the main physiopathological pathways can be crucial, yet the pathogenesis of FD in ESRD remains virtually unknown. Gastroparesis seems to be important, independent of the presence or absence of diabetes. The association of actions to accelerate gastric emptying and to improve depressive feelings should be more effective than traditional treatment algorithms. The hypothesis is that the relief of dyspeptic symptoms would lead to better QOL and nutritional status.

Author details

Paulo Roberto Santos[1,2*]

Address all correspondence to: prsantos@fortalnet.com.br

1 Sobral Faculty of Medicine, Federal University of Ceará, Sobral, Brazil

2 Dialysis Unit, Santa Casa de Sobral Hospital, Sobral, Brazil

References

[1] Zagari R, Fuccio L, Bazzoli F. Investigating dyspepsia. British Medical Journal 2008;337: a1400.

[2] Overland MK. Dyspepsia. Medical Clinics of North America 2014;98: 549-564.

[3] Tack J, Talley NJ, Camilleri M, Holtmann G, Hu P, Malagelada JR, Stanghellini V. Functional gastroduodenal disorders. Gastroenterology 2006;130: 1466-1479.

[4] Rome Foundation. Rome III diagnostic criteria for functional gastrointestinal disorders. http://www.theromefoundation.org/assets/pdf/19_RomeIII_apA_885-898.pdf (accessed 31 August 2014).

[5] Ford AC, Bercik P, Morgan DG, Bolino C, Pintos-Sanchez MI, Moayyedi P. The Rome III criteria for the diagnosis of functional dyspepsia in secondary care are not superior to previous definition. Gastroenterology 2014;46: 932-940.

[6] Shiazian S, Radhakrishnan J. Gastrointestinal disorders and renal failure: exploring the connection. Nature Reviews Nephrology 2010;6: 480-492.

[7] Aro P, Talley NJ, Agréus L, Johansson SE, Bolling-Sternevald E, Storskrubb T, Ronkainen J. Functional dyspepsia impairs quality of life in the adult population. Alimentary Pharmacology & Therapeutics 2011;33: 1215-1224.

[8] Santos PR, Capote Junior JRFG, Cavalcanti JU, Vieira CB, Rocha ARM, Apolônio NAM, Oliveira EB. Quality of life among women with sexual dysfunction undergoing hemodialysis: a cross-sectional observational study. Health and Quality of Life Outcomes 2012;10: 103.

[9] Santos PR. Depression and quality of life of hemodialysis patients living in a poor region of Brazil. Revista Brasileira de Psiquiatria 2011;33: 332-337.

[10] Santos PR, Daher EF, Silva Jr GB, Libório AB, Kerr LR. Quality of life assessment among hemodialysis patients in a single centre: a two-year follow-up. Quality of Life Research 2009;18: 541-546.

[11] Santos PR (2011). Subjective well-being measures of hemodialysis patients. In: Penido MG (ed.) Technical problems in patients on hemodialysis. Rijeka: InTech; 2011. p69-86.

[12] Gabbay E, Meyer KB, Griffith JL, Richardson MM, Miskulin DC. Temporal trends in health-related quality of life among hemodialysis patients in the United States. Clinical Journal of the American Society of Nephrology 2010;5: 261-267.

[13] Cukor D, Cohen SD, Peterson RA, Kimmel PL. Psychosocial aspects of chronic disease: end-stage renal disease as a paradigmatic illness. Journal of the American Society of Nephrology 2007;18: 3042-3055.

[14] Jones MP, Talley NJ, Eslick GD, Dubois D, Tack J. Community subgroups in dyspepsia and their association with weight loss. The American Journal of Gastroenterology 2008;103: 2051-2060.

[15] Salles Jr LD, Santos PR, Santos AA, Souza MHLP. Dyspepsia and gastric emptying in end-stage renal disease patients on hemodialysis. BMC Nephrology 2013;14: 275.

[16] Ravelli AM. Gastrointestinal function in chronic renal failure. Pediatric Nephrology 1995;9: 756-762.

[17] Dumitrascu DL, Barnert J, Kirschner T, Wienbeck M. Antral emptying of semisolid meal measured by real-time ultrasonography in chronic renal failure. Digestive Diseases and Sciences 1995;40: 636-644.

[18] Capelo LR, Cavalcante DM, Leitão IA, Cristino Filho G, da-Silva EAT. Modifications of gastric compliance in dogs related to changes of extracellular fluid volume. Brazilian Journal of Medical and Biological Research 1983;16: 673-676.

[19] Xavier-Neto J, Santos AA, Rola FH. Acute hypervolemia increases the gastroduodenal resistance to the flow of saline in rats. Gut 1990;31: 1006-1010.

[20] Oliveira GR, Gondim FAA, Graça JRV, Xavier-Neto J, Gondim RBM, Santos AA, Rola FH. Acute blood volume expansion delays the gastrointestinal transit of a charcoal meal in awake rats. Brazilian Journal of Medical and Biological Research 1998;31: 835-840.

[21] Gondim FAA, Oliveira GR, Graça JRV, Gondim RBM, Alencar HMP, Dantas RP, Santos AA, Rola FH. Neural mechanisms involved in the delay of gastric empting of liquid elicited by acute blood volume expansion in awake rats. Neurogastroenterology and Motility 1999;11: 93-99.

[22] Graça JRV, Gondim FAA, Rola FH, Santos AA. Variations in gastric compliance induced by acute blood volume changes in anesthetized rats. Brazilian Journal of Medical and Biological Research 2002;35: 405-410.

[23] Macedo GM, Maia APM, Lira GHS, Santos CL, Leal PR, Souza MH, Oliveira RB, Santos AA, Souza MA. Acute blood shedding increases gastric compliance in health subjects. Neurogastroenterology and Motility 2005;17(Suppl 2): 83.

[24] Rome Foundation. Functional dyspepsia module. http://www.romecriteria.org/pdfs/DyspepMode.pdf (accessed 31 August 2014).

[25] Rome Foundation. Rome III Diagnostic Questionnaires. http://www.romecriteria.org/questionnaires/ (accessed 31 August 2014).

[26] Carbone F, Holvoet L, Vandenberghe A, Tack J. Functional dyspepsia: outcome of focus groups for the development of a questionnaire for symptom assessment in patients suffering from postprandial distress syndrome. Neurogastroenterology and Motility 2014;26: 1266-1274.

[27] Mittal SK, Ahern L, Flaster E, Maesaka JK, Fishbane S. Self-assessed physical and mental function of haemodialysis patients. Nephrology Dialysis Transplantation 2001;16: 1387-1394.

[28] Santos PR, Arcanjo FPN. Social adaptability and substance abuse: predictors of depression among hemodialysis patients? BMC Nephrology 2013;14: 12.

[29] Santos PR, Arcanjo FPN. Distance between residence and the dialysis unit does not impact self-perceived outcomes in hemodialysis patients. BMC Research Notes 2012;5: 548.

[30] Santos PR. Evaluation of objective and subjective indicators of death in a period of one year in a sample of prevalent patients under regular hemodialysis. BMC Research Notes 2012;5: 24.

[31] Santos PR. Comparison of quality of life between hemodialysis patients waiting and not waiting for kidney transplant from a poor region of Brazil. Brazilian Journal of Nephrology 2011; 33: 166-172.

[32] Santos PR. Correlation between coping style and quality of life among hemodialysis patients from a low-income area in Brazil. Hemodialysis Internationl 2010;14: 316-321.

[33] Santos PR, Kerr LRFS. Clinical and laboratory variables associated with quality of life in Brazilian haemodialysis patients: a single-centre study. Revista Medica do Chile 2008;136: 1264-1271.

[34] Santos PR. Erectile dysfunction and quality of life in young patients on hemodialysis. Brazilian Journal of Nephrology 2008;30: 132-136.

[35] Santos PR. Relationship between gender and age with quality of life in chronic hemodialysis patients. Revista da Associação Médica Brasileira 2006;52: 356-359.

[36] Santos PR, Coelho MR, Gomes NP, Josué EP. Association of nutritional markers with quality of life in chronic kidney disease patients on hemodialysis. Brazilian Journal of Nephrology 2006; 28: 57-64.

[37] Santos PR. Dyspeptic symptoms are independent predictors of quality of life in end-stage renal disease patients on hemodialysis. In: XVII Paulista Congress of Nephrology, September 18-21, 2013, Bourbon Convention & Spa Resort, Atibaia, Brazil.

[38] Tack J, Bisschops R, Sarnelli G. Pathophysiology and treatment of functional dyspepsia. Gastroenterology 2004;127: 1239-1255.

[39] Bossola M, Muscaritoli M, Tazza L, Panocchia N, Liberatori M, Giungi S, Tortorelli A, Fanelli FR, Luciani G. Variables associated with reduced dietary intake in hemodialysis patients. Journal of Renal Nutrition 2005;15: 244-252.

[40] Santos PR. Dyspepsia: an underestimated problem among end-stage renal disease patients. In: Third International Conference on Nephrology & Therapeutics, June 26-27, 2014, Valencia Conference Centre, Valencia, Spain.

[41] Graybar GB, Tarpey H. Kidney transplantation. In Gelman S (ed.) Anesthesia and organ transplantation. Philadelphia: WB Saunders; 1987. p61-110.

[42] Horváth VJ, Izbéki F, Lengyel C, Kempler P, Várkonyi T. Diabetic gastroparesis: functional/morphologic background, diagnosis, and treatment options. Current Diabetes Reports 2014;14: 527.

[43] Choung RS, Locke GR III, Schleck CD, Zinsmeister AR, Melton LJ III, Talley NJ. Risk of gastroparesis in subjects with type 1 and 2 diabetes in the general population. American Journal of Gastroenterology 2012;107: 82-88.

[44] Strid H, Simrén M, Johansson AC, Svedlund J, Samuelsson O, Björnsson ES. The prevalence of gastrointestinal symptoms in patients with chronic renal failure is increased and associated with impaired psychological general well-being. Nephrology Dialysis Transplantation 2002;17: 1434-1439.

[45] Bytzer P, Talley NJ, Leemon M, Young LJ, Jones MP, Horowitz M. Prevalence of gastrointestinal symptoms association with diabetes mellitus: a population-based survey of 15,000 adults. Archives of Internal Medicine 2001;161: 1989-1996.

[46] Higgins Jr JT, Blair NP. Intestinal transport of water and electrolyte during extracellular fluid volume expansion in dogs. Journal of Clinical investigation 1971;30: 2569-2579.

[47] Levens NR. Control of intestinal absorption by the rennin-angiotensin system. American Journal of Physiology 1985;249: G3-G15.

[48] Lee JS. Relationship between intestinal motility, tone, water absorption and lymph flow in the rat. Journal of Physiology 1983;345: 489-499.

[49] Santos PR. Correlation between hypervolemia and gastric emptying time among end-stage renal disease patients on hemodialysis. In: XVII Paulista Congress of Nephrology, September 18-21, 2013, Bourbon Convention & Spa Resort, Atibaia, Brazil.

[50] Abell TL, Camilleri M, Donokoe K. Consensus recommendation for gastric emptying scintigraphy: a joint of the American Neurogastroenterology and Motility Society and the Society of Nuclear Medicine. American Journal of Gastroenterology 2008;103: 753-763.

[51] Willems M, Quartero O, Numans M. How useful is the paracetamol absorption as a marker of gastric emptying? A systematic literature study. Digestive Diseases and Sciences 2001;46: 2256-2262.

[52] Gentilcore D, Hausken T, Horowitz M. Measurement of gastric empyting of low-and high-nutrient liquids using 3D ultrasonography and scintigraphy in health subjects. Neurogastroenterology & Motility 2006;18: 1062-1068.

[53] Schwizer W, Maecke H, Fried M. Measurement of gastric emptying by magnetic resonance imaging in humans. Gastroenterology 1992;103: 369-376.

[54] Kuo B, McCallum RW, Koch KL. Comparison of a gastric emptying of a non digestible capsule to a radio-labelled meal in healthy and gastroparetic subjects. Alimentary Pharmacology & Therapeutics 2008;27: 186-196.

[55] Ghoos YF, Maes BD, Geypens BJ, Mys G, Hiele MI, Rutgeerts PJ, Vantrappen G. Measurement of gastric emptying rate of solids by means of a carbon-labelled octanoic acid breath test. Gastroenterology 1993;104: 1640-1647.

[56] Monkemuller K, Malfertheiner P. Drug treatment of functional dyspepsia. World Journal of Gastroenterology 2006; 12: 2694-2700.

[57] Moayyedi P, Shelly S, Deeks JJ. Pharmacological interventions for non-ulcer dyspepsia. Cochrane Database of Systematic Reviews 2011;2: CD01960.

[58] Moayyedi P. The efficacy of proton pump inhibitors on functional dyspepsia: a systematic review and economic analysis. Gastroenterology 2004;127: 1329-1337.

[59] Lee KJ, Vos R, Janssens J, Tack J. Influence of duodenal acidification on the sensormotor function of the proximl stomch in humans. American Journal of Physiology-Gastrointestinal and Liver Physiology 2004;286: G278-G284.

[60] Miwa H, Nakajima K, Yamaguchi K, Fujimoto K, Veldhuyzen VAN, Zanten SJ, Kinoshita Y, Adachi K, Kusunoki H, Haruma K. Generation of dyspeptic symptoms by direct acid infusion into the stomach of healthy subjects. Alimentary Pharmacology & Therapeutics 2007;26: 257-264.

[61] Wang WH, Huang JQ, Zheng GF, Xia HH, Wong WM, Liu XG, Karlberg J, Wong BC. Effects of proton pump inhibitors on functional dyspepsia: a meta-analysis of randomized placebo-controlled trials. Clinical Gastroenterology and Hepatology 2007;5: 178-185.

[62] Wysowski DK, Bacsanyi J. Cisapride and fatal arrhythmia. New England Journal of Medicine 1996; 335: 290-291.

[63] Mearin F, Rodrigo L, Pérez-Mota A, Balboa A, Jiménez I, Sebastián JJ, Patón C. Levosulpiride and cisapride in the treatment of dysmotility-like functional dyspepsia: a randomized, double-masked trial. Clinical Gastroenterology 2004;2: 301-308.

[64] Ross EA, Koo LC. Improved nutrition after detection and treatment of occult gastroparesis in nondiabetic dialysis patients. American Journal of Kidney Diseases 1998;31: 62-66.

[65] Hallerback BI, Bommelaer G, Bredberg E, Campbell M, Hellblom M, Lauritsen K, Wienbeck M, Holmgren LL. Dose finding study of mosapride in functional dyspep-

sia: a placebo-controlled, randomized study. Alimentary Pharmacology & Therapeutis 2002;16: 959-967.

[66] Vakil N Laine L, Talley NJ, Zakko SF, Tack J, Chey WD, Kralstein J, Earnest DL, Ligozio G, Cohard-Radice M. Tegaserod treatment for dysmotility-like functional dyspepsia: results of two randomized, controlled trials. American Journal of Gastroenterology 2008;103: 1906-1919.

[67] Talley NJ, Tack J, Ptak T, Gupta R, Giguère M. Itopride in functional dyspepsia: results of two phase III multicenter, randomized, double-blind, placebo-controlled trials. Gut 2008;57: 740-746.

[68] Talley NJ, Verlinden M, Snape W, Beker JA, Ducrotte P, Dettmer A, Brinkhoff H, Eaker E, Ohning G, Miner PB, Mathias JR, Fumagalli I, Staessen D, Mack RJ. Failure of a motilin receptor agonist (ABT-229) to relieve the symptoms of functional dyspepsia in patients with and without delayed gastric emptying: a randomized double-blind placebo-controlled trial. Alimentary Pharmacology & Therapeutics 2000;14: 1653-1661.

[69] Yoshii K, Hirayami M, Nakamura T, Toda R, Hasegawa J, Takei M, Mera Y, Kawabata Y. Mechanism for distribution of acotiamide, a novel gastroprokinetic agent for the treatment of functional dyspepsia, in rat stomach. Journal of Pharmaceutical Sciences 2011;100: 4965-4973.

[70] Hsu YC, Liou JM, Yang TH, Hsu WL, Lin HJ, Wu HT, Lin JT, Wang HP, Wu MS. Proton pump inhibitor therapy versus prokinetic therapy in patients with functional dyspepsia: is therapeutic response predicted by Rome III subgroups? Journal of Gastroenterology 2011; 46: 183-190.

[71] Silang R, Regalado M, Cheng TH, Wesson DE. Prokinetic agents increase plasma albumin in hypoalbuminemic chronic dialysis patients with delayed gastric emptying. American Journal of Kidney Diseases 2001;37: 287-293.

[72] Hojo M, Miwa H, Yokoyama T, Ohkusa T, Nagahara A, Kawabe M, Asaoka D, Izumi Y, Sato N. Treatment of functional dyspepsia with anxiety or antidepressive agents: systematic review. Journal of Gastroenterology 2005;40: 1036-1042.

[73] Otaka M, Jin M, Odashima M, Matsuhashi T, Wada I, Horikawa Y, Komatsu K, Ohba R, Oyake J, Hatakeyama N, Watanabe S. New strategy of therapy for functional dyspepsia using famotidine, mosapride and amitriptyline. Alimentary Pharmacology & Therapeutics 2005;21(Suppl 2): 42-46.

[74] Taraz M, Khatami M, Dashti-Khavidaki S, Akhonzadeh S, Noorbala A, Ghaeli P, Taraz S. Sertraline decreases serum level of interleukin-6 (IL-6) in hemodialysis patients with depression: results of a randomized double-blind, placebo-controlled clinical Trial. International Immunopharmacology 2013;17: 917-923.

[75] Santos PR, Capote Jr JRFG, Cavalcanti JU, Vieira CB, Rocha ARM, Apolônio NAM, Oliveira EB. Sexual dysfunction predicts depression among women on hemodialysis. International Urology Nephrology 2013;45: 1741-1746.

[76] Faramarzi M, Azadfallah P, Book HE. A randomized controlled trial of brief psychoanalytic psychotherapy in patients with functional dyspepsia. Asian Journal of Psychiatry 2013;6: 228-234.

[77] Sebastián-Domingo JJ. La medicina integrative en el manejo de la dyspepsia functional: papel del preparado herbal STW5. Gastroenterología y Hepatología 2014;37: 256-261.

[78] Pilichiewicz AN, Horowitz M, Russo A, Maddox AF, Jones KL, Schemann M, Holtmann G, Feinle-Bisset C. Effects of Iberogast on proximal gastric volume, antro-pyloro-duodenal motility and gastric emptying in healthy men. American Journal of Gastroenterology 2007;102: 1276-1283.

[79] Rosch W, Vinson B, Sassin I. A randomized clinical trial comparing the efficacy of a herbal preparation STW 5 with the prokinetic drug cisapride in patients with dysmotility type of functional dyspepsia. Zeitschrift für Gastroenterologie;40: 401-408.

[80] Lacy BE, Talley NJ, Locke III GR, Bouras EP, DiBaise JK, El-Serag HB, Abraham BP, Howden CW, Moayyedi P, Prather C. Review article: current treatment options and management of functional dyspepsia. Alimentary Pharmacology & Therapeutics 2012;36: 3-15.

[81] Pang B, Zhou Q, Li J, Zhao L, Tong X. Treatment of refractory diabetic gastroparesis: Western medicine and traditional Chinese medicine therapies. World Journal of Gastroenterology 2014;20: 6504-6514.

[82] Xu S, Zha H, Hou X, Gao Z, Zhang Y, Chen JD. Electroacupuncture accelerates solid gastric emptying in patients with functional dyspepsia. Gastroenterology 2004;126: A-437.

[83] O'Grady G, Rgbuji JU, Du P, Cheng LK, Pullan AJ, Windsor JA. High-frequency gastric electrical stimulation for the treatment of gastroparesis: a meta-analysis. World Journal of Surgery 2009;33: 1693-1701.

[84] Chu H, Lin Z, Zhong L, McCallum RW, Hou X. Treatment of high-frequency gastric electrical stimulation for gastroparesis. Journal of Gastroenterology and Hepatology 2012;27: 1017-1026.

[85] Abell T, McCallum R, Hocking M,. Gastric electrical stimulation for medically refractory gastroparesis. Gastroenterology 2003;125: 421-428.

[86] Abell T, Lou J, Tabbaa M, Batista O, Malinowski S, Al-Juburi A. Gastric electrical stimulation for gastroparesis improves nutritional parameters at short, intermediate, and long-term follow-up. Journal of Parenteral and Enteral Nutrition 2003;27: 277-281.

[87] Miller LS, Szych GA, Kantor SB, Bromer MQ, Knight LC, Maurer AH, Fisher RS, Parkman HP. Treatment of idiopathic gastroparesis with injection of botulinum toxin into the pyloric sphincter muscle. American Journal of Gastroenterology 2002;97: 1653-1660.

[88] Lacy BE, Zayat EN, Crowell MD, Schuster MM. Botulinum toxin for the treatment of gastroparesis: a preliminary report. American Journal of Gastroenterology 2002;97: 1548-1552.

[89] Arts J, van Gool S, Caenepeel P, Verbeke K, Janssens J, Tack J. Influence of intra-pyloric botulinum toxin injection on gastric emptying and meal-related symptoms in gastroparesis patients. Alimentary Pharmacology & Therapeutics 2006;24: 661-667.

[90] Arts J, Holvoet L, Caenepeel P, Bisschops R, Sifrim D, Verbeke K, Janssens J, Tack J. Clinical trial: a randomized-controlled crossover study of intrapyloric injection of botinum toxin in gastroparesis. Alimentary Pharmacology & Therapeutics 2007;26: 1251-1258.

[91] Friedenberg FK, Palit A, Parkman HP, Hanlon A, Nelson DB. Botulinum toxin A for the treatment of delayed gastric emptying. American Journal of Gastroenterology 2008;103: 416-423.

Chapter 7

Aspects of Renal Disease Affecting Dental Management — Surgery in Patients Receiving Hemodyalisis

M. Dencheva, E. Deliverska, A. Krasteva,
J. Galabov and A. Kisselova

Additional information is available at the end of the chapter

http://dx.doi.org/10.5772/59930

1. Introduction

Kidneys play several roles in helping maintain physiologic balance; they are therefore important for continuing or regaining homeostasis during and after surgery and anesthesia. The renal system is necessary to support the processes of fluid, electrolyte, and acid-based balance, drug metabolism and elimination, blood pressure control through the renin-angiotensin system, red blood cell production through erythropoietin production, and vitamin D hydroxylation.

2. Main issues regarding the oral health in patients on hemodialysis and those with kidney transplant

The primary role of the dental doctor consists of the early diagnosis or referral of the patient to the right specialist, as the most frequent renal disease a dentist may encounter is the chronic kidney disease [18, 39, 114].

The symptoms that may lead us to the conclusion of constrained renal function vary depending on the extent of the damage and the reaction to the suggested treatment, and are characterized with systemic as well as intraoral findings.

3. Common symptoms at CKD (Chronic Kidney Disease)

Disease	Symptoms
Gastrointestinal	– nausea, vomiting, anorexia, metal taste, malodor, oesophagitis, gastritis, gastrointestinal bleeding
Neuromuscular	– headache, peripheral neuropathy, paralysis, sleep disturbances, numbness of limbs, convulsions correlating with level of the azotemia
Hematoimmunologic	– normocytic and normochrome anemia, coagulopathy, low resistance to infections, low production of erythropoietin, lymphocytopenia
Endocrine metabolic	– renal osteodystrophy (osteomalacia, osteosclerosis, fibrous cysts), secondary hyperparathyroidism, disturbed growth, decreased libido, amenorrhea, thyroid dysfunction
Cardio vascular	– cardiomyopathy, arrhythmia, pericarditis, high blood pressure, difficulty in breathing, congestive heart failure
Dermatologic	– paleness, itching, signs of scratching because of the itch, increased photosensitive pigmentation, uremic white spots, brown coloring of the nails- Fig.1, signs of water retention, limb heaviness, edema of the ankles
Respiratory	– Kussmaul breathing because of acidosis, pulmonary edema, dyspnea

Table 1. Symptoms at CKD [18, 125]

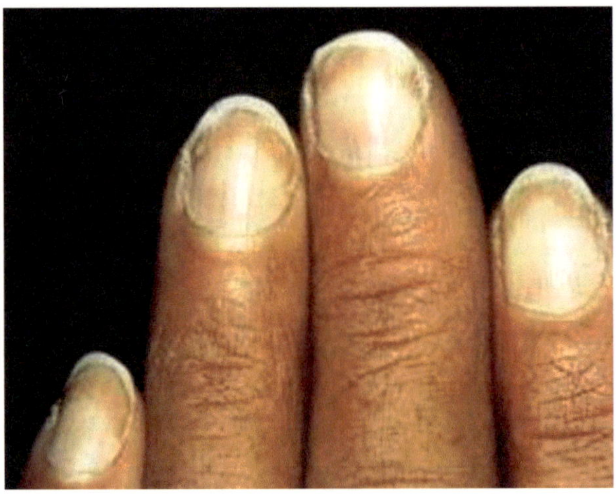

Figure 1. Brown coloring of nails

Renal osteodystrophy or renal bone disease is one of the most prominent signs of CKD and may occur in one or several combined forms. As a result of the increase of the level of phosphates in blood plasma, the decrease of calcium in blood plasma and the failure of processing of 25-hydroxycholecalciferol into the active and necessary 1.25 dihydroxycholecalciferol, an

http://dx.doi.org/10.5772/59930

increase of the parathormone (PTH) occurs. This leads to secondary hyperparathyroidism. Because of the increase of the non-mineralized bone matrix progressive bone changes may be observed - osteomalacia, lytic lesions followed by bone fibrosis. Renal osteodystrophy in kids leads to a delay in skeletal growth and a tendency for spontaneous fractures.

Most frequent orofacial signs of renal osteodystrophy are bone demineralization, lower trabeculation, lower density of the cortical bone, calcifications in soft tissues, radiolucent fibrocystic lesions, and complicated bone healing following extraction. Regarding the teeth and parodontal tissues we may observe delayed eruption, enamel hypoplasia (fig.2), loss of lamina dura, widening of the periodontal space, severe periodontal destruction, tooth mobility, denticles, obliteration of pulp chamber, and giant-cell lesions of the type "brown tumors"[78, 85].

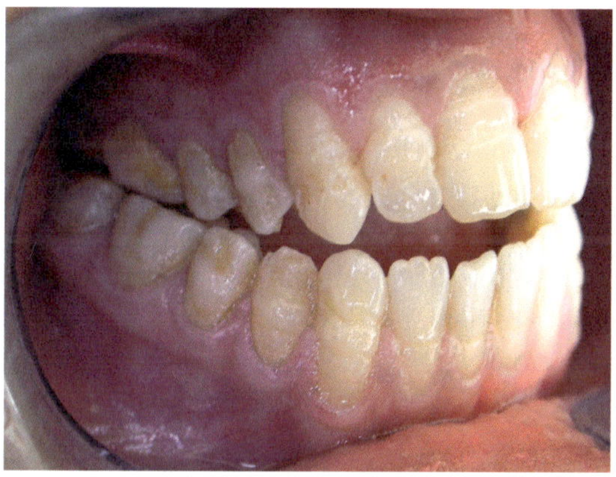

Figure 2. Hypoplasia and open bite in a female patient on hemodialysis

Nephrotic syndrome is observed in patients with glomerular diseases. It includes proteinuria (over 3.5 gr), hypoalbuminemia, hyperlipidemia, lipiduria, and edema. Causes may vary: sugar diabetes, chronic lupus erythematosus, or membrane glomerulonephritis. Increased level of blood coagulation factor VIII may lead to hypercoagulation and increased risk of thrombosis. Such patients may suffer catabolic processes, bacterial, fungal and viral infections [53, 66].

It should be noted that a significant part of the patients with renal disorders may also suffer from diabetes [14]. It is less probable for a dentist to diagnose diabetes, but patients whose dental status alters unexpectedly as rapidly as in progressive parodontitis, fungal eczemas, abscesses, high fluid intake, rapid weight loss, mouth dryness and halitosis [28, 29] may be suspicious. Those symptoms impose the appointment of definite examinations, which may help to set the latter diagnosis.

Renal disorders almost invariably cause anemia as a result of the kidneys' inability to produce erythropoietin. Fibrosis of marrow and the increased loss of erythrocytes are additional factors which increase the development of the disease. Anemia leads to fatigue, loss of concentration, tissue hypoxia, and paleness of the oral mucosa. In patients with advanced and untreated uremia, yellow-brownish coloring of the skin and mucosa because of the accumulation of carotene-like substances [4, 125] may be observed.

4. Intraoral findings typical for patients on hemodialysis and patients with kidney transplant

- Almost mandatory findings for each patient on hemodialysis are uremic breath and altered taste in the oral cavity. They occur as a result of the increased concentration of urea in saliva and its following transformation to ammonia [18, 60, 113, 121]. It is possible, however, for similar complaints to be registered in patients with normal values for blood and urine, for example after transplantation, and this is caused by the higher corrosion potential, combined with insufficient and personal and professional oral hygiene [90].
- Xerostomia could be explained with lowered fluid intake, as a side effect of antihypertensive or other medicaments, possible alterations in the salivary glands due to autoimmune or age-related changes [25, 26, 27, 28, 41, 47, 52, 73, 91, 92]. The study of Bots et al. [12] proves that in patients on hemodialysis the saliva quantity (stimulated and non-stimulated) is temporarily lowered but after transplantation and recovery of the renal function it is restored to normal values. With the same patients they register drop in pH from 7.36 to 6.74 probably because of the lower concentration of urea in saliva and the following decrease of hydrolysis and by the transformation of oral flora to ammonia [16].
- Oral mucosa findings, reported in patients with CKD, with the exception of uremic stomatitis (fig.3), are unusual and vary, as a result of the main disease, as well as the intake of drugs: white plaques, macules, nodules, erythematous plaques, fibro-epithelial polypus, ulceration, geographic tongue (fig.4), lichen planus, red fibrous tongue, fiber leukoplakia, and papilloma [21, 38, 76]. We may notice pale oral mucosa because of anemia, but also red-orange coloring of the skin following the deposition of carotene-like substances [71, 92, 110].

Cervero et al. [18] described 4 types of uremic stomatitis (erythematous, ulcerative, haemorrhagic and hyperkeratotic). The lesions are painful, situated on the ventral surface of the tongue, on the floor of the oral cavity and the buccal mucosa. Most frequently the cause is untreated CKD. It emerges because of inflammation and the chemical influence of ammonia or ammonia components, formed by the hydrolysis of the urea (over 30mmol/L intraoral) [95] in the saliva by urease. Kellet [58] reports about four patients with chronic renal insufficiency suffering white painless plaques. They are not subject to treatment, and they disappear in up to 2 or3 weeks after regulating the level of blood urea. Long [71] defines two types of uremic stomatitis: I type - generalized or localized erythema with grey-white pseudomembrane coating the removal of which doesn't lead to bleeding or ulceration, and type II- after removing the coating of the surface is ulcerating [3, 27, 58, 71].

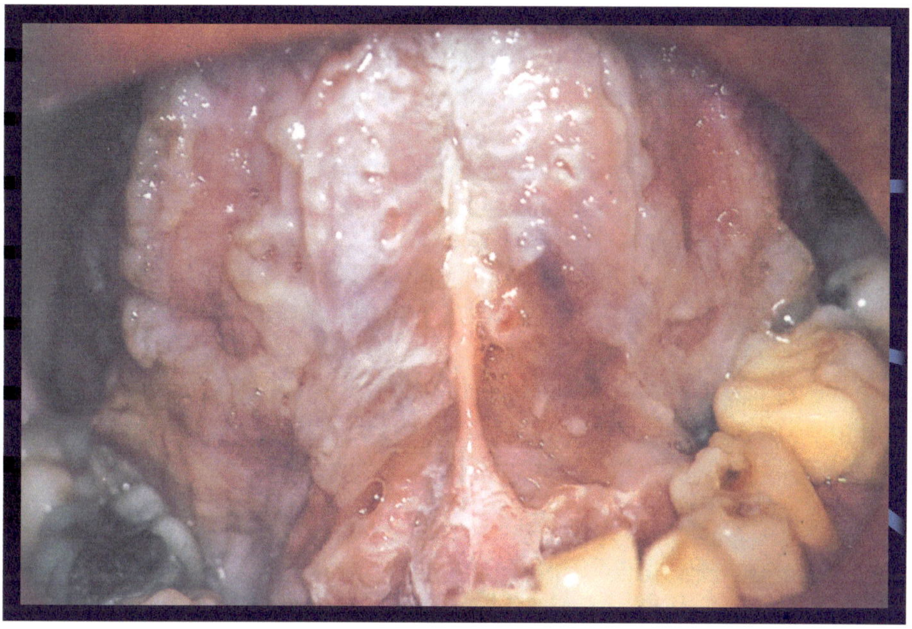

Figure 3. Uremic stomatitis

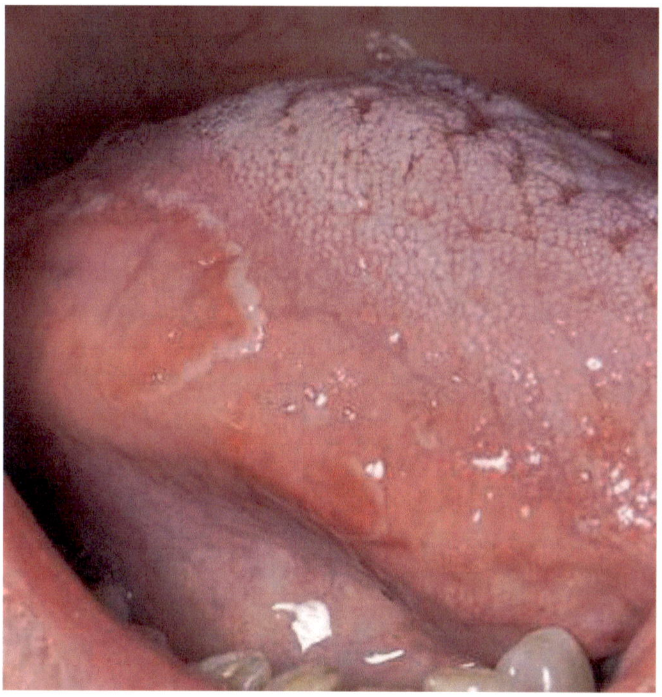

Figure 4. Geographic tongue

- Mac-Donald [74], Peneva et al. [87] found delay in the eruption of the permanent teeth with statistically significant difference in children born with the disease and lasting for life in comparison to healthy children.

Peneva et al. [85] explored the incidence of tooth decay among 30 children on hemodialysis and defined that children on dialysis suffer less frequently from decay compared to healthy children. They also found that, decay resistance is higher at children with earlier beginning of the disease and longer duration.

Shu et al. [105] explored the correlation between decay and urease activity of the tooth plaque in 25 caries-free participants and 8 participants with decays. They found that in the caries-free subjects urease activity of the dental plaque is significantly higher than this in patients with caries. They suggested that the loss of alkalizing potential of the tooth biofilm is in positive correlation with the incidence of tooth decay. Meanwhile they didn't establish statistically significant difference in the salivary urease activity.

- Takeuchi et al. [111] researched the oral microbial flora in patients with renal disease and its influence on caries and parodontal pathology. They discovered significantly higher count of parodontal and decay pathogens in patients with renal disease. This fact in turn defines the higher risk of tooth decay and parodontal disease compared to healthy samples.

Most researches regarding the oral status of patients with CKD, on hemodialysis or transplanted, are made with a control group consisting of healthy patients. For the first time a long-term, two- year research by Bots et al. [13] compares xerostomia, the sense of thirst, saliva secretion and the general oral health of patients with renal failure to those of a group of transplanted patients. Using DMFT, DMFS- indexes they find that the teeth affected by decay don't differ statistically in the group of patients on hemodialysis from those of the control group with transplanted patients. In this research, the scholars expressly note the increased necessity of examining the oral status of patients expecting transplantation.

Gavalda et al. [41] examined 105 patients on hemodialysis. They diagnosed mucosal, salivary, dental and periodontal findings in the oral cavity. They didn't find significant difference between the value of the index referring to the decay incidence in patients on hemodialysis and healthy samples, but they established such at indexes reflecting the amount of calculus and tooth plaque.

Bayraktar et al. [8] found elevated incidence of tooth caries in their control healthy group compared to group of patients on hemodialysis, but that rise is not statistically significant. Rustemeyer et al. [97] didn't find statistically significant difference of the dental health of the groups in their research either, but they noted the tendency for higher value of DMFT in the groups expecting renal transplantation (=14,9), liver transplantation (=14,5), valve transplantation (=15,2) and the control group (=13,8).

In the scientific literature, the issue of prevention and early dental intervention in patients on dialysis has become extremely pertinent, with a marked emphasis on the requirement for an interdisciplinary approach towards these patient groups [11, 30, 61].

http://dx.doi.org/10.5772/59930

Hypoplasia- there are cases where ESRD evolved in childhood. Pulp obliteration is due to violations in calcium and phosphoric exchange [60, 74, 81, 86, 90].

1. It's been proven that **parodontitis** may contribute to the development of common inflammation processes and systemic diseases such as atherosclerosis and cardiovascular diseases [22, 109]. Gingival pathogens may damage system circulation in the body by one of two connected mechanisms:

2. They provoke liver enzyme activity, influencing IL-6 and C-reactive protein, which in its turn activates the system of the complement and cause the deposition of calcium connections and aggregation of LDL and very LDL cholesterol.

3. *P. gingivalis* damages human endothelial cells and helps the formation of atheromatous plaques [11, 22, 60, 65, 84, 112].

Fisher [37] in his research defines parodontal disease as an "unconventional risk factor for the development of chronic renal disease". Pejcic et al. [84] took part into the discussion about the role of periodontitis as a risk factor for general diseases. Authors such as Klassen and Krassko [62] and Al Wahadni and Al Omari [2] report prevalence of gingival and parodontal diseases in patients on hemodialysis. There are authors who don't find increase in parodontal indexes with such patients [13, 55, 81]. Kshisageret et al. [68] note the significance of parodontal health in end-stage renal failure. They carried out a retrospective cohort research and followed the correlation between parodontal diseases and the mortality rate of patients with severe cardiovascular disease, such as patients with CKD. They established define that the mortality rate in the group of the patients with medium to severe periodontitis and cardiovascular disease is five times higher for the 18- month period of the research.

Using parodontal diagnostics, that includes CPITN, PI, PBI (papillary bleeding index), CAL (clinical attachment level), Borawski et al. examine patients on hemodialysis, patients on peritoneal dialysis, patients in the pre-dialysis stage, patients with advanced periodontitis and average patients (randomly selected). The research shows a much higher incidence of parodontitis development in patients with renal disease in comparison to average patients. Periodontal disease is practically most severe in patients on hemodialysis, less severe in patients on peritoneal dialysis and moderate in patients in the pre-dialysis stage.

Relatively little is known about the **long term** effect of dialysis treatment on oral health. A research carried out by a group of Turkish scientists, Bayraktar et al. [8], proves the necessity of sanitation, because of the negative results that occur with time onto oral health of this patient group. The publications of Graig [44], Donald [31], and Davidovich [23, 24] testify to the two-way relation between end-stage CKD and the severity of parodontal inflammation, which can be proved by examining the levels of C-reactive protein.Bayractar et al. [8], led by the fact that problems with oral health may have a negative influence over patients in end-stage CKD, launched a survey comparing the parodontal and dental status of patients with renal failure and a healthy control group. They established that there isn't a statistically significant difference between the measured pocket depths (PPD) of the two groups, but the values of the plague index (PI), the calculus index (CSI), and the gingival index (GI) show significant statistical difference. A positive correlation was established between the duration of dialysis procedures more than 3 years and missing teeth, the gingival index and pocket depth.

The research of Davidovich [24] shows for the first time the relation between the duration of dialysis and parodontal diseases in children. The results present a significant loss of epithelial attachment in patients with end-stage CKD compared to healthy patients. A positive correlation was established between the severity of parodontal status and bad oral hygiene, the uremic status, and the duration of the kidney disease.

- Regarding the cause of commonly reported gingival inflammation in patients with CKD, controversial data in literature exists. Nunn et al. [81], Tollefsen & Jonasen [118, 119], and Ertugrul et al. [36] report reduction in gingivitis because of immunosuppressants and uremia. Naugle et al. [79] reveal conflicting data. Furthermore, Kitsou et al. [62] reproduce experimental gingivitis following the protocol of Löe. Oral hygiene is discontinued for 28 days. The authors report they haven't found differences in the gingival indexes between the group of 6 patients on hemodialysis and one of 6 patients without renal problems and conclude that chronic uremia doesn't contribute to the defensive mechanisms of parodontal tissue against tooth plaque. Davidovich et al. [24] report a statistically significant difference comparing the duration of the dialysis and CKD and gingival and parodontal changes. They report that uremia and immunosuppression reduce but don't eliminate an inflammation response of the gingiva and periodontium against tooth plaque. Another condition accompanying end-stage renal failure is diabetes. Chuang et al. [21] compared the oral health of 45 patients suffering from diabetes and undergoing hemodialysis treatment to that of 83 patients without diabetes but on hemodialysis. They reported lower saliva secretion and lower pH connected with higher caries levels in the diabetes group, but they didn't observe differences in gingival inflammation and the presence of parodontitis. In the research of Borawski et al. [11] the need is noted of treatment through CPITN for patients on hemodialysis and transplanted renal patients.

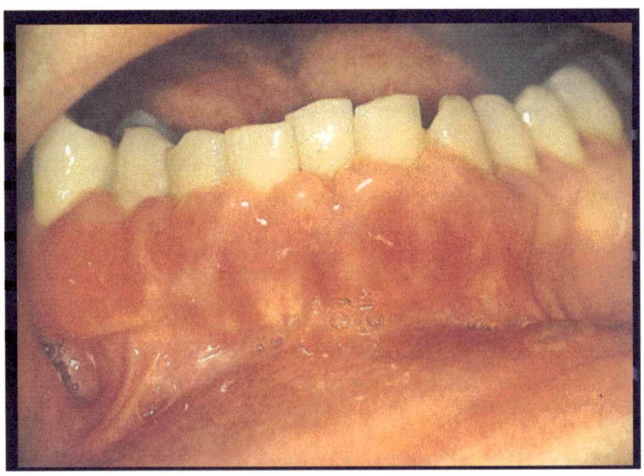

Figure 5. Cyclosporine induced gingival hyperplasia

- Another finding in patients with end-stage liver failure, is drug-induced **gingival hyperplasia (DIGH)** (fig.5). Its mechanism of occurrence is multifactorial and has not yet been fully explained. The intake of antihypertensive and immunosuppressive drugs gives evidence in the oral cavity [42, 50, 104, 115]. Such overgrowth is usually observed in the early posttransplantation period (4 m) and in combination with insufficient oral hygiene or previously damaged periodontium [1, 30, 89, 112].The sole influence of cyclosporine remains controversial in the specialized literature. Data varies from 25 to 81% depending on methods used [104]. R. A. Seymour [103] compares the influence of azathioprine on gingiva to that of cyclosporine and finds that azathioprine has no damaging effect on the gingiva. J. A. James [57] reports the absence of gingival changes when using tacrolimus (6,4%) and cyclosporine (17,9%) on the third month after immunosuppression, excluding patients with accompanying antihypertensive therapy. Their study shows that tacrolimus also induces gingival hyperplasia, but to a lesser extent [3]. James [56] takes into consideration 4 cases of swapping cyclosporine with tacrolimus, combined with professional care of periodontist. In only one case a full regression of the gingival overgrowth occurs. J. A. James [57] compares gingival hyperplasia among 25 patients taking tacrolimus, and 26 control group patients and doesn't find a statistically significant difference. This gives him the grounds to distinguish tacrolimus as an alternative to cyclosporine A, when a severe case of gingival hyperplasia is present.

Researches made by Davidovich [24] and Thorp et al. 116] confirmed the findings of Nunn et al. [81] about gingival overgrowth in transplanted patients on immunosuppression with cyclosporine A and less frequently occurring one in patients taking tacrolimus.

Radwan- Oczko et al. [94] sought a connection between gingival hyperplasia, immunosuppressive drugs and the growth factor β1 (TGF β1), which is considered a key cytokine in fibrogenesis. They didn't prove any statistically significant relation between gene expression of TGF β1, gingival hyperplasia and treatment with cyclosporine A and tacrolimus.

Djemileva [30] and Gera [42] believe that shared responsibility in maintaining oral health in the long process of treatment of these patients is a crucial factor as well as the possible switch of immunosuppressants. The studies of Somacarrera et al. [108], Ellis et al. [34], and J. Smith et al. [106] are taken as evidence corroborating the supposition that maintaining sufficient oral hygiene leads to a decrease of gingival hyperplasia.

- **Malignancy.** The suppression of the immune system in transplanted patients may predispose the formation of malignant entities. Two types of malignant formations that prevail in patients with kidney transplantation have been reported: cancer of the cervix and squamous cancer of the skin [10, 17, 66, 88, 100]. Malignancy may also include Kaposi's sarcoma, renal cancer, and lymphomas.

- **Candidiasis** is particularly specific for the early post-transplantation period: from 0 to 6 months. It is caused first by the immunosuppressive action of the drugs and the impact on oral homeostasis and second by the decrease of saliva secretion- medications for hypertension, and dialysis procedures [32, 49, 78, 99].

4.1. A dental treatment approach to patients on hemodialysis and transplanted

Assuming susceptibility of the patients on hemodialysis and those with a renal transplant to infections, it proves necessary to pick the right antibiotics for each dental procedure, that may cause longer bacteraemia [97, 120]. A number of studies prove the need of antibiotic protection at risky dental manipulations, even though according to Lockhart et al. [70], washing one's teeth is comparable to tooth extraction as a possible cause for bacteraemia [122, 123]. It's necessary to have in mind the possibility of contamination of parodontal tissues through various means of personal oral hygiene [72, 93].

The American Heart Association in its recommendations for the prevention of bacterial endocarditis from 2007 [123] divides the dental procedures into such hazardous for bacteraemia: all procedures connected with manipulation of the gingival tissue and the periapical region of the teeth, or perforation of the oral mucosa, and these where antibiotic prophylaxis is not necessary: routine anesthesia through non-infected tissue, radiographs, and bleeding from trauma of the oral mucosa. In a similar way, D. Tong [119, 120] made a division of the dental procedures (table 2).

High risk category
Tooth extraction
Periodontal procedure that includes surgery, Ultrasound scaling
Root probing
Implant placing and tooth reimplantation
Endodontic instrumentation or surgery beyond root apex
Subgingival application of antibiotic fibers and bands
Initial placing of orthodontic rings but not brackets
Intraligamentary local anesthesia
Preventive cleaning of teeth or implants with expected bleeding
Procedures where prophylaxis is not needed
Dental restorations with or without a retraction cord
Local anesthesia (excluding intraligamentary)
Intracanal endodontic procedures after placing implants and build-ups
Rubber dam placing
Post-operative suture removal
Placement of orthodontic and prosthetic constructions
Taking of dental impressions
Teeth fluoridation
Radiographs
Adjustment of orthodontic constructions
Replacement of milk teeth

Table 2. Dental procedures with a compelling antibiotic prophylaxis in patients at risk

4.2. Dental treatment approaches in the pre- and post-operative periods

i. Most authors are unanimous that in the pre-transplantation period preventive sanitation of all foci is necessary [5, 6, 11, 12, 27, 46, 64, 82, 84, 96, 97, 98]. To the initial dental diagnostics that includes standard dental examination and parodontal examination the methods of the complex oral and focal diagnostics could be added, which may define the dominant and latent foci that early in the pre-transplantation period so that a treatment plan for the post-transplantation period can be devised. Dental doctors should be aware of the degree of renal insufficiency and the current medical status of the patient. Consultation with the patient's general doctor should be made and lab tests should be performed, especially before surgical dental interventions. The intake of systemic antibiotics in the pre-transplantation period is contraindicated [82], not counting life-threatening situations. Heavily damaged decayed teeth and such with radiograph changes and symptoms should be extracted. A mass teeth extraction procedure is to be performed on patients with bad oral hygiene and advanced periodontal disease, and on those unmotivated to maintain sufficient oral hygiene. Surgical sanitation is followed by prosthetic restoration [54].

It is necessary **to treat all newly emerged dental conditions** without waiting for the clinical symptoms to develop. Moreover, to fulfil the requirements for sufficient dental health, a patient should have a sufficient knowledge. Several studies take notice of the fact that patients suffering from CKD don't maintain sufficient oral hygiene and it should be improved [7, 43].

Infection control is a complex issue regarding patients with end-stage renal disease. If an invasive dental procedure is required, a consultation with the treatment doctor must be made. The current health status of the patients is consulted, as well as the possible need of antibiotic premedication, usage of local anesthetics and other drugs. Prescribing medicaments to patients with renal insufficiency should be approached with care and in full accordance with their current medical and renal condition [19, 20, 53, 67] (table 3).

Antibiotic	Normal renal function	Glomerular filtration 10–50 ml/min	Glomerular filtration <10 ml/min
Amoxicillin	8 h	8–12 h	12–18
Ampicillin	6 h	6–9 h	9–12
Cephalexin	6 h	6 h	6–12 h
Clindamycin	8 h	8 h	8 h
Doxycycline	12–24 h	12–24 h	12–24 h
Erythromycin	6 h	6 h	6 h
Metronidazole	8 h	8 h	12–16 h

Table 3. Antibiotic premedication for patients suffering from CKD, adap. J. W. Little, D. A. Falace et al [66]; J. A. Ship [105]

W. M. Bennett et al. [9] propose a change in dosage for patients on hemodialysis with emerged tooth infection:

- Penicillin 500 mg p. o. every 6 hours after dialysis;
- Amoxicillin 500 mg p. o. every 24 hours after hemodialysis;
- Ampicillin 250 mg – 1 g p. o. every 12-24 hours after hemodialysis;
- Erythromycin 250 mg p.o. every 6 hours optional only after dialysis;
- Clindamycin 300 mg p.o. every 6 hours optional only after dialysis.

According to data from Tong and Walker [120] in Australia and New Zealand, 53% of dental doctors follow the instructions of AHA for the prevention of bacterial endocarditis. One of the most frequently used patterns for premedication is taking a 2g Amoxicillin or 600 mg Clindamycin (in cases of Penicillin allergy) one hour before a dental procedure: for kids 50mg/kg oral intake 30-60 minutes before the procedure.

A survey in two Swedish provinces reveals that the most frequently prescribed antibiotics to kidney transplanted patients when performing scaling, tooth extraction and root canal treatment are Amoxicillin, Penicillin, Clindamycin [33].

The issue of antibiotic prevention of bacterial endocarditis has undergone considerable development in the past 10 years. In 2007 AHA published an amendment to the recommendations from 1997. AHA (2007) narrows significantly the diseases whose dental treatment is indicative for antibiotic prevention. In the recommendations patients with dialysis shunts are classified in class 3, level C on account of the possibility for the development of bacterial endocarditis during dental treatment. This means that there are indications, supported with evidence or general agreement, that the procedures/treatment are not necessary, ineffective and in some cases even damaging. The level of evidence is C, in other words the recommendations are based only on an established consensus of views of experts, on separate cases or on accepted standards of treatment. Despite this fact, these patients are defined as "unique" in view of the higher risk of infections of the venous shunt, because of their immunocompromised status and the increased count of *S. aureus* [5]. Around 22% of the arteriovenous shunts get infected, which leads to antibiotic intake or to changes in the intake plan. The pathogens linked with the infection occurring in the application of the vascular approach are 53% S. aureus and 20.3% coagulase-negative staphylococci. In the AHA guide [5] to non-valvular cardiovascular equipment a regime of antibiotic prophylaxis of patients with hemodialysis shunts and organ transplants is not mentioned. The same opinion is maintained by Pallsh [83]. Lockhart et al. [69] methodically examine the efficiency of antibiotic premedication in dental practice. They divide patients taking antibiotics in 8 groups. One of the groups consists of patients with hemo- and peritoneal dialysis: with kidney dialysis shunts (hemodialysis and peritoneal). The authors found little or no scientific evidence on issues relating tothe usage of antibiotic prophylaxis before dental procedures in these 8 groups of patients.

Until now no clear evidence has been provided that during invasive dental treatment of patients with advanced renal, liver or heart condition antibiotic prevention is needed, but most dental centers and authors follow the instructions of the AHA [123], pointing out two main reasons: shunt infection risk [101] or the possible development of infectious endocarditits [109] (table 4).

Condition	Antibiotic	Prescription	
Standard prophylaxis	Amoxicillin	Adults 2.0mg	Kids 50 mg/kg
Inability for oral intake	Ampicillin	2g i.m. or i.v.	50 mg/kg i.m. or i.v.
Penicillin allergy	Clindamycin	600mg	20 mg/kg
	Cephalexin* or cefadroxil	2 gr	50 mg/kg
	Azithromycin or Clarithromycin	500 mg	15 mg/kg
Penicillin allergy and inability for oral intake	Clindamycin	600 mg i.m. or i.v.	20 mg i.m. or i.v.
	Cefazolin	1 gr i.m. or i.v.	50 mg/kg i.m. or i.v.

* Or other first or second generation cephalosporins in equivalent doses for adults and children

Table 4. Antibiotic premedication according to AHA's recommendations

Patients awaiting transplantation undergo antibiotic premedication from the moment they are moved into the operation theater. The duration of the antibiotic treatment is usually with a duration of up to 3 days. In the best case scenario the antibiotic intake should be determined on the basis of the bacterial flora present, the kind of transplantation and patient-specific features [107]. For example a kidney transplanted patient may be prescribed Cefazolin and Ampicillin-sulbactam to cope with the uropathogens and staphylococci. In patients with chronic dental infections, frequent or continuous bacteraemia may occur, which in its turn may trigger acute or chronic inflammation in other organs [61].

De Rossi and Glick [27] systematize a few guidelines for a recommended dental approach to patients on hemodialysis. They also follow AHA's recommendations, but they think that the antibiotic of choice should be Vancomycin, which must be flowed on the day of the dialysis before an invasive dental procedure, since its action on the organism lasts for the next 7 days. What follows is a radical approach with the extraction of the tootth.

With better medical care, the expectations of the patients for better and longer life are justified.

Hemostatic agents

Standard tests for suspected coagulopathy include [45]:

1. Bleeding time (BT).
2. Prothrombin time (PT).
3. Partial thromboplastin time (PTT).

4. Platelet count (table 8).

5. INR (International Normalised Ratio).

Lockhart et al. [68] define several points which need to be considered before invasive dental procedure is initiated on patients with CKD. The first issue to consider is the analysis of what is described above, as well as the influence of the platelet count on the expected post-operative bleeding (table 5).

Platelet count (на µl)	Diagnose	Effect
150 000-450 000	Normal	Rare but possible operative bleeding
100 000–150 000	Mild thrombocytopenia	
50 000–100 000	Moderate thrombocytopenia	Increased possibility for bleeding during dental manipulation but unusual.
25 000–50 000	Severe thrombocytopenia	Expected problematic bleeding Spontaneous bleeding at <10 000
<25 000	Life-threatening condition	Invasive procedures only at emergency and blood transfusion

Table 5. Platelet count and its effect on post-operative bleeding

They define hemostasis in the oral cavity as a multifactorial process, which is not well studied yet. To a greater extent the insufficient use of lab tests may confound the appointed anticoagulation therapy and the risk for the patient could be greater than post-operative bleeding.

Meechan and Greenwood [76] propose that in cases of platelet count lower than $50*10^9/L$ an urgent invasive procedure is needed. The latter could be performed after substitute platelet transfusion 30 minutes before operation. In practice this approach is used quite rarely because of the risk of immune sensitization. Patients on hemodialysis undergo heparinisation 3 times a week before procedures, but heparin has a short half-life (around 5 hours), that's why as a precaution it's accepted that it is best for any dental procedures to be performed on the day after dialysis [30, 59]. On the other hand, the longer the time since the last dialysis, the greater the chance for prolonged bleeding during invasive dental procedures because of uremia.

As a result of thrombocytic dysfunction, even with relatively good blood indicators, profuse bleeding could be expected during invasive dental procedures [53, 80]. The treatment of these patients requires a preventive strategy for oral and parodontal surgery that includes:

- the ability and the knowledge to perform atraumatic surgery;
- the use of sutures, compression bandages and local or systemic hemostatic agents. Assuming different reference books that propose different patterns for hemostasis and according to Bulgarian experience in this direction, most frequently used medicaments are as follow:

EAK, amp. 40% 20 ml	I.v. very slow 1 amp.
Pamba, amp. 1% 5 ml	I.m., I.v. 1–2 amp./24 h.
Vit. K, amp. 1% 1ml	I.m, I.v.
Metadiol	5–10 mg oral/24 hours
Phytonadione	5–10 mg oral/24 hours
Tranexamic acid	10–12,5 mg/kg 2 times a day, p.o.
Desmopressin	03 mg/kg i.v. for 30 min single dose
Conjugated estrogen	0,6 mg/kg i.v. or 2,5–25 mg p.o. for 5 days

Cryoprecipitates are less frequently used because of the risk of disease transmission [40, 67, 80].

6. Post transplantation period (fig. 6)

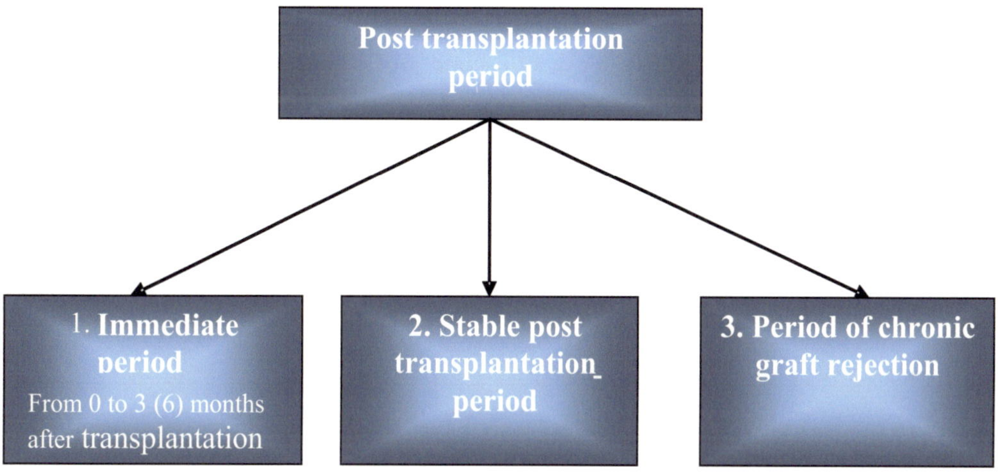

Figure 6. Schematic depiction of the post transplantation period

Dental treatment after transplantation can be differentiated in 3 periods - **immediately** after transplantation to the 3rd month after transplantation, **stable** post-transplantation period, and the period of **chronic graft rejection** [45, 67]. Diaz [54] defines the immediate after transplantation period till the 6th month following the operation.

Through the immediate period the possibility for post-operative complications, dominating opportunistic virus and fungal infections, the risk of acute graft rejection is greater. Therefore dental interference is not advisable, excluding any emergencies [53, 67, 82, 117].

Muzyka et al. [78] and J. B. Epstein [35] find that the most used antifungal agent in the initial treatment plan of surface forms of oral candidiasis is Nystatin, applied locally as well as clotrimazole. Parenteral administration of Amphotericin B is associated with increased nephrotoxicity, especially in combination with cyclosopin or aminoglycoside antibiotics. A diluted parenteral solution of Amphotericin B for mouth rinse is successfully used in USA [15]. Ketoconazole is part of the imidazole group, but in combination with cyclosporine it may lead to increased level of Cyclosporin A [32, 49, 99, 124].

The recommendations for dental treatment in the immediate after-transplantation period are the following:

- Avoiding routine dental treatment, and if such is needed, conservative treatment methods should be used;
- Meticulous oral hygiene that includes mouth rinse solutions containing chlorhexidine. Djemileva [30] points out that the simultaneous use of toothpastes containing sodium laurylsulfate may inactivate the chlorhexidine which is part of some mouth rinse solutions and gels.

Dental rehabilitation of patients on hemodialysis and transplanted patients would be more successful, if the methods of complex focal diagnostics and treatments are applied. They are non-invasive and provide atraumatic and aseptic work techniques, combining thermal diagnostics and a laser treatment approach.

Author details

M. Dencheva[2], E. Deliverska[1*], A. Krasteva[2], J. Galabov[2] and A. Kisselova[2]

*Address all correspondence to: elitsadeliverska@yahoo.com

1 Department of Oral and Maxillofacial Surgery, Faculty of Dental Medicine, Medical University, Sofia, Turkey

2 Department of imaging and oral Diagnostics, Faculty of Dental Medicine, Medical University, Sofia, Turkey

References

[1] Al Nowaiser, A., V. S. Lucas, M. Wilson, G. L. Roberts, R. S. Trompeter. Oral health and caries related microflora in children during the first three months following renal transplantation. Int J Pediatr Dent, 2004, 14, 2: 118–126 (9).

[2] Al Wahadni, A., M. A. Al Omari. Dental diseases in a Jordanian population on renal dialysis. Quintessence Int, 2003; 34: 343–347.

[3] Asante-Korang, A., G. J. Boyle, S. A. Webber, S. A. Miller, F. J. Fricker. Experience of FK506 immune suppression in pediatric heart transplantation: a study of long-term adverse effects. J Heart Lung Transplant, 1996;15: 415–22.

[4] Azmanova, V., L. Brankova, I. Ivanov, L. Videnov, P. Karaboicheva. Atlas of oral diseases. Medicine, C., 1992.

[5] Baddour, L., M. Bettmann, A. Bolger, A. Epstein, P. Ferriere et al. Nonvalvular cardiovascular device-related infections. Circulation, 2003; 108; 2015–2031.

[6] Barnett, M. The oral-systemic disease connection. An update for the practicing dentist. JADA, 2006, vol. 137, 5S–6S.

[7] Bayraktar, G., C. Kurtulus, R. Kazancioglu et al. Effect of educational level on oral health in peritoneal and hemodialysis patients. International Journal of Dentistry (2009)Article ID 159767,5 pages

[8] Bayraktar, G., I. Kurtulus, A. Duraduryan et al. Dental and periodontal findings in hemodyalisis patients. Oral Disiase, 2007; 13: 393–7.

[9] Bennett, W. M. et al. Drug prescribing in renal failure, 1999, 2nd ed. Philadelphia, American College of Physicians.

[10] Birkeland, S. A. et al. Cancer risk after renal transplantation in the Nordic countries, 1964–1986. Int J Cancer, 1995: 60: 183–189.

[11] Borawski, J., M. Wilczynska-Borawska, W. Stokowska, M. Mysliwiec. The periodontal status of pre – dialysis chronic kidney disease and maintenance dialysis patients. Nephrol Dial Transplant, 2007; 22: 457–464.

[12] Bots, C. P., H. S. Brand, Ihg. Poorterman. Oral and salivary changes in patients with end stage renal disease (ESRD): a two year follow – up study. British dental Journal, 2007; 10; 10–38.

[13] Bots, C., J. Poorteman, H. Brand, H. Kalsbeek, B. Amerongen, E. Veerman, A. Nieuw Amerongen. The oral health status of dentate patients with chronic renal failure undergoing dialysis therapy. Oral Dis, 2006; 12: 176–180.

[14] Brancati, F. et al. Risk of end-stage renal disease in diabetes mellitus. A prospective cohort study of men screened for MRFIT. JAMA, 1997, 278: 2069–2074.

[15] Brandell, R., S. L. Chase, J. R. Cohn. Treatment of oral candidiasis with amphotericin B solution. Clin Pharm, 1988; 7: 70–2.

[16] Burne, R. A., R. E. Marquis. Alkalai production by oral bacteria and protection against dental caries. FEMS Microbiol Lett, 2000; 193: 1–6.

[17] Caillard, S., L.Y. Agodoa, E.M.Bohen, K.C. Abbott. Myeloma, Hodgkin disease, and lymphoid leukemia after renal transplantation: characteristics, risk factors and prognosis. Transplantation, 2006, 27; 81 (6): 888–95.

[18] Cervero, A. J., J. V. Bagan, Y. J. Soriano, R. P. Roda. Dental management in renal failure: Patients on dialysis. Med Oral Patol Oral Cir Bucal, 2008 Jul 1: 13 (7): E 419–27.

[19] Chainani-Wu, N., T. Wu. Immunosuppressants. CDA Journal, 2006, vol. 36, 10, 775–779.

[20] Chavez, E. Systematic review of the medication list: A resource for risk assessment and dental management. CDA Journal, October 2008, vol. 36; 10: 739–745.

[21] Chuang, S. F., J. M. Sung, S. C. Kuo, J. J. Huang, S. Y. Lee. Oral and dental manifestations in diabetic and nondiabetic uremic patients receiving hemodialysis. OOOOE, 2005, 99: 6; 689–695.

[22] Craig, R. G. Interactions between chronic renal disease and periodontal disease. Oral Dis, 2008 Jan; 14 (1): 1–7.

[23] Davidovich, E., M. Davidovits, E. Eidelman, Z. Schvarz, E. Bimstein. Pathophysiology, therapy, and oral implications of renal failure in children an adolescents: an update. Pediatr Dent., 2005 Mar–Apr; 27 (2): 98–106.

[24] Davidovich, E., Z. Schwarz, M. Davidovitch, E. Eidelman, E. Bimstein. Oral findings and periodontal status in children, adolescents and young adults suffering from renal failure. J Clin Periodontol, 2005; 32: 1076–1082.

[25] Davies, A., K. Broadley, D. Beighton. Xerostomia in patients with advanced cancer. Journal of pain and symptom management, 2001 October, vol. 22; 4: 820–825.

[26] De la Rosa Garcia, E. et al. Oral mucosa symptoms, signs and lesions, in end stage renal disease and non end – stage renal disease diabetic patients. Med Oral Patol Oral Cir Bucal., 2006 Non 1; 11 (6): E 467–73, Synder, S., B. Pendrgraph. Detection and evaluation of chronic kidney disease. Am Fam Physican, 2005 Nov 1; 72 (9): 1723–32.

[27] De Rossi, S., M. Glick. Dental considerations for the patient with renal disease receiving hemodialysis. JADA, vol. 127, 1996, 211–219.

[28] Djemileva, T. Xerostomia (dryness in mouth). Publ., АЦЕР, 1998.

[29] Djemileva, T. Parodontal diseases. Publ. „АЦЕР", C., 1999, 367.

[30] Djamileva, T.,Bolqrova,T. Gingival hyperplasia during system intake of calcium antagonists, immunosuppressants and hydantoins,. Publ. „АЦЕР", C., 2007, 118.

[31] Donald, G. Vidt. Inflammation in renal disease. Am J Cardiol, 2006; 97 [supp]: 20A–27A.

[32] Dongari-Bogtzoglou, A. et al. Oral Candida infection and colonization in solid organ transplant recipients. Oral Microbiol Immunol, 2009 Juni; 24 (3): 249–254.

[33] Ellervall, E., F. Bjorklund, M. Rohlin, E. Vinge, K. Knutsson. Antibiotic prophylaxis in oral health care: administration strategies of general dental practitioners. Acta Odontologica Scandinavica, 2005; 63: 321–329.

[34] Ellis, J. S., R. A. Seymour, J. J. Taylor, J. M. Thomason. Prevalence of gingival overgrowth in transplant patients immunosuppressed with tacrolimus. J Clin Periodontol, 2004, 31: 126–131.

[35] Epstein, J. B. Antifungal therapy in oropharyngeal mycotic infections. Oral Surg Oral Med Oral Pathol, 1990; 69: 32–41.

[36] Ertugrul, F., C. Elbek-Cubukcu, E. Sabah, S. Mir. The oral health status of children undergoing hemodialisis treatment. Turk J Pediat, 2003: 45; 108–113.

[37] Fisher, M., G. Taylor. A prediction model for chronic kidney disease includes periodontal disease. J Periodontol, 2009, 1, 80, 16–23.

[38] Franca, C. M., M. Domingues-Martins, A. Volpe et al. Severe oral manifestations of chronic graft-vs.-host disease. JADA,Vol. 132, August 2001.

[39] Friedlander, A. et al. Restless legs syndrome. JADA, June 2006, vol. 137, 755–761.

[40] Gacina, P., D. Carzavec, V. Stancic, V. Pejsa. Dental procedures in patients receiving oral anticoagulant therapy. Acta clin Croat, 2006, 45 (2): 101–104.

[41] Gavalda, C., J. Bagan, C. Scully, F. Silvestre, M. Milian, Y. Jimenez. Renal haemodialysis patients: oral, salivary, dental and periodontal findings in 105 adult cases. Oral Dis, 1999; 5: 299–302.

[42] Gera, I., T. Keglevich. A case history of a kidney transplant patient with ciclosporin – induced gingival overgrowth combined with chronic periodontitis. Perio, 2007; 12: 287–293.

[43] Gheith, O. A., S. Ali-El Saadany et al. Compliance with recommended life style behaviours in kidney transplant recipients. Does it matter in living donor kidney transplant? IJKD, 2006; 2: 216–26.

[44] Graig, R., P. Kotanko, A. Kamer, N. Levin. Periodontal diseases – a modifiable source of systemic inflammation for the end-stage renal disease patient on haemodialysis Therapy. Nephrol Dial Transplant, 2007, 22: 312–315.

[45] Gudapati, A., P. Aahmed, R. Rada. Dental management of patients with renal failure. Gen Dent., 2002 Nov-Dec; 50 (6): 508–10.

[46] Guggenheimer, J., D. Mayher, B. Eghtesad. A survey of dental care protocols among US organ transplant centers. Clinical Transplantation, 2005; 19: 15–8.

[47] Guggenheimer, J., P. Moore. Xerostomia.Etiology, recognition and treatment. JADA, vol. 134, 2003.

[48] Gurkan, A., T. Kose, Gul. Atilla. Oral health status and oral hygiene habits of an adult Turkish population on dialysis. Oral Health Prev Dent, 2008, 6, 1:37–43.

[49] Hamid, M., C. Dummer, L. Pinto. Systemic conditions, oral findings and dental management of chronic renal failure patients: general considerations and case report. Braz Dent J, 2006, 17 (2): 166–170.

[50] Hassell, T. M., A. F. Hefti. Drug-induced gingival overgrowth: old problem, new problem. Crit Rev Oral Biol Med, 1991; 2: 103–37.

[51] Heeger, P. Frontiers in nephrology: Tolerance. J Am Soc Nephrol, 2007, 18: 2240–2241.

[52] Helenius, L., J. Meurman, I. Helenius, K. Kari, J. Hietanen, R. Suuronen at al. Oral and salivary parameters in patients with rheumatic diseases. Acta Odontologica Scandinavica, 2005; 63: 284–293.

[53] Herr, R., R. Cydulka. Emergency care of the compromised patient. 1994, 808.

[54] http://www.usc.edu/hsc/dental/dhnet/papers/coral149.html

[55] Jaffe, E. C., G. J. Roberts, C. Chantler, J. E. Carter. Dental findings in chronic renal failure. Br Dent J, 1986; 160: 18–20.

[56] James, J., S. Boomer, A. Maxwell, P. Hull, C. Short at al. Reduction in gingival overgrowth associated with conversion from cyclosporine A to tacrolimus. J Clin Periodontol, 2000; 27: 144–148.

[57] James, J., S. Jamal, P. Hull, T. Macfariane, B. Campbell at al. Tacrolimus is not associated with gingival overgrowth in renal transplant patients. J Clin Periodontol, 2001; 28: 848–852.

[58] Kellett, M. Oral white plaques in uraemic patients. B Dent J, 1983; 154: 366.

[59] Kerr, A. R. Update on renal disease for the dental practitioner. Oral Surg Oral Med Oral Pathol, 2001; 92: 9–16.

[60] Kho, H. S., S. W. Lee, S. C. Chung, Y. K. Kim. Oral manifestations and salivary flow rate, pH, and buffer capacity in patients with end-stage renal disease undergoing hemodialisis. Oral Surg Oral Med Oral Pathol Oral Radiol Endod, 1999, 88: 316–319.

[61] Kiselova-Yaneva, A. Dental allergology and focal diagnostics. Gutenberg, C., 2001, 327 c.

[62] Kitsou, V. K., A. Konstantinidis & K. C. Siamopoulus. Chronic renal failure and periodontal disease. Renal failure, 2000, 22; 307–318.

[63] Kozarov, E. V., B. R. Dorn, C. E. Shelburne et al. Human atherosclerotic plaque contains viable invasive Actinobacillus actinomicetemcomitans and Porphyromonas gingivalis. Arteroscler Thromb Vasc Biol, 2005; 25: e17–e18.

[64] Krennmair, G., J. Auer et al. Odontogenic infection sources in patients scheduled for cardiac valve replacement. Oral Health Prev Dent., 2007: 2: 153–159.

[65] Kshirsager, A. et al. Periodontal disease adversely affects the survival of patients with end- stage renal disease. Kidney International, 2009, 75, 746–751.

[66] Little, J. W., D. A. Falace et al. Dental management of the medically compromised patient, seventh ed., St. Louis, Mo., Mosby Elsevier, 2008.

[67] Little, J., D. Falace, G. Miller, N. Rhodus. Dental Management of the Medically Compromised Patient. Sixth edition, Chapter 9, 2002, 617.

[68] Lockhart, P. B., J. Gibson, S. H. Pond, J. Leitch. Dental management considerations for the patient with an aquired coagulopathy. Part 1: Coagulopathies from systemic disease. British Dental Journal, 2003; 195: 439–445.

[69] Lockhart, P., B. Loven, M. Brennan, Ph. Fox. The evidence base for the efficacy of antibiotic prophylaxis in dental practice. J Am Dent Assoc, 2007, 4, 458–474.

[70] Lockhart, P., M. Brennan, H. Sasser P. Fox at al. Bacteremia associated with toothbrushing and dental extraction. Circulation, 2008; 117; 3118–3125.

[71] Long, R., L. Hlousek, J. Doyle. Oral manifestations of systemic diseases. Dermatol Clin, 1998, 65: 309–315.

[72] Malmberg, E., D. Birkhed et al. Microorganisms on tootbrushes at day – care centers. Acta Odontol Scand, 1994: 52: 93–98.

[73] Marton, K., M. Madlena, J. Banoczy, G. Varga at al. Unstimulated whole saliva flow rate in relation to sicca symptoms in Hungary. Oral Diseases, 2008, 14, 472–477.

[74] Mc Donald, P., Avery, D. Стоматология детей и подростков. Пер. с англ. М., Медицинское информационное агентство, 2003. 766 с.

[75] Mccartan, B. E., C. E. Mccreary. Oral lichenoid drug eruptions. Oral Dis, 1997; 3: 58–63.

[76] Meechan, J. G., M. Greenwood. General medicine and surgery for dental practitioners Part 9: Haematology and patients with bleeding problems. BDJ, 2003 September, vol. 195; 305–310.

[77] Mihailova, Hr.,Nikolov, V. Maxillofacial changes during hemodialysis and secondary hyperparathyroidism. Dental management, C., 1999–2000, issue XXVII, 59–64.

[78] Muzyka, B., M. Glick. A review of oral fungal infections and appropriate therapy. JADA, 1995, vol. 126.

[79] Naugle, K., M. L. Darby, D. B. Bauman, L. T. Lineberger, R. Powers. The oral health status of individuals on renal dialysis. Ann Periodontol, 1998, 3: 197–205.

[80] Nishide, N., T. Nishikawa, N. Kanamura. Extensive bleeding during surgical treatment for gingival overgrowth in patient on haemodialysis. A case report and review of the literature. Australian dental journal, 2005; 50: 4.

[81] Nunn, J. H., J. Sharp, H. J. Lambert, N. D. Plant, M. G. Coulthard. Oral health in children with renal disease. Pediatr Nephrol, 2000; 14: 997–1001.

[82] Otten, J. E. Zahnsanierung vor und nach Organstransplantation. Wissenschaftliche Stellungnahme der DGZMK, 1998.

[83] Pallasch, Th. Perspectives on the 2007 AHA endocarditis prevention guidelines. CDA Journal, July 2007, vol. 35; 7: 50–513.

[84] Pejcic, A., S. Pesevska, I. Grigorov, M. Bojovic. Periodontitis as a risk factor for general disorders. Acta Fac Med Naiss, 2006; 23 (2): 59–63.

[85] Peneva, M., Anadolska, A., Apostolova, D. Tooth decay in children suffering CKD. Dentistry, C., 3, 1989, 6–9.

[86] Peneva, M., Anadolska, A., Apostolova, D. Oral status in children with CKD. Dentistry, C., 3, 1988, 72–76.

[87] Peneva, M., Anadolska, A., Apostolova, D. Eruption of permanent teeth in children with CKD. Dentistry, C., 2, 1989, 8–11.

[88] Penn, I. Occurrence of cancers in immunosuppressed organ transplant recipients. Clin Transpl, 1998: 147–157.

[89] Pernu, H. E., L. M. Pernu, K. R. Huttunen, P. A. Nieminen, M. L. Knuuttila. Gingival overgrowth among renal transplant recipients related to immunosuppressive medication and possible local background factors. J Periodontol., 1992; 63: 548–53.

[90] Petrunov, B., Dimitrov, V., Kiselova-Yaneva, A.Clinical immunology, allergology, dental clinical allergology. C., Apco, 2009, 276.

[91] Porter, S. R., A. Hegarty, C. Scully. An update of the etiology and management of xerostomia. Oral Surg Oral Med Oral Pathol Oral Radiol Endod, 2004, 97: 28–46.

[92] Proctor, R., N. Kumar, A. Stein, D. Moles, S. Porter. Oral and dental aspects of chronic renal failure. J Dent Res., 2005 Mar; 84 (3): 199–208.

[93] Quirynen, M., M. De Soete, M. Pauwels et al. Bacterial survival rate on tooth – and interdental brushes in relation to the use of toothpaste. J Clin Periodontol, 2001: 28: 1160–1114.

[94] Radwan-Oczko, M., M. Boratynska, M. Zietec, T. Dobosz. Transforming growth factor – β1gene expression and cyclosporine A – induced gingival overgrowth: a pilot study. J Clin Periodontol, 2008; 35: 371–378.

[95] Ross, W. F., P. L. Salisbury. Uremic stomatitis associated with undiagnosed renal failure. Gen Dent, 1994; 9/10: 410–412.

[96] Rustemeyer, J., A. Bremerich. Necessity of surgical dental foci treatment prior to organ transplantation and heart valve replacement. Clin Oral Invest, 2007, 11: 171–174.

[97] Rustemeyer, J., M. Black, A. Bremerich. Stellenwert der dentalen und parodontalen Fokusssanierung vor Organtransplantationen und Herzklappenersatz. Transplantazionsmedizin, 2006; 18: 24.

[98] Sarachev, E. Connection between some joint diseases and foci of odontogenic origin. Journal of IMAB – Annual Proceeding (Scientific papers), 2006, book 2.

[99] Segal, B., G. Nikolaus et al. Prevention and early treatment of invasive fungal infection in patients with cancer and neutropenia and in stem cell transplant recipients in the era of newer broad-spectrum antifungal agents and diagnostic adjuncts. Clinical Infectious Diseases, 2007; 44: 402–9.

[100] Seymour, R. A., J. M. Thomason, A. Nolan. Oral lesions in organ transplant patients. J Oral Path Oral Med, 1997; 26: 297–304.

[101] Seymour, R. A., J. M. Whitworth. Antibiotic prophylaxis for endocarditis, prosthetic joints, and surgery. Dent Clin North Am, 2002; 46 (4): 635–51.

[102] Seymour, R., D. Smith, S. Rogers. The comparative effects of azathioprine and cyclosporine on some gingival health parameters of renal transplant patients. J. Clin Periodontol, 1987; 14: 610–613.

[103] Seymour, R., D.J. Jacobs. Cyclosporin A and the gingival tissues. Journal of clinical periodontology, 1992; 19: 1–11.

[104] Seymour, R., M. Rudralingam. Oral and dental adverse in drug reactions. Periodontology, 2000, vol. 46, 2008, 9–26.

[105] Shu, M., E. Morou-Bermudez et al. The relationship between dental caries status and dental plaque urease activity. Oral microbiology and Immunology, 2007, 22: 1: 61–66.

[106] Smith, J., G. Wong et al. Sonic tooth brushing reduces gingival overgrowth in renal transplant recipients. Pediatr Nephrol, 2006, 21: 1753–1759.

[107] Soave, R. Prophylaxis strategies for solid-organ transplantation. Clinical Infectious Diseases, 2001; 33 (suppl 1): S26–31.

[108] Somacarrera, M. L., G. Hernandez, J. Acero, B. S. Moskow. Factors related to the incidence and severity of cyclosporine – induced gingival overgrowth in transplant patients. A longitudinal study. J Periodontol, 1994; 65: 671–5.

[109] Sowell, Sb. Dental care for patients with renal failure and renal transplantationen. J am dent assoc, 1982; 104 (2): 171–7.

[110] Summers, S. A., W. M. Tilakaratne, F. Fortune, N. Ashman. Renal disease and the mouth. Am J Med, 2007; 120 (7): 568–73.

[111] Takeuchi, Y., H. Ishikawa, M. Inda, O. Shinozuka, M. Umeda, Ts. Yamazaki. Study of the oral microbial flora in patients with renal disease. Nephrology, 2007; 12 (2), 182–190.

[112] Taylor, B. A. Management of drug – induced gingival enlargement. Australien Prescriber, 2003, vol. 26, 1.

[113] Temnqlov, N. Urea-pharmacology, clinics and therapeutic aspects. Grafik OOD, Varna, 2004, 78.

[114] Terasaki, P. I., J. M. Cecka, D. W. Gertson, S. Takemoto. High survival rates of kidney transplants from spousal and living unrelated donors. N Engl J Med, 1995; 10: 333–6.

[115] Thomason, J. M., R. A. Seymour. The prevalence and severity of cyclosporin and nifedipine – induced gingival overgrowth. J Clin Periodontol, 1993; 20: 37–40.

[116] Thorp, M., A. DeMattos, W. Bennett, J. Barry, D. Norman. The effect of conversion from cyclosporine to tacrolimus on gingival hyperplasia, hirsutism and cholesterol. Transplantation, 2000, 69 (6): 1218–20.

[117] Toivonen, H. J. Anaesthesia for patients with a transplanted organ. Acta Anaesthesiologica Scandinavica, 2000; 44: 812–833.

[118] Tollefsen, T. & R. Johansen. Periodontal status of prospective and renal transplant patients. Comparison with systemically healthy subjects. Journal of periodontal research, 1985 a), 20, 220–226.

[119] Tong, D., B. Rothwell. Antibiotic prophylaxis in dentistry: A review and practice recommendations. JADA March 2000, vol. 131: 366–374.

[120] Tong, D., R. Walker. Antibiotic prophylaxis in dialysis patients undergoing invasive dental treatment. Nephrology, 2004; 3: 167–170.

[121] Vanholder, R., E. Shepers, N. Meert, N. Lameire. What is uremia? Retention versus oxidation. Blood Purif, 2006; 24: 33–38.

[122] Villaciaran, J., C. Paya. Prevention of infections in solid organ transplant recipients. Transplant Infectious Disease, 1999; 1: 50–64.

[123] Wilson, W., K. Taubert, M. Gewitz et al. Prevention of infective endocarditis. Guidelines from American Heart Association. Circulation, 2007; 115; &NA.

[124] Zaiton, H. End stage renal disease: The oral component. BDJ, 2006, 201, 180.

[125] Zlatkov, N., Andreev, N. Skin manifestations of internal diseases. Wolkohim, C., 1994, 263.

Chapter 8

Prevention and Management of Nosocomial Pneumonia in Hemodialysis Patients

Shu Wakino, Hitoshi Minakuchi,
Hajime Inamoto and Hiroshi Itoh

Additional information is available at the end of the chapter

http://dx.doi.org/10.5772/59731

1. Introduction

Infectious disease is one of the main complications in the patients on long-term hemodialysis. Various clinical features, including multiple comorbidities, frequent hospitalization, and immunosuppression, rendered these patients susceptible to nosocomial infections. Furthermore, hemodialysis frequently results in chronic wasting, inflammation, uremia and gastrointestinal disturbances, all of which contribute to the increasing frailty of the patient. In their weakened state, these patients are susceptible to infectious complications such as aspiration pneumonia. In this section, we discuss these aspects of hemodialysis based on the recent our clinical observations.

1.1. Background of infectious disease in maintenance hemodialysis patients

Infectious diseases are significant causes of morbidity and mortality among patients with end-stage renal disease (ESRD), which is ranked as the second leading cause of death in Japanese maintenance hemodialysis (MHD) patients, following cardiovascular diseases. An increased susceptibility to infections has been ascribed partly to old age, a high prevalence of diabetes, defective phagocytic function of granulocytes, and frequent exposure to potential infectious risk factors during the hemodialysis therapy including endotoxin [1]. Anemia and malnutrition also contribute to the immune-compromised status of MHD patients. In addition, MHD patients are suffering from protein-energy wasting (PEW), making them susceptible to sarcopenia due to increased muscle protein degradation. Malnutrition causes impaired immune function and poor wound healing.

In addition, MHD patients usually have problems other than infections, such as cardiovascular or muscle-skeletal disorders. These patients are frequently hospitalized for surgical procedures or reasons other than infection, where they were treated with various kinds of antibiotics over a long period. These typical clinical courses undergone by MHD patients are known to influence the clinical characteristics and microbiological features of pneumonia.

2. PEW and Frailty in MHD patients

As MHD patients get older, they are affected more severely by age-related problems as compared to their counterparts in the general population. Two of the most significant problem are frailty and protein energy wasting (PEW) [2]. This phenomenon is clinically relevant because many manifestations of frailty and PEW are strong risk factors that affect quality of life, morbidity, and mortality. Frailty can be defined as a biological syndrome of decreased resistance to stressors caused by cumulative declines across multiple physiological systems which, ultimately, results in vulnerability to adverse outcomes. Frailty implies decreased body energy, protein reserves and reduced strength. Frailty is a common occurrence in CKD as well as MHD patients. A simple criterion for frailty can be the presence of three or more of the following abnormalities; unintentional weight loss, self-reported exhaustion, measured weakness, slow walking speed, and low physical activity. On the other hand, PEW is defined as the loss of somatic and circulating body protein and energy reserves. The comorbidity of infectious disease is also subject to the influence of these conditions. For instance, sarcopenia and osteopenia puts the patient at risk for falls as well as contracting pneumonia. In regards to aspiration pneumonia (AP), sarcopenia often causes difficulty in swallowing, which leads to unrecognized aspiration. Coordinated muscle movement and optimal muscle strength play an important role in the well-organized swallowing movement. Aspiration status was partly dependent on the lower anterior and posterior esophageal muscle and tongue strength [3]. These muscle strength was imparired by the decline in the global physical status. In ESRD patients under MHD, muscle and energy wasting are prominent, which influences the mortality and morbidity [2]. The tissue changes in muscle varies from morphological, electrophysiological and metabolic alterations. These malign changes of muscles lead to muscle weakness and finally to myopathy [4]. Additionally, atrophy of type II fibers was observed in the patients with MHD in several studies. These functional and structural muscle impairments in both systemic and/or oropharyngeal muscle strength are derived from the PEW state in MHD patients. Impaired immune function is associated with PEW in MHD [5]. In addition to an increased susceptibility to infections and poor wound healing, PEW leads to an impaired immune function which affects the gastrointestinal tract malfunction and aberrant microbiota population. These intestinal changes cause malabsorption and malnutrition [6], accelerating further the immune dysfunction. Deterioration in intestinal structure also leads to the enhancement of bacterial translocation in the intestine, leading to systemic inflammation and PEW state.

PEW involves several mechanisms, including the activation of oxidative stress, the inflammatory response, and the dialysis measure itself. Several markers of PEW and the resultant malnutrition have been associated with the incidence and death rates in patients with MHD [2]. Biochemical markers like lower serum albumin, prealbumin and cholesterol levels [7] are linked to malnutrition with higher fatality in dialysis patients. Serum transferrin, creatinine and bicarbonates [8] as well as hemoglobin levels, lymphocytes counts and white blood cell counts are also shown to be associated with malnutrition. We previously reported that serum creatatinine, albumin and total cholesterol levels are independent risk factors for contracting AP and its corresponding mortality rate. We also identified serum inorganic phosphorus (IP) as the main predictors of dietary intake in MHD patients [9]. Since 24-hour creatinine excretion and serum creatinine levels are associated with muscle mass [10], creatinine decline over time are related to the level of malnutrition as well as sarcopenic changes after admission [10]. It was reported that, in a cohort of 121,762 MHD patients, serum creatinine decline, and lower body mass, lower muscle mass and weight loss are associated with higher mortality in MHD patients [11]. It was also reported that among these clinical parameters, a decline in serum creatinine is suggested to be a stronger predictor of fatality than weight loss in MHD patients [12]. Our study is in consistent with the results of this large cohort study in that creatinine decline rate as well as albumin decline rate are good predictive indicator for morbidity and mortality of AP [9].

3. Respiratory infection in hemodialysis

Pneumonia is the second most common cause of severe infection in the MHD population. Regarding infectious diseases, it has been reported that approximately 20% of infectious deaths in MHD patients are attributed to pneumonia. The mortality of pulmonary infections in MHD patients has been reported to be 14 to 16 times higher than in the general population [13]. *Streptococcus pneumonia*, seasonal influenza and bacterial pneumonia secondary to influenza have been leading causes for community-acquired pneumonia in MHD. A vaccination is available for the prevention of pneumonia from *Streptococcus pneumonia as is same with the case in* the general population. Current guidelines recommend the vaccination of all MHD patients and revaccination after 5 years since a more rapid decline in the antibody titer was observed compared to that of the general population.

4. Nosocomial pneumonia

We surveyed 1803 MHD patients admitted to our university hospital between April 2001 and March 2007 [14]. We investigated basic patient characteristics and clinical characteristics of nosocomial pneumonia. The distribution of patient age indicated that about 70% of the patients were over 60 years old. The average length of hospitalization was 28.1 days, ranging from one day to 478 days, which was longer than the average for our hospital (14.2 days). Patients were admitted to different departments for a variety of reasons. We isolated 391 microorganisms from the sputa of 138 patients that were suspected of respiratory tract infections. These include *Candida albicans (C. albicans)*, methicillin-resistant *Staphyloccocus aureus* (MRSA), and *Staphy-*

loccocus epidermidis which were the leading three isolates. Among these patients, 47 were diagnosed with pneumonia and 57 pathogens were isolated. From the sputa specimen of pneumonia patients, MRSA and *C. albicans* were most frequently isolated. *Stenotrophomonas maltophilia* (*S. maltophilis*) was also isolated and found to be resistant to older generation cephalosporins, carbapenems, and quinolones. However, new fluoroquinolones, such as levofloxacin, were found to be affective. Among the 138 patients suspected of respiratory tract infections, 15 out of 23 patients infected with *S. maltophilia* died, resulting in the highest mortality among all patients with nosocomial pneumonia examined. With this survey, we concluded that MHD patients suffered from nosocomial pneumonia with multi-drug resistant pathogens. Consequently, *S. maltophilia*-related infections are associated with a high mortality rate and should be taken very seriously.

5. AP in MHD patients

Of the different types of pneumonia, AP is of particular interest due to its recent increase in occurrence in the aged MHD population. Aged patients are susceptible to dysphagia caused by neurological dysfunctions due to cerebral infarctions, cognitive deficits, and muscle weakness. Since HD patients are susceptible to sarcopenia and malnutrition, these changes increases the risk of development of AP. We recently reported on the clinical characteristics of AP in MHD patients [9]. We surveyed consecutive MHD patients with nosocomial AP who were admitted to our university hospital between April 2007 and December 2008. We determined hospitalized MHD patients as a high-risk population for AP, and we revealed that the mortality rate of HD patients with AP was high. We analyzed the risk factors for AP and found that the rate of decline of serum creatinine and albumin levels indicative of the decrease in muscle mass and malnutrition were of predictive value for the contraction of AP. We also found that he AP patients fed via nasal tube feeding or oral intake tended to survive.

6. Management of nosocomial pneumonia

Based on the clinical backgrounds, MHD patients suffered from nosocomial pneumonia with multi-drug resistant pathogens. Significantly, we reported that *S. maltophilia*-related infections should be taken seriously due to the associated high mortality rate. In addition, we stressed the clinical importance of AP for MHD patients suffering from PEW. Various treatment options to prevent AP were advocated, including oral hygiene, altered food viscosity, and positioning [9]. Medications for this purpose include angiotensin-converting enzyme inhibitors and amantadine. In our study, early initiation of tube feeding appears to provide more favorable outcomes in light of intestinal conditions or fluid restrictions in HD patients. Parenteral nutrition directly affects the total body fluid volume and is prone to volume overload as compared to tube feeding. In addition, malnutrition and sarcopenia lead to silent aspiration where the symptoms are not always clinically evident. Since hospitalized patients with hemodialysis often progress to a state of malnutrition, the patients should be considered to have silent aspiration and treated with tube feeding.

7. Conclusions

Various backgrounds including multiple comorbidities, PEW or frailty, impaired immune response, infectious diseases and pneumonia were prevalent in MHD patients. Our surveillance revealed that MHD patients suffered from nosocomial pneumonia with multi-drug resistant pathogens. *S. maltophilia*-related infections should be very seriously in light of the associated high mortality rate. Based on the PEW condition, both the contraction and mortality rates of nosocomial AP were high among HD patients.

Author details

Shu Wakino*, Hitoshi Minakuchi, Hajime Inamoto and Hiroshi Itoh

*Address all correspondence to: shuwakino@z8.keio.jp

Department of Internal Medicine, School of Medicine, Keio University, Tokyo, Japan

References

[1] Vanholder R, Ringoir S. Infectious morbidity and defects of phagocytic function in end-stage renal disease: a review. *J Am Soc Nephrol* 1993;3:1541-54.

[2] Johansen KL, Shubert T, Doyle J *et al.* Muscle atrophy in patients receiving hemodialysis: effects on muscle strength, muscle quality, and physical function. *Kidney Int.* 2003 Jan;63(1):291-7.

[3] Butler SG, Stuart A, Leng X *et al.* The relationship of aspiration status with tongue and handgrip strength in healthy older adults. *J Gerontol A Biol Sci Med Sci.* 2011;66:452-8.

[4] Sawant A, Garland SJ, House AA, Overend TJ. Morphological, electrophysiological, and metabolic characteristics of skeletal muscle in people with end-stage renal disease: a critical review. *Physiother Can.* 2011;63:355-76.

[5] Chinen J, Shearer WT. Secondary immunodeficiencies, including HIV infection. *J Allergy Clin Immunol* 2008;121:S388-92.

[6] El Solh AA, Saliba R. Pharmacologic prevention of aspiration pneumonia: a systematic review. *Am J Geriatr Pharmacother* 2007;5:352-62.

[7] Degoulet P, Legrain M, Réach I *et al.* Mortality risk factors in patients treated by chronic hemodialysis. Report of the Diaphane collaborative study. *Nephron* 1982;31:103-10.

[8] Pifer TB, McCullough KP, Port FK *et al.* Mortality risk in hemodialysis patients and changes in nutritional indicators: DOPPS. *Kidney Int* 2002;62:2238-45.

[9] Minakuchi H, Wakino S, Hayashi K, Inamoto H, Itoh H. Serum creatinine and albumin decline predict the contraction of nosocomial aspiration pneumonia in patients undergoing hemodialysis. Ther Apher Dial. 2014 Aug;18(4):326-33.

[10] Harita N, Hayashi T, Sato KK *et al.* Lower serum creatinine is a new risk factor of type 2 diabetes: the Kansai healthcare study. *Diabetes Care.* 2009 Mar;32(3):424-6.

[11] Kalantar-Zadeh K, Streja E, Molnar MZ *et al.* Mortality prediction by surrogates of body composition: an examination of the obesity paradox in hemodialysis patients using composite ranking score analysis. *Am J Epidemiol.*2012;175:793-803.

[12] Kalantar-Zadeh K, Kilpatrick RD, Kuwae N *et al.* Revisiting mortality predictability of serum albumin in the dialysis population: time dependency, longitudinal changes and population-attributable fraction. Nephrol Dial Transplant. 2005;20:1880-8.

[13] Slinin, Y., R.N. Foley, and A.J. Collins, Clinical epidemiology of pneumonia in hemodialysis patients: the USRDS waves 1, 3, and 4 study. Kidney Int 2006, 70(6): 1135-41.

[14] Wakino S, Imai E, Yoshioka K et al. Clinical importance of *Stenotrophomonas maltophilia* nosocomial pneumonia due to its high mortality in hemodialysis patients. Ther Apher Dial. 2009 Jun;13(3):193-8.

Chapter 9

Renal Cell Carcinoma in End-Stage Renal Disease

Yasukazu Nakanishi, Fumitaka Koga,
Hiroshi Fukushima, Toru Motoi and Ken-ichi Tobisu

Additional information is available at the end of the chapter

http://dx.doi.org/10.5772/59378

1. Introduction

Acquired cystic disease of the kidney (ACDK) was first described in patients dying from Brights disease by John Simon in 1847 [1]. It was rediscovered and reported in 1977 in a study of 14 kidneys in 30 hemodialysis patients, and six of the 14 patients had renal cell carcinoma (RCC) [2]. Miller et al. subsequently reported a large autopsy series of 155 hemodialysis patients in which ACDK was noted in 58% and RCC in 2% of patients [3].

ACDK must be distinguished from other acquired renal cystic diseases including simple renal cysts that develop as age advances, and the cystic changes found with primary hyperaldosteronism that causes hypokalemia. It must be distinguished from hereditary autosomal-dominant polycystic disease, and from cystic kidney disease such as Von-Hipple-Lindau disease, tuberous sclerosis, medullary cystic disease, autosomal recessive polycystic disease, and medullary sponge kidney [4]. ACDK is defined as the presence of more than three cysts in either or both of the kidneys or the presence of cysts occupying more than 25% of the renal parenchyma in patients with end-stage renal disease (ESRD) [5, 6]. ACDK increases in prevalence and severity with increasing years on dialysis: 20% of patients dialyzed for 1 to 3 years have ACDK, compared with greater than 90% of patients dialyzed for 5 to 10 years [7]. Time spent on hemodialysis is the most important key features of developing ACDK and increasing risk for RCC [8, 9]. The most important predisposing factor for ACDK is a duration of dialysis of 5 to 10 years or longer [6, 10]. Reportedly, the incidence of ACDK in peritoneal dialysis is almost equal to that in hemodialysis patients [11, 12].

In the current practice, periodic screening for RCC is recommended for dialysis patients because of high incidence of RCC. Screening is recommended from the start of hemodialysis. Ultrasonography (US), one of standard screening tools of RCC in dialysis patients, sometimes fails to distinguish RCC from hemorrhagic cysts [13]. The usefulness of magnetic resonance imaging (MRI) without the use of contrast material has been reported for the detection of RCC in patients with ACDK [14]. The principle treatment strategy for RCC in dialysis patients is radical nephrectomy (RN). Long-term dialysis patients are at high risk for cardiovascular events [4]. Therefore, less invasive surgery is preferable to avoid postoperative systemic complications. Pathologically, clear and papillary RCC had been considered as common histological types of renal cancer arising from acquired cystic disease (ACD) [15, 16]. Recently, a novel standard pathologic entity of ACD-associated RCC has been established [10, 17-19].

In this chapter, we overview the upated topics on RCCs in ESRD patients, particularly focusing on screening and diagnosis, minimally invasive surgery, and pathology.

2. Epidemiology of RCC in hemodialysis patients

Patients with ESRD on dialysis have more than 100 times greater risk of RCC than age-matched healthy controls [20-22]. In a series of 831, 804 dialysis patients followed up for an average of 2. 5 years, 2, 053 (0. 25%) patients were diagnosed as having RCC, representing a 3. 6-fold increased risk over the general population [23]. Kojima et al. reported that in a cohort of 2, 624 patients 81. 8% developed ACDK during a median dialysis time of 11 years and that 1. 68% developed RCC [24]. The risk is considered to be progressively higher in patients with a longer duration of dialysis. According to some recent publications, a long duration of dialysis (> 10y) has a stronger association with ACD-associated RCC than other subtypes of RCC [25-27]. In a multicenter retrospective study by Neuzillet et al. , RCC developing in patients with ESRD has many favorable clinical, pathologic, and outcome features compared with RCC in patients without ESRD.

According to a multicenter retrospective study, more patients diagnosed as having RCC are young and asymptomatic in the ESRD group than the non-ESRD counterpart [28]. Denton et al. reported that of 260 patients who underwent ipsilateral native nephrectomy at the time of transplantation, 11 (4. 2%) diagnosed as RCC with short duration of hemodialysis, and age was significant risk factor of RCC [11]. In ESRD patients, modality of dialysis does not appear to associate with the incidence of RCC; the incidence of RCC is almost same in patients on hemodialysis and those on peritoneal dialysis. Savaji et al. reported the annual incidence of RCC was estimated to be 130 per 100, 000 patients on peritoneal dialysis [29].

3. Imaging studies for screening and diagnosing RCC in ESRD

As mentioned above, ESRD patients are at greatly high risk for developing RCC. In addition, prognosis is better for asymptomatic patients than symptomatic ones among those with ESRD-associated RCC [30]. Since early intervention may prolong cancer free survival [13, 31], periodic imaging studies are considered to be important for detection of RCC in its early stage. Sarasin et al. [32] recommended evaluation strategies with either computed tomography (CT) or US every three years for all patients on dialysis and annually for those with ACDK. To date, screening for RCC is recommended for ESRD patients.

3. 1. Ultrasonography (US)

Past studies evaluating the prevalence of RCC in patients with ACDK were based on US diagnosis. US is the most widely used screening tool for RCC in patients with ESRD. On US-based screening, RCC was identified in native kidneys in 3. 8% and 3. 9% of ESRD patients of pre- and post-transplantation, respectively [33, 34], which represents a 100-fold increase in prevalence compared to the general population. Gulanikar et al. [33] reported that sensitivity of US screening for the diagnosis of RCC was 36. 3% in ESRD patients.

Because ESRD kidney shows heterogeneous and hyperechoic parenchymal echo-texture and irregular parenchymal contour associated with uneven parenchymal atrophy and compensatory hypertrophy, it would be more difficult to detect RCC on US in ESRD kidneys than in non-ESRD kidneys. Compensatory hypertrophy sometimes produces a mass effect or compresses the pelvo-calyceal systems and thus closely mimics renal neoplasm [35]. US has disadvantage of operator-dependence and often fails to distinguish RCC from hemorrhagic cyst [13].

Among several diagnostic parameters of US, Kim et al. reported the possibility of usefulness of resistive index (RI), which is calculated as (peak systolic velocity – end-diastolic velocity) / peak-systolic velocity on renal Doppler sonography, in detection of RCC in ESRD kidneys. RCC arising in ESRD kidneys shows significantly lower RI values than the background renal parenchyma [36]. Speculated theoretical background is as follows; because tumor vessels generally lack smooth muscle layer, diastolic flow of the tumor vessels is higher than that of the normal vessels, resulting in lower RI values in tumor tissues compared to the non-neoplastic counterparts.

3. 2. Computed Tomography (CT)

Contrast-enhanced computed tomography (CECT) is the most widely used modality for the detection of RCC associated with ACDK (Fig. 1). Takebayashi et al. [37] demonstrated that early enhanced helical CT could detect RCC better than delayed enhanced CT in ESRD patients with and without ACDK because the cortex of the ESRD kidneys shows minimal enhancement in the early phase, rendering higher differences in the attenuation values between the RCC and the atrophic parenchyma. However, as ESRD patients require life-long follow-up, screening with CECT may be burdensome in that it uses ionizing radiation and poses a risk for contrast-induced nephropathy.

3. 2. 1. Bosniak renal cyst classification system

Schwarz et al. [38] recommended a CT-based screening and management protocol in transplant recipients, incorporating the Bosniak Renal Cyst Classification System. The Bosniak renal cyst classification system was initially reported in 1986 based on CT scan findings [39]. The Bosniak system consists of four categories, ranging from simple to complex cysts. Forty-two-59% of category III and 90-100% of category IV lesions were proven to be malignancy [40-42].

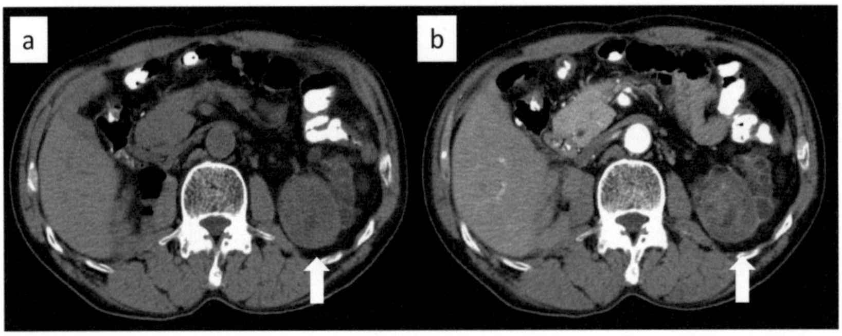

Figure 1. CT images of a 65-year-old man with ACD-associated RCC. a: Unenhancement CT shows multiple small cysts and a mass (arrow). b: At early enhancement phase, the mass (arrow) is slightly and heterogenously enhanced.

Category I. —Simple benign cysts showing homogeneous water content, and a sharp interface with adjacent renal parenchyma, without wall thickening, calcification, or enhancement.

Category II. — Cystic lesions with one or two thin (≤1 mm thick) septations or thin, fine calcification in their walls or septa and hyperdense benign cysts with all the features of category I cysts except for homogeneously high attenuation. A benign category II lesion must be 3 cm or less in diameter and have one quarter of its wall extending outside the kidney, without contrast enhancement.

Category IIF. — Minimally complicated cysts that need follow-up. This group is not well defined by Bosniak originally and consists of lesions that are not classified into category II. There are some suspicious features that deserve follow-up.

Category III. — True indeterminate cystic masses that need surgical evaluation but prove to be benign in many cases. They may show uniform wall thickening, a multilocular nature with multiple enhancing septa, thick or irregular peripheral calcification. Hyperdense lesions that do not fall into category II are classified in this group.

Category IV. —Lesions with uneven or contrast-enhanced thick wall, contrast-enhanced or large nodules in the wall, or clearly solid components in the cystic lesion.

3. 3. Magnetic Resonance Imaging (MRI)

Recently, MRI is one of topics in diagnosis of ESRD-related RCC. Some studies have reported the usefulness of diffusion-weighted MRI in differentiating RCC from benign cyst, without the use of contrast material [43-46]. Diffusion-weighted imaging (DWI) is a non-invasive functional modality using strong bipolar gradients to create a sensitivity of the signal to the thermally-induced Brownian motion of water molecules and in vivo measurement of molecular diffusion [47]. This imaging technique has been applied to the diagnosis of cancer [48]. The apparent diffusion coefficient (ADC) is a quantitative parameter of the degree of diffusion, which is calculated from several DWI images of different *b* values. RCC showed a tendency toward higher signal intensities (SIs) with lower ADC values on DWI obtained at high *b* values than benign cysts (Fig. 2). Akita et al. [14] reported 10 RCCs containing viable parts in the pathologic specimens showed high signal areas on DWI (at high *b* values). Solitary RCC with no macroscopic degeneration was visualized as a homogenous high SI on DWI and as a homogenous iso SI on T2-weighted image (T2WI). They also reported that the mean ADC of ACD-associated RCCs was lower than the value of clear cell RCCs. Several researchers reported T1-weighted image (T1WI) is useful for discriminating between RCC and hemorrhagic cyst. Hemorrhagic cyst shows homogeneous high SIs or fluid-iron levels on T1WI [13, 49].

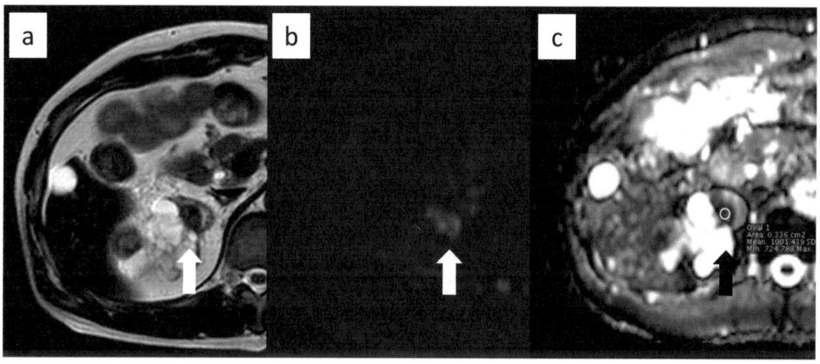

Figure 2. MRI images of a 71-year-old man with ACD-associated RCC. a: Axial T2WI shows a heterogenous signal intensity mass (arrow). b: DWI shows heterogenous high signal intensity mass (arrow). c:ADC map demonstrates the tumor (arrow) with ADC value of 1. 00 $\times 10^{-3}$ mm^2/s.

4. Surgical Treatment

The principle strategy for RCC in dialysis patients is radical nephrectomy (RN). On a nationwide survey in the United States, ESRD-associated RCC patients undergoing RN showed improved survival compared with those not receiving RN [50]. RN is the established surgical approach for conventional RCC. This surgical procedure originally included early vascular control of the renal hilum, removal of the kidney with the Gerota's fascia, removal of the ipsilateral adrenal gland, and a regional lymph node dissection. Although the true benefits of adrenalectomy and regional lymph dissection in patient without enlarged nodes have been a subject of continuing controversy, the principles of early vascular control and removal of the kidney with a wide margin of Gerota's fascia remain the standard of care.

The surgical risk of patients with ESRD is classified as physical status 3 or greater, according to the American Society of Anesthesiologist (ASA) classification [51]. ASA physical status is reported to be a predictor of postoperative outcomes [52]. Therefore, safer and less invasive surgery is recommended for ESRD-associated RCC patients to avoid postoperative systemic complications. Reported series of minimally invasive RN in ESRD patients are listed in Table. 1.

Operation	Authors(publication year)	Number of renal units	Approach		Mean EBL (ml)	Mean OT (min)
			TP	RP		
LRN	Yamashita et al. (2012) [61]	39	1	38	157	240
LRN	Sanli et al. (2010) [62]	20	4	16	111	133
LRN	Bird et al. (2010) [60]	16	16	0	153	unknown
LRN	Ghasemian et al. (2005) [63]	20	20	0	164	390
LRN	Gulati et al. (2003) [59]	6	4	2	120	294
LRN	Iwamura et al.(2001) [58]	6	0	6	58	162
GasLESS	Masuda et al. (2011) [72]	57	0	57	218	170

LRN, laparoscopic radical nephrectomy; GasLESS, gasless laparoendoscopic single-port surgery; TP, transperitoneal; RP, retroperitoneal; EBL, estimated blood loss; OT, operative time.

Table 1. Surgical outcomes of minimally invasive surgery for renal cell carcinoma in ESRD patients.

4. 1. Laparoscopic surgery

Laparoscopic radical nephrectomy (LRN) is a minimally invasive surgical procedure for malignant tumors of the kidney. Clayman et al. first described the successful laparoscopic nephrectomy in 1991 [53]. This was one of the greatest milestones in the history of minimally invasive surgery in that a large solid organ could be removed without an incision of equal or greater size. The utility of the laparoscopic procedures has been verified at many institutions with far less morbidity when compared to open surgery. Many kidney surgeries are currently available laparoscopically [54] via transperitoneal or retroperitoneal approach. Transperitoneal approach has advantages of being a very familiar approach with easily recognizable anatomy and a much larger working space. Some investigators mentioned that advantages of retroperitoneal LRN include quicker access to the renal hilum, easier dissection in obese individuals, the avoidance of intraperitoneal injury, and less interference with respiratoty and hemodynamic functions [55]. In regard to the best approach for performing RN, both retroperitoneal and transperitoneal approaches showed similar oncological outcomes in the two randomized control studies [56, 57]. For RCCs in ESRD patients, LRN also showed feasible and acceptable surgical outcomes [58-62], including bilateral cases [63].

4. 2. Gasless Laparoendoscopic Single-port surgery (GasLESS)

Gasless laparoendoscopic single-port surgery (GasLESS) is gasless (no CO_2 gas insufflation) single-port retroperitoneoscopic surgery that was initiated in the late 1990s in Japan. GasLESS is also referred to as minimum incision endoscopic surgery. Kihara et al. first described GasLESS radical nephrectomy (GasLESS-RN); initially minimum incision of 4 or 5 cm is made on the tip of the 12th rib. The length of incision, which narrowly permits extraction of the kidney http://dx.doi.org/10. 5772/59378

with perinephric fat, depends on the size of the specimen (Fig. 3). A wide working space is then made through the port by separating anatomical planes extraperitoneally and displacing the peritoneum and the kidney using retractors specialized for GasLESS [64-67]. This operation was certified by the Japanese government as an advanced surgery in 2006, and it has been covered by the Japanese universal health insurance system since 2008. Because of gasless surgery, GasLESS-RN is safely performed for patients with respiratory and circulatory comorbidities compared to LRN. Indeed, feasibility, safety and favorable surgical outcomes of GasLESS-RN were reported for RCC patients [68] [69] including ESRD-associated RCC patients [61, 62]. GasLESS-RN is also indicated for RCC patients on continuous ambulatory peritoneal dialysis because the peritoneum remains intact after GasLESS-RN. Recently, GasLESS-RN incorporates a three-dimentional endoscope and a head mounted display system (3D-HMD system), which enhances safety of surgical procedures and facilitates their fluidity via a coin-sized tiny single port [60] (Fig. 4).

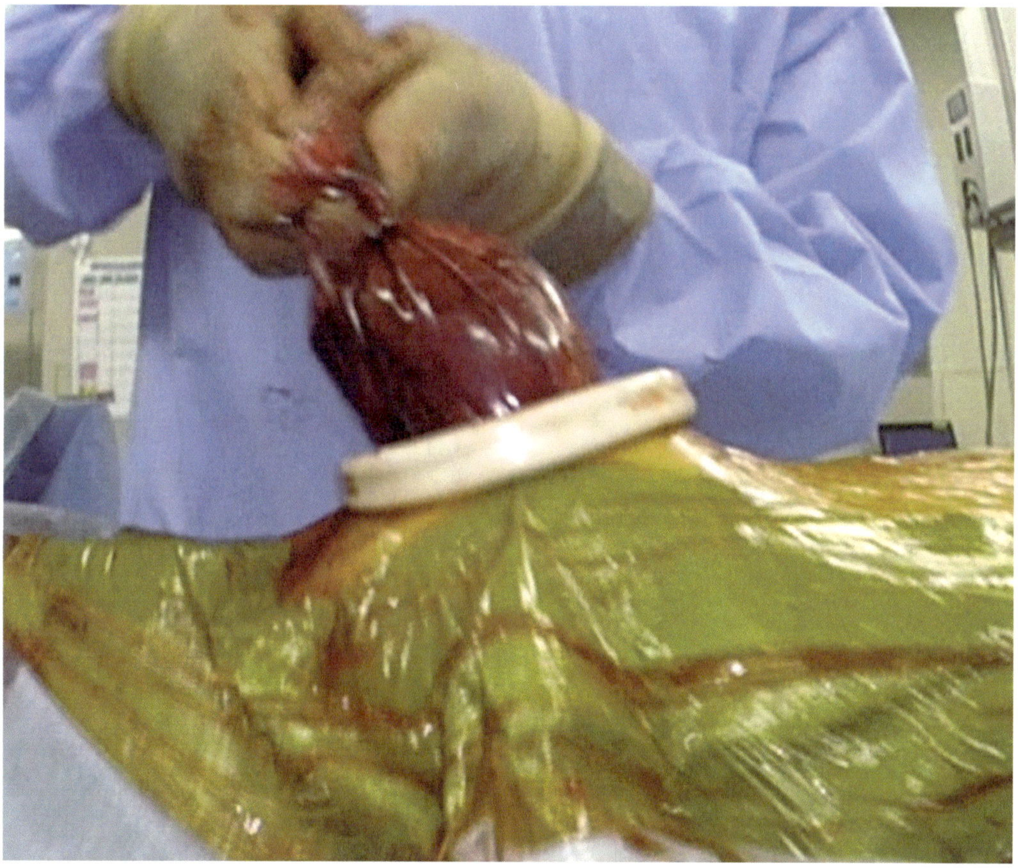

Figure 3. Extraction of a surgical specimen of ACD-associated RCC via a single port in a 65-year-old man treated with GasLESS RN.

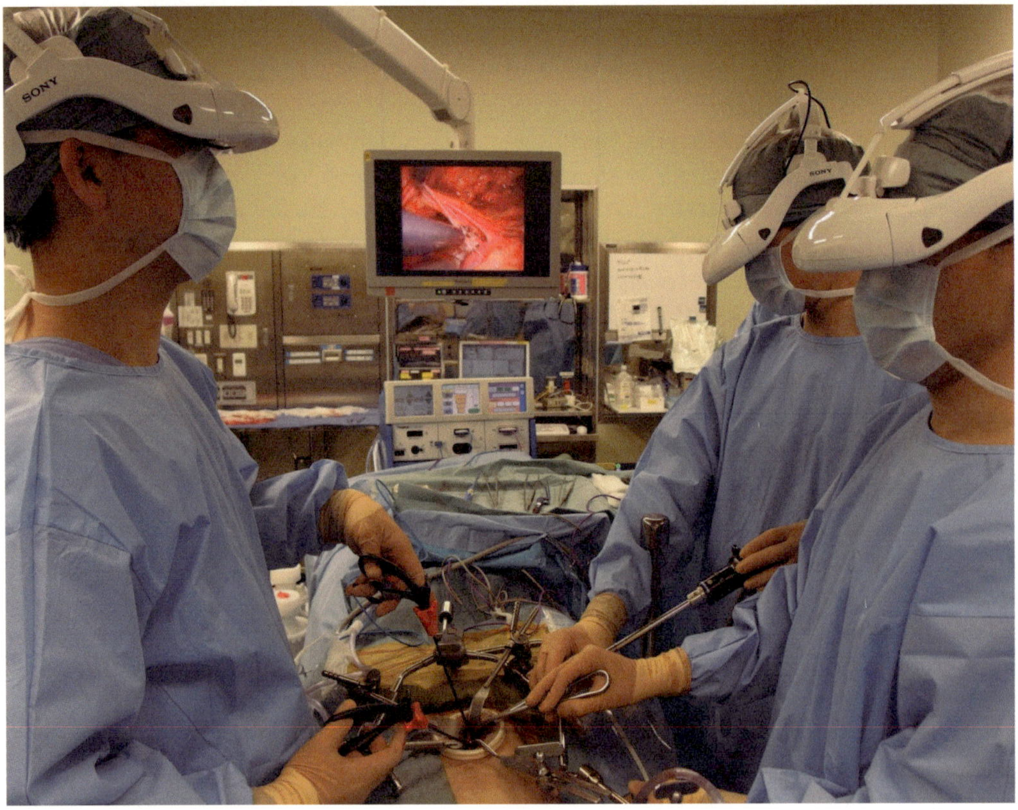

Figure 4. Scenery of GasLESS via a coin-sized port using the 3D-HMD system.

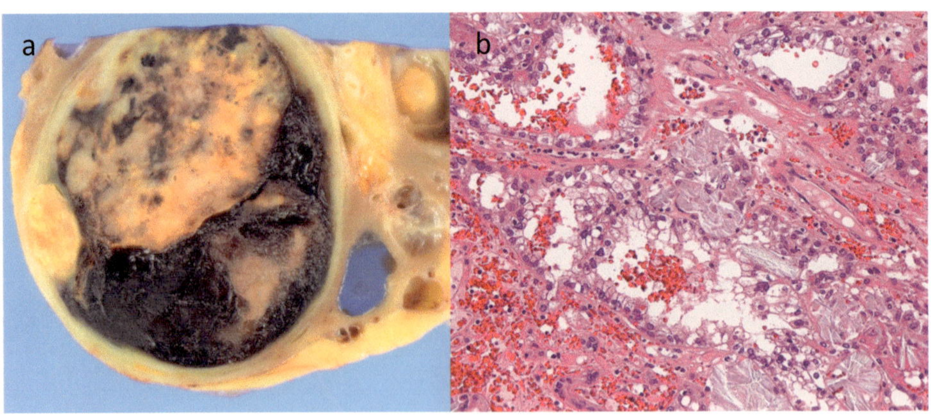

Figure 5. Pathology of ACD-associated RCC in a 65-year-old man. a: Macrophotograph. b: Microphotograph. The tumor tissue contains oxalate crystals.

4. 3. Robotic Radical Nephrectomy

At present, the affirmative opinion for robotic radical nephrectomy has not been published. Hemal et al. [70] reported a prospective comparison of robotic and laparoscopic radical nephrectomy for non-ESRD RCCs. They concluded that there were no benefits of robotic radical nephrectomy observed over LRN for localized RCC.

4. 4. Partial nephrectomy

Partial nephrectomy (PN) is a standard of care for small RCC in patients without ESRD. PN offers better postoperative renal function than RN. RCC in ESRD patients has not yet been reported. However, PN would be beneficial for ESRD patients who have small RCC and still maintain urine production. These patients would have to strictly restrict water intake due to reduced urine output when they undergo RN, which impairs their quality of life. PN might be a viable option for a subset of ESRD patients considering their postoperative quality of life.

5. Pathology

Many investigators had considered for a long time that clear cell or papillary RCC is a common histological type of renal cancer arising from ACDK [15, 16]. However, a new disease entity of ACD-associated RCC showing characteristic histologic features has been established.

5. 1. Characteristics of Histological Types

Papillary RCC was previously reported to be the most common histological subtype found in ACDK in dialysis patients, accounting for 42-71% of cases [15, 17, 71]. Since the establishment of the current histological classification, ACD–associated RCC is the most common histological type of RCC occurring in ESRD kidneys [19]. ACD-associated RCC was found in 36% of surgically resected ESRD kidneys [10]. Some investigators reported that histological patterns of RCC change according to the duration of dialysis. ACD-associated RCC was the major histological subtype in those on dialysis for 10 years or longer [26, 72].

Clear cell (tubulo) papillary RCC was also initially reported in patients with ESRD [10]. However, the majority of cases reported subsequently were not associated with ACDK [73-76]. Reportedly, clear cell papillary RCC comprises less than a few percent of all RCCs [75, 77].

5. 1. 1. ACD-associated RCC

Diagnostic criteria for ACD include the presence of cystic structures occupying at least 25% of the renal parenchyma or greater than three cysts per kidney [78]. ACD-associated RCC appears as a nodule arising from cystic wall, occasionally completely filling the cyst, or as a solid mass separate from the cyst (Fig. 5a). Non-cystic tumors are well circumscribed and may be surrounded by a thick fibrous capsule showing dystrophic calcification. The cut surface of the tumor varies from grey tan to yellowish or brownish and hemorrhage or necrosis is occasionally seen [25]. Multifocality and bilaterality are seen in >50% and >20% of the cases, respectively [10].

Microscopically, ACD-associated RCC is defined as a tumor having eosinophilic or oncocytic cytoplasm and is frequently associated with intratumoral oxalate crystal deposition [10, 17, 79] (Fig. 5b). Some investigators suggest that many microcysts maybe formed by intracyto-palsmic vacuoles mainly due to degenerative change. These crystals are multicolored under polarized microscopic observation. Papillary, tubular, cribriform or solid growth pattern may also be seen. Nuclear grade is frequently classified as Fuhrman grade 3 [10, 17, 25]. Clear cell change, sarcomatoid change or rhabdoid features may be present in some cases [10, 80, 81]. Immunohistochemically, neoplastic cells of ACD-associated RCC are positive for α-methyl-acyl-coenzyme A racemase (AMACR), CD10, CD57, GST-α, vinculin and c-met, but negative for cytokeratin 7 (CK7) and high molecular weight cytokeratins [10, 25, 27, 81-83].

5. 1. 2. Clear Cell Papillary RCC

Clear cell papillary RCC is seen in ESRD patients without ACDK. The tumors appear well circumscribed and usually well encapsulated. The cut surface is tan-white to yellow with grossly apparent fibrotic areas and ranges from completely solid to predominantly cystic.

Microscopically, clear cell papillary RCC have variable tubular/acinar, papillary, and cycti-carchitectures [10, 74, 75]. The tumor cells have clear cytoplasm. Nuclear grade is often classified into Fuhrman grade 1 or 2. In contrast to ACD-associated RCC, clear cell papillary RCC is positive for CK7 but negative for AMACR and CD10 [74, 75].

6. Etiology of RCC in ESRD

Genetic profiles are distinct from classic papillary RCC or clear cell RCC. Gain of chromosomes 1, 2, 3, 6, 7, 10, 16, 17 and Y are observed in ACD-associated RCC [81, 82, 84-86]. Deletion of 3p25, +7, -Y are absent in clear cell papillary RCC [74].

The developing process of ACDK and RCC in long dialysis patients is still unclear. Several researchers reported the role of cytokine activation. Phosphorylated c-jun, the activated c-jun, which is a critical component of the AP-1 transcription factors that consist of homo- or heterodimers of basic region-leucine zipper proteins, is positive on staining of atypical hyperplastic cells in ACDK [87]. The concentration such as IL-6, -8, and VEGF is significantly high in the cystic fluid of ACDK [88]. Possibility of the relationship of calcium oxalate crystal and tumorigenesis has also been reported [17, 79, 89]. Immunohistochemical expression of oxidative stress markers, such as iNOS, 8-OHdG, and COX-2, are more frequently observed in ESRD-associated RCC than in conventional RCCs [90], since patients on dialysis are affected by oxidative stress which is caused by an imbalance between the production of reactive oxygen species and the cells ability to neutralize the reactive intermediates [91, 92].

7. Prognosis

ACD-associated RCC patients appearto show relatively good prognosis because of a low incidence of advanced disease [26]. In ACD-associated RCC patients treated with RN, asymptomatic patients diagnosed on screening show more favorable prognosis than symptomatic patients [30]. Ishikawa et al. reported the actual five year survival rate was 79. 7% and cancer-specific survival rate was 91. 7% for surgically treated 662 cases of ESRD-associated RCC [93]. Neuzillet et al. reported that ESRD-associated RCC seems to exhibit many favorable clinicopathologic features and prognosis compared with conventional RCC [28]. Shrewsberry et al. reported that there was no difference in overall or cancer specific mortality between non-metastatic RCC patients with ESRD and those without ESRD when the patients underwent RN [94]. Several cases of ACD-associated RCC with sarcomatoid change [10] and rhabdoid features [95] have been reported to behave in an aggressive fashion.

8. Conclusions

ESRD patients on dialysis are at high risk for development of RCC. Periodic screening for RCC is recommended for these patients. MRI without use of contrast material would be useful for screening RCC in ESRD patients. ACD-associated RCC and clear cell papillary RCC are the current standard histological spectrum of RCCs arising from the kidney with ESRD. For patients with ESRD-associated RCC in early stage, less invasive surgical treatment is preferable to avoid postoperative systemic complications. Prognosis of ESRD-associated RCC patients is generally favorable when treated in early stage.

Author details

Yasukazu Nakanishi[1], Fumitaka Koga[1*], Hiroshi Fukushima[1], Toru Motoi[2] and Ken-ichi Tobisu[1]

*Address all correspondence to: f-koga@cick. jp

1 Department of Urology, Tokyo Metropolitan Cancer and Infectious diseases Center Komagome Hospital, Honkomagome, Tokyo, Japan

2 Department of Pathology, Tokyo Metropolitan Cancer and Infectious diseases Center Komagome Hospital, Honkomagome, Tokyo, Japan

References

[1] Simon, J. , *On sub-acute inflammation of the kidney.* Med Chir Trans, 1847. 30: p. 140 2-164.

[2] Dunnill, M. S. , P. R. Millard, and D. Oliver, *Acquired cystic disease of the kidneys: a hazard of long-term intermittent maintenance haemodialysis.* J Clin Pathol, 1977. 30(9): p. 868-77.

[3] Miller, L. R. , et al. , *Acquired renal cystic disease in end-stage renal disease: an autopsy study of 155 cases.* Am J Nephrol, 1989. 9(4): p. 322-8.

[4] Fick, G. M. and P. A. Gabow, *Hereditary and acquired cystic disease of the kidney.* Kidney Int, 1994. 46(4): p. 951-64.

[5] Ishikawa, I. , *Uremic acquired renal cystic disease. Natural history and complications.* Nephron, 1991. 58(3): p. 257-67.

[6] Farivar-Mohseni, H. , et al. , *Renal cell carcinoma and end stage renal disease.* J Urol, 2006. 175(6): p. 2018-20; discussion 2021.

[7] Matson, M. A. and E. P. Cohen, *Acquired cystic kidney disease: occurrence, prevalence, and renal cancers.* Medicine (Baltimore), 1990. 69(4): p. 217-26.

[8] Ishikawa, I. , et al. , *Ten-year prospective study on the development of renal cell carcinoma in dialysis patients.* Am J Kidney Dis, 1990. 16(5): p. 452-8.

[9] Ishikawa, I. , *Present status of renal cell carcinoma in dialysis patients in Japan: questionnaire study in 2002.* Nephron Clin Pract, 2004. 97(1): p. c11-6.

[10] Tickoo, S. K. , et al. , *Spectrum of epithelial neoplasms in end-stage renal disease: an experience from 66 tumor-bearing kidneys with emphasis on histologic patterns distinct from those in sporadic adult renal neoplasia.* Am J Surg Pathol, 2006. 30(2): p. 141-53.

[11] Denton, M. D. , et al. , *Prevalence of renal cell carcinoma in patients with ESRD pre-transplantation: a pathologic analysis.* Kidney Int, 2002. 61(6): p. 2201-9.

[12] Ishikawa, I. , et al. , *Comparison of severity of acquired renal cysts between CAPD and hemodialysis.* Adv Perit Dial, 1991. 7: p. 91-5.

[13] Levine, E. , *Renal cell carcinoma in uremic acquired renal cystic disease: incidence, detection, and management.* Urol Radiol, 1992. 13(4): p. 203-10.

[14] Akita, H. , et al. , *Renal cell carcinoma in patients with acquired cystic disease of the kidney: assessment using a combination of T2-weighted, diffusion-weighted, and chemical-shift MRI without the use of contrast material.* J Magn Reson Imaging, 2014. 39(4): p. 924-30.

[15] Ishikawa, I. and G. Kovacs, *High incidence of papillary renal cell tumours in patients on chronic haemodialysis.* Histopathology, 1993. 22(2): p. 135-9.

[16] Truong, L. D. , et al. , *Renal neoplasm in acquired cystic kidney disease.* Am J Kidney Dis, 1995. 26(1): p. 1-12.

[17] Sule, N. , et al. , *Calcium oxalate deposition in renal cell carcinoma associated with acquired cystic kidney disease: a comprehensive study.* Am J Surg Pathol, 2005. 29(4): p. 443-51.

[18] Petrolla, A. A. and G. T. Maclennan, *Renal cell carcinoma associated with end stage renal disease.* J Urol, 2006. 176(1): p. 345.

[19] Srigley, J. R. , et al. , *The International Society of Urological Pathology (ISUP) Vancouver Classification of Renal Neoplasia.* Am J Surg Pathol, 2013. 37(10): p. 1469-89.

[20] Choyke, P. L., *Acquired cystic kidney disease.* Eur Radiol, 2000. 10(11): p. 1716-21.

[21] Hora, M., et al., *Tumours in end-stage kidney.* Transplant Proc, 2008. 40(10): p. 3354-8.

[22] Vamvakas, S., U. Bahner, and A. Heidland, *Cancer in end-stage renal disease: potential factors involved -editorial.* Am J Nephrol, 1998. 18(2): p. 89-95.

[23] Maisonneuve, P., et al., *Distribution of primary renal diseases leading to end-stage renal failure in the United States, Europe, and Australia/New Zealand: results from an international comparative study.* Am J Kidney Dis, 2000. 35(1): p. 157-65.

[24] Kojima, Y., et al., *Renal cell carcinoma in dialysis patients: a single center experience.* Int J Urol, 2006. 13(8): p. 1045-8.

[25] Enoki, Y., et al., *Clinicopathological features and CD57 expression in renal cell carcinoma in acquired cystic disease of the kidneys: with special emphasis on a relation to the duration of haemodialysis, the degree of calcium oxalate deposition, histological type, and possible tumorigenesis.* Histopathology, 2010. 56(3): p. 384-94.

[26] Nouh, M. A., et al., *Renal cell carcinoma in patients with end-stage renal disease: relationship between histological type and duration of dialysis.* BJU Int, 2010. 105(5): p. 620-7.

[27] Sassa, N., et al., *Renal cell carcinomas in haemodialysis patients: does haemodialysis duration influence pathological cell types and prognosis?* Nephrol Dial Transplant, 2011. 26(5): p. 1677-82.

[28] Neuzillet, Y., et al., *Renal cell carcinoma (RCC) in patients with end-stage renal disease exhibits many favourable clinical, pathologic, and outcome features compared with RCC in the general population.* Eur Urol, 2011. 60(2): p. 366-73.

[29] Savaj, S., et al., *Renal cell carcinoma in peritoneal dialysis patients.* Int Urol Nephrol, 2003. 35(2): p. 263-5.

[30] Ishikawa, I., et al., *Renal cell carcinoma detected by screening shows better patient survival than that detected following symptoms in dialysis patients.* Ther Apher Dial, 2004. 8(6): p. 468-73.

[31] Heinz-Peer, G., et al., *Role of magnetic resonance imaging in renal transplant recipients with acquired cystic kidney disease.* Urology, 1998. 51(4): p. 534-8.

[32] Sarasin, F. P., et al., *Screening for acquired cystic kidney disease: a decision analytic perspective.* Kidney Int, 1995. 48(1): p. 207-19.

[33] Gulanikar, A. C., et al., *Prospective pretransplant ultrasound screening in 206 patients for acquired renal cysts and renal cell carcinoma.* Transplantation, 1998. 66(12): p. 1669-72.

[34] Doublet, J. D., et al., *Renal cell carcinoma of native kidneys: prospective study of 129 renal transplant patients.* J Urol, 1997. 158(1): p. 42-4.

[35] Cho, C., G. W. Friedland, and R. S. Swenson, *Acquired renal cystic disease and renal neoplasms in hemodialysis patients.* Urol Radiol, 1984. 6(3-4): p. 153-7.

[36] Kim, S. Y. , et al. , *Usefulness of resistive index on spectral Doppler ultrasonography in the detection of renal cell carcinoma in patients with end-stage renal disease.* Ultrasonography, 2014. 33(2): p. 136-42.

[37] Takebayashi, S. , et al. , *Using helical CT to evaluate renal cell carcinoma in patients undergoing hemodialysis: value of early enhanced images.* AJR Am J Roentgenol, 1999. 172(2): p. 429-33.

[38] Schwarz, A. , et al. , *Renal cell carcinoma in transplant recipients with acquired cystic kidney disease.* Clin J Am Soc Nephrol, 2007. 2(4): p. 750-6.

[39] Bosniak, M. A. , *The current radiological approach to renal cysts.* Radiology, 1986. 158(1): p. 1-10.

[40] Aronson, S. , et al. , *Cystic renal masses: usefulness of the Bosniak classification.* Urol Radiol, 1991. 13(2): p. 83-90.

[41] Siegel, C. L. , et al. , *CT of cystic renal masses: analysis of diagnostic performance and interobserver variation.* AJR Am J Roentgenol, 1997. 169(3): p. 813-8.

[42] Curry, N. S. , S. T. Cochran, and N. K. Bissada, *Cystic renal masses: accurate Bosniak classification requires adequate renal CT.* AJR Am J Roentgenol, 2000. 175(2): p. 339-42.

[43] Zhang, J. , et al. , *Renal masses: characterization with diffusion-weighted MR imaging--a preliminary experience.* Radiology, 2008. 247(2): p. 458-64.

[44] Taouli, B. , et al. , *Renal lesions: characterization with diffusion-weighted imaging versus contrast-enhanced MR imaging.* Radiology, 2009. 251(2): p. 398-407.

[45] Sandrasegaran, K. , et al. , *Usefulness of diffusion-weighted imaging in the evaluation of renal masses.* AJR Am J Roentgenol, 2010. 194(2): p. 438-45.

[46] Cova, M. , et al. , *Diffusion-weighted MRI in the evaluation of renal lesions: preliminary results.* Br J Radiol, 2004. 77(922): p. 851-7.

[47] Le Bihan, D. , et al. , *Diffusion MR imaging: clinical applications.* AJR Am J Roentgenol, 1992. 159(3): p. 591-9.

[48] Koh, D. M. and D. J. Collins, *Diffusion-weighted MRI in the body: applications and challenges in oncology.* AJR Am J Roentgenol, 2007. 188(6): p. 1622-35.

[49] Mosetti, M. A. , et al. , *Autosomal dominant polycystic kidney disease: MR imaging evaluation using current techniques.* J Magn Reson Imaging, 2003. 18(2): p. 210-5.

[50] Stiles, K. P. , et al. , *Renal cell carcinoma as a cause of end-stage renal disease in the United States: patient characteristics and survival.* Kidney Int, 2003. 64(1): p. 247-53.

[51] Dripps, R. D. , A. Lamont, and J. E. Eckenhoff, *The role of anesthesia in surgical mortality.* JAMA, 1961. 178: p. 261-6.

[52] Wolters, U. , et al. , *ASA classification and perioperative variables as predictors of postoperative outcome.* Br J Anaesth, 1996. 77(2): p. 217-22.

[53] Clayman, R. V. , et al. , *Laparoscopic nephrectomy: initial case report.* J Urol, 1991. 146(2): p. 278-82.

[54] Cadeddu, J. A. , et al. , *Laparoscopic nephrectomy for renal cell cancer: evaluation of efficacy and safety: a multicenter experience.* Urology, 1998. 52(5): p. 773-7.

[55] Nadu, A. , et al. , *Ventilatory and hemodynamic changes during retroperitoneal and transperitoneal laparoscopic nephrectomy: a prospective real-time comparison.* J Urol, 2005. 174(3): p. 1013-7.

[56] Desai, M. M. , et al. , *Prospective randomized comparison of transperitoneal versus retroperitoneal laparoscopic radical nephrectomy.* J Urol, 2005. 173(1): p. 38-41.

[57] Nambirajan, T. , et al. , *Prospective, randomized controlled study: transperitoneal laparoscopic versus retroperitoneoscopic radical nephrectomy.* Urology, 2004. 64(5): p. 919-24.

[58] Iwamura, M. , et al. , *Retroperitoneoscopic radical nephrectomy by the posterior lumber approach for renal-cell carcinoma associated with chronic renal failure.* J Endourol, 2001. 15(7): p. 729-34.

[59] Gulati, M. , et al. , *Laparoscopic radical nephrectomy for suspected renal cell carcinoma in dialysis-dependent patients.* Urology, 2003. 62(3): p. 430-6.

[60] Bird, V. G. , et al. , *Transperitoneal laparoscopic radical nephrectomy for patients with dialysis-dependent end-stage renal disease: an analysis and comparison of perioperative outcome.* Urology, 2010. 75(6): p. 1335-42.

[61] Yamashita, K. , F. Ito, and H. Nakazawa, *Perioperative outcomes of laparoscopic radical nephrectomy for renal cell carcinoma in patients with dialysis-dependent end-stage renal disease.* Ther Apher Dial, 2012. 16(3): p. 254-9.

[62] Sanli, O. , et al. , *Laparoscopic nephrectomy in patients undergoing hemodialysis treatment.* JSLS, 2010. 14(4): p. 534-40.

[63] Ghasemian, S. R. , et al. , *Bilateral laparoscopic radical nephrectomy for renal tumors in patients with acquired cystic kidney disease.* J Laparoendosc Adv Surg Tech A, 2005. 15(6): p. 606-10.

[64] Kihara, K. , et al. , *Portless endoscopic radical nephrectomy via a single minimum incision in 80 patients.* Int J Urol, 2004. 11(9): p. 714-20.

[65] Kihara, K. , et al. , *Gasless single-port access endoscopic surgery in urology: minimum incision endoscopic surgery, MIES.* Int J Urol, 2009. 16(10): p. 791-800.

[66] Kihara, K. , et al. , *Minimum incision endoscopic surgery (MIES) in Japanese urology: results of adrenalectomy, radical nephrectomy and radical prostatectomy.* Aktuelle Urol, 2010. 41 Suppl 1: p. S15-9.

[67] Kihara, K. , et al. , *New three-dimensional head-mounted display system, TMDU-S-3D system, for minimally invasive surgery application: procedures for gasless single-port radical nephrectomy.* Int J Urol, 2012. 19(9): p. 886-9; author reply 890.

[68] Kageyama, Y. , et al. , *Endoscopic minilaparotomy radical nephrectomy for chronic dialysis patients.* Int J Urol, 2002. 9(2): p. 73-6.

[69] Sakura, M. , et al. , *Sequential bilateral minimum incision endoscopic radical nephrectomy in dialysis patients with bilateral renal cell carcinomas.* Int J Urol, 2007. 14(12): p. 1109-12.

[70] Hemal, A. K. and A. Kumar, *A prospective comparison of laparoscopic and robotic radical nephrectomy for T1-2N0M0 renal cell carcinoma.* World J Urol, 2009. 27(1): p. 89-94.

[71] Dhillon, J. , et al. , *Mucinous tubular and spindle cell carcinoma of the kidney with sarcomatoid change.* Am J Surg Pathol, 2009. 33(1): p. 44-9.

[72] Masuda, H. , et al. , *Renal cell carcinoma in dialysis patients with end stage renal disease: focus on surgery and pathology.* Hemodialysis-Different Aspects. Intech, Rijeka, Croatia, 2011: p. 31-44.

[73] Bhatnagar, R. and B. A. Alexiev, *Renal-cell carcinomas in end-stage kidneys: a clinicopathological study with emphasis on clear-cell papillary renal-cell carcinoma and acquired cystic kidney disease-associated carcinoma.* Int J Surg Pathol, 2012. 20(1): p. 19-28.

[74] Gobbo, S. , et al. , *Clear cell papillary renal cell carcinoma: a distinct histopathologic and molecular genetic entity.* Am J Surg Pathol, 2008. 32(8): p. 1239-45.

[75] Aydin, H. , et al. , *Clear cell tubulopapillary renal cell carcinoma: a study of 36 distinctive low-grade epithelial tumors of the kidney.* Am J Surg Pathol, 2010. 34(11): p. 1608-21.

[76] Adam, J. , et al. , *Clear-cell papillary renal cell carcinoma: 24 cases of a distinct low-grade renal tumour and a comparative genomic hybridization array study of seven cases.* Histopathology, 2011. 58(7): p. 1064-71.

[77] Tickoo, S. K. and V. E. Reuter, *Differential diagnosis of renal tumors with papillary architecture.* Adv Anat Pathol, 2011. 18(2): p. 120-32.

[78] Pope, J. C. , M. O. Koch, and R. F. Bluth, *Renal cell carcinoma in patients with end-stage renal disease: a comparison of clinical significance in patients receiving hemodialysis and those with renal transplants.* Urology, 1994. 44(4): p. 497-501.

[79] Rioux-Leclercq, N. C. and J. I. Epstein, *Renal cell carcinoma with intratumoral calcium oxalate crystal deposition in patients with acquired cystic disease of the kidney.* Arch Pathol Lab Med, 2003. 127(2): p. E89-92.

[80] Kuroda, N. , et al. , *Sarcomatoid acquired cystic disease-associated renal cell carcinoma.* Histol Histopathol, 2008. 23(11): p. 1327-31.

[81] Kuroda, N. , et al. , *Acquired cystic disease-associated renal cell carcinoma with gain of chromosomes 3, 7, and 16, gain of chromosome X, and loss of chromosome Y.* Med Mol Morphol, 2010. 43(4): p. 231-4.

[82] Pan, C. C. , et al. , *Immunohistochemical and molecular genetic profiling of acquired cystic disease-associated renal cell carcinoma.* Histopathology, 2009. 55(2): p. 145-53.

[83] Ahn, S. , et al. , *Acquired cystic disease-associated renal cell carcinoma: further characterization of the morphologic and immunopathologic features.* Med Mol Morphol, 2013. 46(4): p. 225-32.

[84] Cossu-Rocca, P. , et al. , *Acquired cystic disease-associated renal tumors: an immunohistochemical and fluorescence in situ hybridization study.* Mod Pathol, 2006. 19(6): p. 780-7.

[85] Kuroda, N. , et al. , *Acquired cystic disease-associated renal cell carcinoma: an immunohistochemical and fluorescence in situ hybridization study.* Med Mol Morphol, 2011. 44(4): p. 228-32.

[86] Kuntz, E. , et al. , *Oligoarray comparative genomic hybridization of renal cell tumors that developed in patients with acquired cystic renal disease.* Hum Pathol, 2010. 41(9): p. 1345-9.

[87] Oya, M. , et al. , *C-jun activation in acquired cystic kidney disease and renal cell carcinoma.* J Urol, 2005. 174(2): p. 726.

[88] Ito, F. , et al. , *Cytokines accumulated in acquired renal cysts in long-term hemodialysis patients.* Urol Int, 2000. 65(1): p. 21-7.

[89] Dry, S. M. and A. A. Renshaw, *Extensive calcium oxalate crystal deposition in papillary renal cell carcinoma: report of two cases.* Arch Pathol Lab Med, 1998. 122(3): p. 260-1.

[90] Hori, Y. , et al. , *Oxidative stress and DNA hypermethylation status in renal cell carcinoma arising in patients on dialysis.* J Pathol, 2007. 212(2): p. 218-26.

[91] Huang, X. B. , et al. , *Increased expression of 8-hydroxydeoxyguanosine in acquired cystic disease of the kidney.* Nephron, 1999. 81(4): p. 458-9.

[92] Huang, X. B. , et al. , *Inducible nitric oxide synthase localization in acquired cystic disease of the kidney.* Nephron, 1999. 81(3): p. 360-1.

[93] Ishikawa, I. , *Prognosis in dialysis patients complicated with renal cell carcinoma (in Japanese with English abstract).* J Jpn Ass Soc Dial Ther, 2002. 35: p. 287-93.

[94] Shrewsberry, A. B. , et al. , *Renal cell carcinoma in patients with end-stage renal disease has favorable overall prognosis.* Clin Transplant, 2014. 28(2): p. 211-6.

[95] Kuroda, N. , et al. , *Acquired cystic disease-associated renal cell carcinoma with sarcomatoid change and rhabdoid features.* Ann Diagn Pathol, 2011. 15(6): p. 462-6.

Section 2

Mechanical Aspects of Dialysis

Chapter 10

Dialysis Membranes — Physicochemical Structures and Features

Akihiro C. Yamashita and Kenji Sakurai

Additional information is available at the end of the chapter

http://dx.doi.org/10.5772/59430

1. Introduction

When functions of the living kidney decrease down to under survival level, patients are required to be treated with a system that supports kidney functions. There are several such treatment modalities available, including peritoneal dialysis (PD), hemodialysis (HD), hemofiltration (HF), hemodiafiltration (HDF), hemoadsorption (HA), and their advanced derivatives, among which the most popular treatment system is HD. The artificial kidney device used in HD is called "hemodialyzer" or more simply "dialyzer" that includes membrane to separate the waste products and excess water from blood.

Artificial kidney is also expected to correct pH that is usually acidic before treatment by balancing electrolytes in addition to removing waste products and excess water. All these functions are dependent upon the permeability of the membrane used in a dialyzer and since the quality of treatment is strongly dependent on the performance of the dialyzer, many materials have been proposed as a candidate of the membrane. We have currently several commercial materials available, including natural polymers and synthetic polymeric ones.

In this chapter, dialysis membrane and its materials are extensively discussed from the physicochemical points of view, including microscopic views taken by scanning electron microscope (SEM), mathematical expressions of membrane transport, fundamental *in vitro* experiments as well as *in vivo* trials or clinical experiences.

2. Basic principles and history of dialysis membrane

2.1. Law of diffusion

Dialysis is a phenomenon at which two different fluids (usually liquids) are separating flowing on either side of the membrane (usually counter-currently) and the solute of interest in higher concentration transports across the membrane due to concentration gradient in accordance with the Fick's 1-st law of diffusion, i.e.,

$$J_{Ax} = -D_{Ax}\frac{\partial C_A}{\partial x} \tag{1}$$

where x is the co-ordinate in the diffusion direction [m], J_{Ax} is the mass flux of solute A in x direction [kg/(s m^2)], D_{Ax} is the diffusion coefficient of A in x direction [m^2/s], and C_A is the concentration of A [kg/m^3]. Dialysis, therefore, is one of separation techniques of the solute of interest by using the membrane and is applied elsewhere in many industrial as well as laboratory situations. Letting C_{A0} and C_{AL} to be the concentrations of A at x=0 and x=L, respectively (Figure 1), Eq.(1) is integrated in a straight-forward manner to get,

$$J_{Ax} = \left(\frac{D_{Ax}}{L}\right)(C_{A0} - C_{AL}) \equiv k_M \times (C_{A0} - C_{AL}) \tag{2}$$

where k_M is the membrane permeability [m/s] defined by (D_{Ax}/L). From Eq.(2), one would alternately mention that the rate of diffusion is proportional to the concentration difference between either side of the membrane. The value of k_M is discussed in section 4.

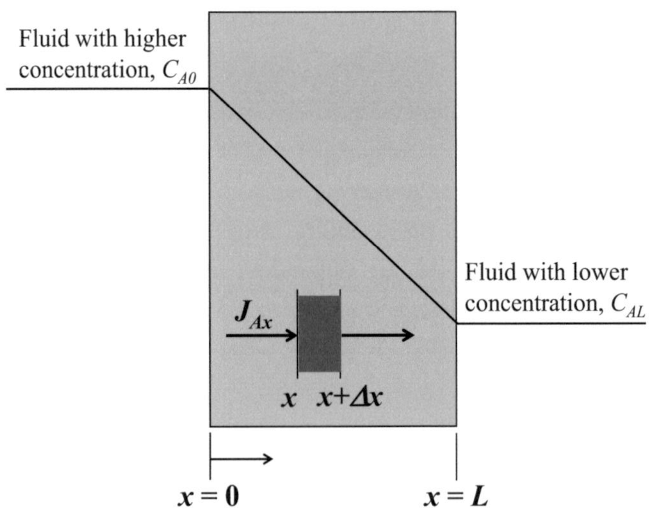

Figure 1. Diffusion across a piece of membrane assuming no existence of boundary film adjacent to either side of the membrane.

2.2. Dawn of hemodialysis

Application of dialysis to blood purification, hemodialysis (HD), was first performed for canines reported by Abel *et al.* in 1914 [1]. A chemical substance (sodium salicylate) was added to the subject as a marker prior to the experiment, mimicking the clinical situation of kidney failure in which waste products accumulate in the human body. Then the marker substance was removed by the dialyzer that included the membrane made of collodion. The dialyzer included 16 collodion tubes whose length was 40 cm that is 1.5 times longer than a currently available normal commercial model and the diameter was about 8 mm that is approximately 40 times larger than a popular hollow fiber membrane currently utilized worldwide. Since the collodion was too fragile to perform dialysis experiments, many other membranes cast from natural materials were examined whether or not they were suited as a separation membrane. Finally collodion was replaced by cellophane, and the first clinical trial was performed by Kolff *et al.* in 1943 with a rotating drum dialyzer, designed and assembled by themselves [2]. Separation performance of these dialysis membranes, however, was not discussed extensively at that time because mechanical strength of the materials was more important for performing experiments or treatments than the permeability of the membrane.

2.3. Development of commercial dialysis membranes

Cuprophan® is a registered name of the membrane made of cuprammonium rayon made from cellulose dissolved in cuprammonium solution, produced by Enka Co. in West Germany, later Membrana in Polypore Co., Germany. Another cuprammonium rayon membrane with nearly the same chemical and physical structures was developed by Asahi-Kasei Co. (Tokyo, Japan) termed Bemberg®, followed by Terumo (Tokyo, Japan). These membranes were also called regenerated cellulosic (RC) membrane since they were cast from cellulose or cotton fibers. Chemical modifications were made for RC membranes mostly because of improving their biocompatibility by replacing their hydroxyl group(s) with acetate group(s). They are called cellulose acetate (CA), cellulose diacetate (CDA), and cellulose triacetate (CTA) in accordance with the number of introduction of acetate groups to the cellulose backbone. Although RC membranes are no longer commercially available, CA, CDA, and CTA membranes still have fairly good market share since they have much higher solute and hydraulic permeabilities as well as better biocompatibility than original RC membranes.

The first synthetic polymeric membrane was developed in 1969 by Rhône-Poulenc (France) and was named AN-69®, since the main material of the membrane was acrylonitrile (AN). The brand name of the dialyzer assembled with a flat sheet AN-69® membrane was RP-6® and it was also the first dialyzer sterilized by the gamma-ray irradiation. Although the production company of AN-69® membrane has been changed over time from Rhône-Poulenc to Hospal, Gambro, and Baxter, dialyzers with AN-69® membrane are still available worldwide, especially in the field of acute kidney injury (AKI) therapy since it has strong adsorption characteristic to specific substances such as inflammatory cytokines.

The first dialyzer with a cellulosic hollow fiber membrane was developed by chemical engineers, Stuart and Lipps in 1967 [3] in Massachusetts Institute of Technology (Boston, MA, U.S.A.), and the commercial product was available in 1972 from Cordis-Dow Co. (Miami, FL,

U.S.A.). The basic structure of the hollow-fiber dialyzer is the same as the one of multi-tube heat exchanger that is compact and has large surface area. Because of these advantages, dialyzers with hollow fiber membrane have been become widely used. The first dialyzer with a synthetic polymeric hollow fiber membrane sterilized by gamma-ray was introduced by Toray Co. (Tokyo, Japan), in which polymethylmethacrylate (PMMA) was used as a main material of the membrane [4].

In order to improve solute and hydraulic permeabilities as well as biocompatibilities, many synthetic polymeric membranes have been introduced to the market since early 1980's, and currently these membranes are the main stream. Among them, polysulfone (PSf) and the like (including polyethersulfone (PES), polyarylethersulfone (PAES), etc.) have the highest market share over the world. Since these membranes are made from petroleum, they are hydrophobic in nature. Then most of these membranes include so-called hydrophilic agent that also plays a role of pore-forming agent when cast. The role of the hydrophilic agent is discussed later from the chemical (section 3), mass transport (section 4), and biological (section 5) points of view.

3. Chemical structures of dialysis membrane

3.1. Main material of the membrane

Chemical structure of the dialysis membrane usually refers to the chemical structural formula of the main material(s) of the dialysis membrane. Most chemical structural formulae of the main material of the membrane are tabulated in Table 1, including both natural and synthetic polymers. Among them AN-69®, ethylenevinylalcohol (EVAL) co-polymer, polyester polymer alloy (PEPA, Nikkiso Co., Tokyo, Japan, Figure 2) include two main materials. Actually PMMA is also a stereo complex co-polymer of two kinds of PMMA, isotactic and syndiotactic. Isotactic PMMA has acetate groups on only one side of the main chain, resulting a curled structure, whereas syndiotactic PMMA has acetate groups alternately on either side of the main chain, resulting a fairly straight structure. Combining these two polymers, membranes with low to high hydraulic permeability has been brought to realization [4].

3.2. Hydrophilic agent

In general, cellulosic membranes are hydrophilic in nature, including original RC and its derivatives such as CA, CDA, and CTA in which hydroxyl group(s) are replaced by acetate group(s). On the contrary, since synthetic polymeric membranes are originated from petroleum, generally speaking they are hydrophobic in nature. Blood coagulation usually occurs soon after blood interacts with hydrophobic materials. Most synthetic polymeric membranes, therefore, include so-called hydrophilic agent such as polyvinylpyrrolidone (PVP) to make membrane hydrophilic. Figure 2 includes the chemical structure of PVP together with two other polymers (polyarrylate and polyethersulfone). PEPA is composed of these two polymers with or without PVP, the former shows little hydrophobicity, while the latter has strong adsorptive characteristic to various proteins due to its hydrophobicity (see section 4).

http://dx.doi.org/10.5772/59430

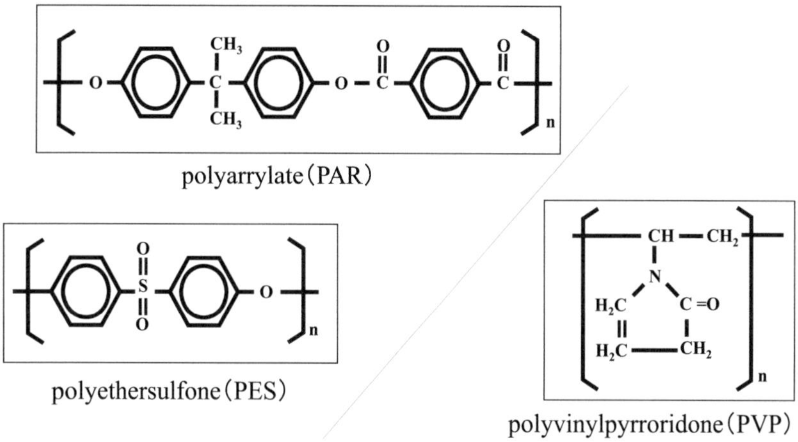

Figure 2. Chemical structures of polyester polymer alloy (PEPA) composed of PES and PAR with polyvinylpyrroridone (PVP).

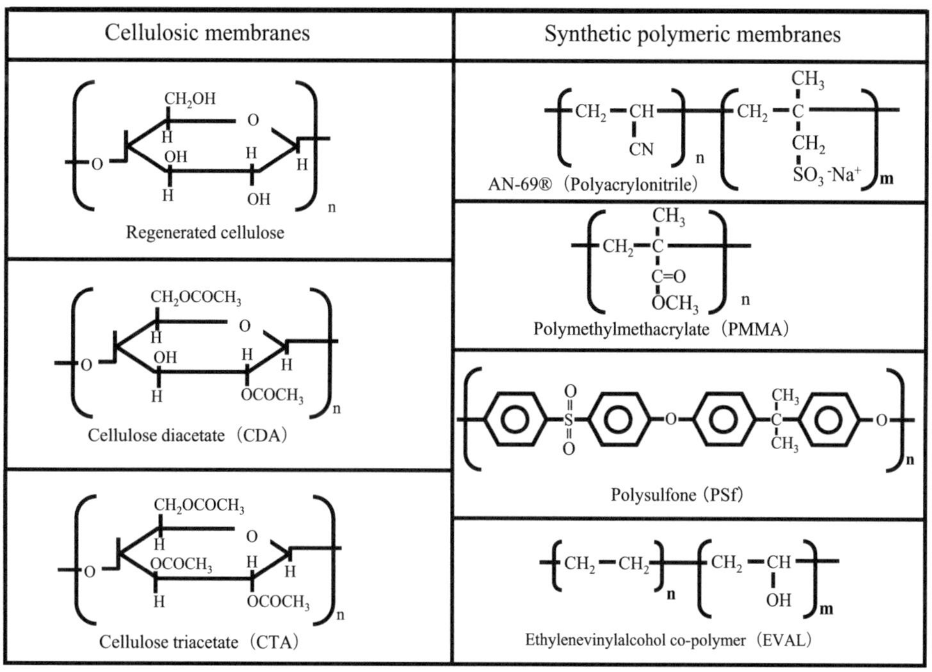

Table 1. Chemical structures of cellulosic and synthetic polymeric membranes for blood purification.

Since PVP is water-soluble, excess amount of PVP may be rinsed out from the membrane after cast that forms pores for solute and water transport. Therefore PVP is also known as a pore-forming agent. Namely, it should be understood that PVP residues in or on the membrane after rinse behave as a hydrophilic agent. Both an average and a distribution of molecular weight of PVP are important as well as the amount of PVP used in the membrane. Moreover, PVP may be cross-linked together and to the main material of the membrane by irradiating gamma-ray in the final sterilization process. With this procedure, PVP should be tightly attached together and/or on the membrane that does not allow PVP to behave as a "cushion" (cushion effect) to the blood corpuscles [5].

Acrylic acid is specifically chosen for polyacrylonitrile (PAN, Asahi Kasei, different from AN-69®) as a hydrophilic agent, whereas no hydrophilic agent is used in PMMA, EVAL and the original PEPA in which micro-layer separation technology plays a significant role in casting procedure.

4. Physical structure of dialysis membrane

4.1. Homogeneous and asymmetry membrane

Physical structures can be demonstrated in the following two ways, i.e., microscopic view analysis and a theoretical analysis based on mathematical models. Microscopic views are usually taken by a scanning electron microscope (SEM). Recently the microscope technology has been advancing drastically and a field-emission SEM (FE-SEM) that has much higher resolutions can be utilized widely.

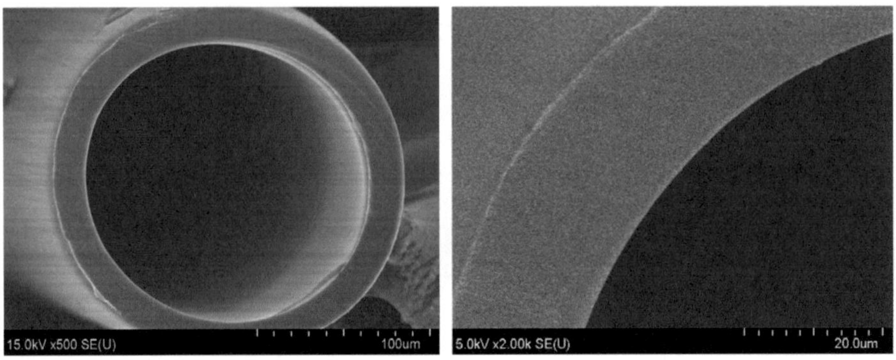

Figure 3. A cross-sectional view of EVAL hollow fiber membrane (Asahi-Kasei, Tokyo, Japan) taken by FE-SEM.

Figure 3 is a FE-SEM of intersection of EVAL membrane (Asahi-Kasei). It is entirely a dense membrane and the entire thickness contributes to the transport resistance for solutes and water. Membranes of this kind are usually called "homogeneous." Besides EVAL, PMMA, and AN-69®, most cellulosic membranes are homogeneous. Figure 4 shows a cross-sectional view of PSf membrane (Toray). One should realize that a dense thin layer exists on the inner surface of the membrane, called "skin layer" from which the density is gradually decreasing in the radial direction. Since most part excluding the skin layer is known to have little resistance for solute and water transport, it is called the "support layer" (Figure 5). The support layer, however, has an important role for the membrane to have enough mechanical strength with little resistance for transport. Membranes of this kind are called "asymmetry." Most synthetic polymeric membranes (except for PMMA, EVAL, and AN-69®) are asymmetry. In general, although the physical thickness of synthetic polymeric membranes is thicker (approximately 35 μm) than that of cellulosic membranes (approximately 15 μm), the thickness that contributes to the separation (Δx) of the former is approximately 0.5-2 μm that is much thinner than the latter. As mentioned before, synthetic polymeric membranes are main stream these days because much higher solute and hydraulic permeabilities are achieved with the thinner Δx.

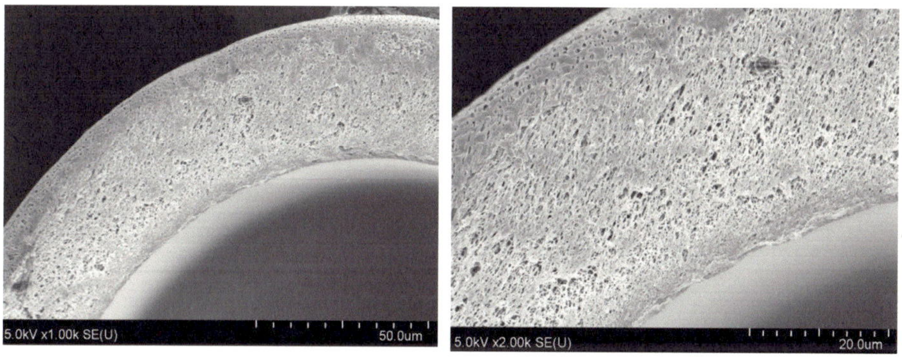

Figure 4. A cross-sectional view of PSf hollow fiber membrane (Toray, Tokyo, Japan) taken by FE-SEM.

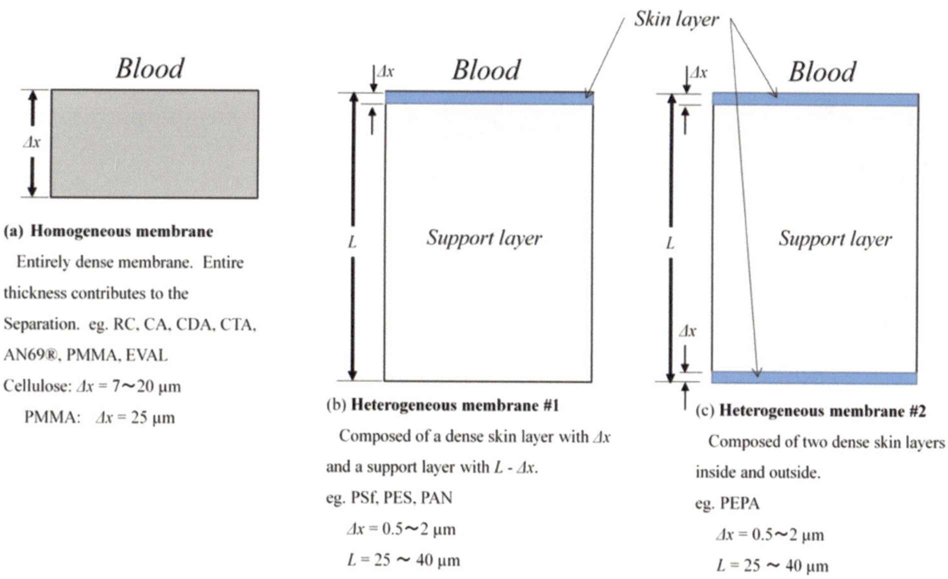

Figure 5. Cross-sectional views of dialysis membranes.

4.2. Pore theory

The pore theory is often used to analyze and to design physical structures of the membrane. The original pore theory was introduced by Pappenheimer *et al.* [6] to analyze the Glomerular filtration in the living kidney (Figure 6), and was later modified by Verniory *et al.* [7], introducing steric hindrance effect. Sakai [8] further modified the model by introducing the tortuosity for transporting across the membrane. Followings are the equations for modified pore theory.

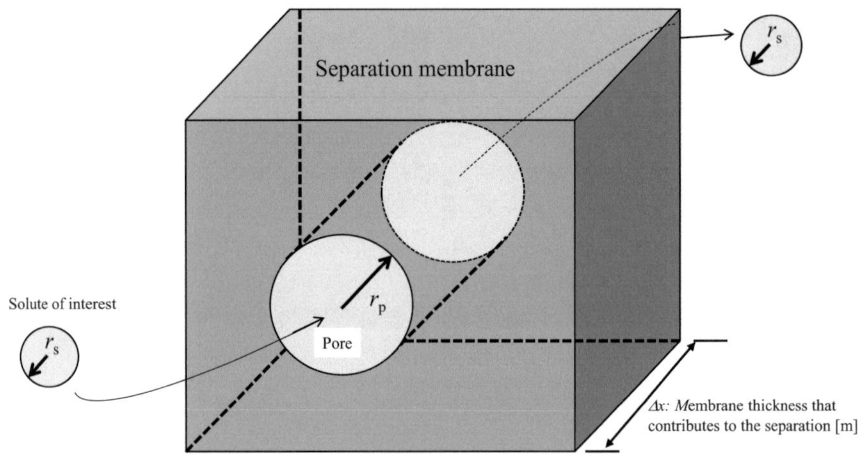

Figure 6. Pore theory (pore diffusion model). Assuming pores whose radius is uniformly r_p [m] with a membrane thickness of Δx [m], through which a solute of interest whose radius is r_s [m] is passing.

$$k_M = D_w \times f(q) \times S_D \times \left(\frac{A_k}{\tau \times \Delta x}\right) \tag{3}$$

$$L_p = \left(\frac{r_p^2}{8\mu}\right) \times \left(\frac{A_k}{\tau \times \Delta x}\right) \tag{4}$$

$$q = \frac{r_s}{r_p} \tag{5}$$

$$\sigma = 1 - g(q) \times S_F \tag{6}$$

$$S_D = (1 - q)^2 \tag{7}$$

$$S_F = 2(1 - q)^2 - (1 - q)^4 \tag{8}$$

$$f(q) = \frac{1 - 2.1050q + 2.0865q^3 - 1.7068q^5 + 0.72603q^6}{1 - 0.75857q^5} \tag{9}$$

$$g(q) = \frac{1 - (2/3)q^2 - 0.20217q^5}{1 - 0.75857q^5} \tag{10}$$

where k_M is the membrane permeability [m/s] (see also section 1), D_w is the diffusion coefficient for the solute of interest in pure water [m²/s], A_k is the surface porosity of the membrane [-], Δx is the membrane thickness that contributes to the transport resistance [m], r_s is the solute radius [m], r_p is the pore radius of the membrane [m], L_p is the hydraulic permeability of the membrane [m² s/kg], σ is the Staverman's reflection coefficient [-], τ is the tortuosity of the membrane [-], q is the ratio of r_s to r_p [-], S_D, S_F, $f(q)$, and $g(q)$ are the dimensionless stereo correction factors defined as functions of q. The pore theory can be applied to the situation in which $q < 0.8$ is satisfied.

From Eqs.(3) and (4), it is clear that $A_k/(\tau \Delta x)$ is an important factor both for solute and water transport because both k_M and L_p include this value. Figure 7 shows two examples of L [m] x L [m] portions of the membrane, i.e., membrane (A) with four pores with the same radius of a [m], and membrane (B) with one pore with a radius of $2a$. Then the surface porosity can be calculated, respectively for membranes (A) and (B) with subscripts (A) and (B), i.e.,

$$A_{k(A)} = \frac{4 \times \pi a^2}{L^2} = \frac{4\pi a^2}{L^2}$$

$$A_{k(B)} = \frac{\pi (2a)^2}{L^2} = \frac{4\pi a^2}{L^2}$$

$$\therefore \; A_{k(B)} = A_{k(A)}$$

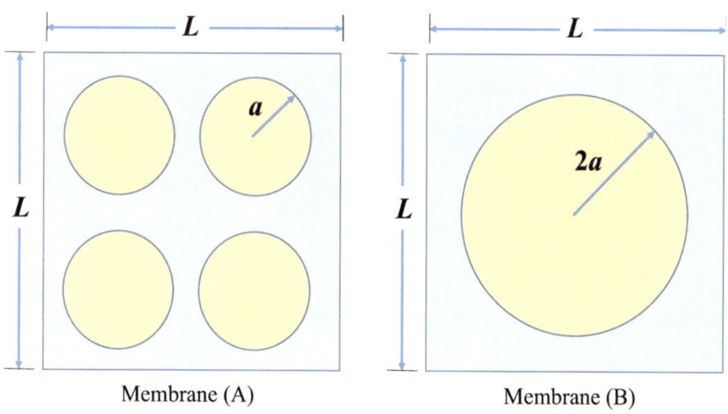

Figure 7. Portions of two modeled membranes with the same surface porosity.

Then one would realize that membranes (A) and (B) have the same surface porosities, although the situations are quite different in terms of the pore diameter.

Example)

Compare the two membranes (A) and (B) that have the same surface porosity (Figure 7), tortuosity and the thickness in terms of

i. hydraulic permeability

ii. solute permeability

under the following two conditions

a. r_s is negligibly small compared with a

b. $r_s = a/3$

Solution) As stated above, A_k, τ, and Δx are the same in two membranes, $A_k/(\tau\ \Delta x)$ is just a constant.

i. Recalling Eq. (4) to get,

$$L_{p(A)} = \left(\frac{a^2}{8\mu}\right) \times \left(\frac{A_k}{\tau \times \Delta x}\right)$$

$$L_{p(B)} = \left(\frac{(2a)^2}{8\mu}\right) \times \left(\frac{A_k}{\tau \times \Delta x}\right) = \left(\frac{4a^2}{8\mu}\right) \times \left(\frac{A_k}{\tau \times \Delta x}\right)$$

$$\therefore\ L_{p(B)} = 4\ L_{p(A)}$$

Therefore, the membrane (B) has four times higher hydraulic permeability than the membrane (A).

ii. Since $q=0$ may reasonably be applied in this case, recalling Eqs.(7)-(10) to get,

$S_D = S_F = f(q) = g(q) = 1$

in both membranes (A) and (B). Therefore Eq.(3) may be simplified as follows,

$$k_{M(A)} = k_{M(B)} = D_w \times (1) \times (1) \times \left(\frac{A_k}{\tau \times \Delta x}\right) = D_w \times \left(\frac{A_k}{\tau \times \Delta x}\right)$$

Consequently, there is no difference between membranes (A) and (B) in terms of transport of small solutes.

iii. Recalling Eq.(5),

$$q_{(A)} = \frac{r_s}{r_p} = \frac{a/3}{a} = \frac{1}{3}$$

$$q_{(B)} = \frac{r_s}{r_p} = \frac{a/3}{2a} = \frac{1}{6}$$

Then recalling Eqs.(7) and (9) with q values calculated above,

$$S_{D(A)}=(1-q_{(A)})^2=0.8889$$

$$S_{D(B)}=(1-q_{(B)})^2=0.9722$$

$$f(q_{(A)})=0.3707$$

$$f(q_{(B)})=0.6587$$

Then from Eq.(3),

$$k_{M(A)} = D_w \times (0.3707) \times (0.8889) \times \left(\frac{A_k}{\tau \times \Delta x}\right) = 0.3295 \times D_w \times \left(\frac{A_k}{\tau \times \Delta x}\right)$$

$$k_{M(B)} = D_w \times (0.6587) \times (0.9722) \times \left(\frac{A_k}{\tau \times \Delta x}\right) = 0.6404 \times D_w \times \left(\frac{A_k}{\tau \times \Delta x}\right)$$

$$\therefore\ k_{M(B)}=1.94\ k_{M(A)}$$

Finally one would conclude that the membrane (B) has almost two times higher solute permeability than the membrane (A) for those solutes whose $r_s=a/3$.

Chemical characteristic determines the hydrophilicity and hydrophobicity of the material, whereas physical structure determines the pore sizes as well as the thickness that contributes to the transport resistance. Therefore, both chemical and physical features are important for designing dialysis membrane.

5. Performance of dialysis membrane

In this section, we discuss the performances under *in vitro* ultrafiltration experiments and those under on-line HDF in clinical situations because the former is suited for evaluation of maximal performance of the membrane and the latter takes a responsibility of the real performance under advanced clinical situations.

5.1. Aqueous *in vitro* ultrafiltration experiment

Six filters (dialyzers), one with PSf (PS-1.6UW, Fresenius-Kawasumi Co., Tokyo, Japan) and other five with PEPA (Nikkiso Co., Tokyo, Japan) were investigated (Table 2). Since both PSf and PEPA are hydrophobic in nature, these membranes include PVP for anti-thrombosis purpose, except for one dialyzer that includes PEPA membrane with no additives (FLX). Amount of PVP used in the membrane is semi-quantitatively shown as (+++), (++), (+), and (-), respectively for “most”, “much”, “small” and “none”.

#	name of products	abbreviated names	Surface area [m²]	membrane materials	hydrophilic agent	pore size info	membrane make
1	PS-1.6UW	PS	1.6	PSf	PVP (+++)	(Not available)	Fresenius Medical Care, Badhonburg, Germany
2	FLX-15GW	FLX	1.5	PEPA	PVP (-)	standard	Nikkiso Co., Tokyo, Japan
3	FDX-15GW	FDX	1.5	PEPA	PVP (+)	standard	Nikkiso Co., Tokyo, Japan
4	FDY-15GW	FDY	1.5	PEPA	PVP (+)	larger	Nikkiso Co., Tokyo, Japan
5	FDX-150GW	new FDX	1.5	PEPA	PVP (++)	standard	Nikkiso Co., Tokyo, Japan
6	FDY-150GW	new FDY	1.5	PEPA	PVP (++)	larger	Nikkiso Co., Tokyo, Japan

Table 2. Technical specification of investigated ultrafilters

The time courses of the sieving coefficient ($s.c._4$) [9, 10] for albumin of PS-1.6UW dialyzer were shown in Figure 8. Strong time-dependent patterns were found with peak values approximately at 10 minutes after starting experiments. The lower the albumin concentration, the higher the $s.c._4$ values was found with longer time for achieving steady-state.

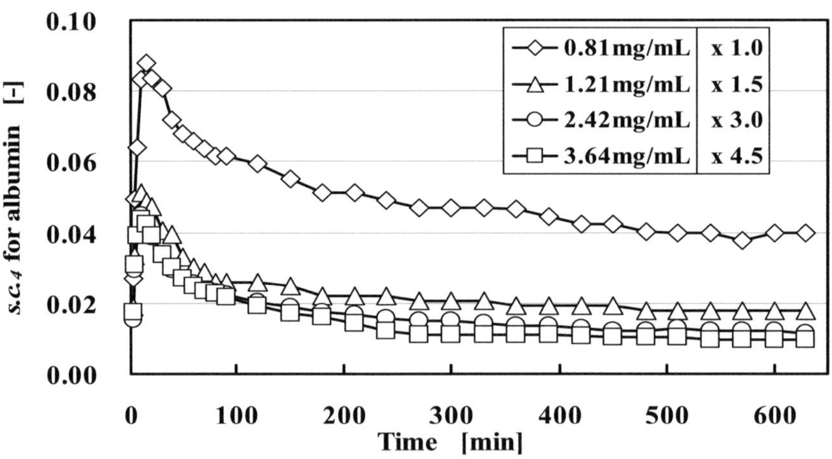

Figure 8. Time courses of the sieving coefficient for albumin under various concentrations of albumin in PS-1.6UW (PSf membrane) Q_{Bi}=200 mL/min, Q_F=10 mL/min, Volume of test sol'n=2.0 L.

The time courses of $s.c._4$ for albumin of three PEPA filters with albumin concentration of 3.64 mg/mL are shown in Figure 9. The $s.c._4$ gradually increased in these PEPA with PVP(-) or

PVP(+) and never took peak values. Membranes used in FLX and FDX basically have the same pore sizes and the only difference is that the latter contained PVP, which concludes that PVP directly influences the membrane transport of albumin. By enlarging the pore diameter by approximately 5 % in FDY with the same PVP content, the $s.c._4$ increased with the enlargement accordingly.

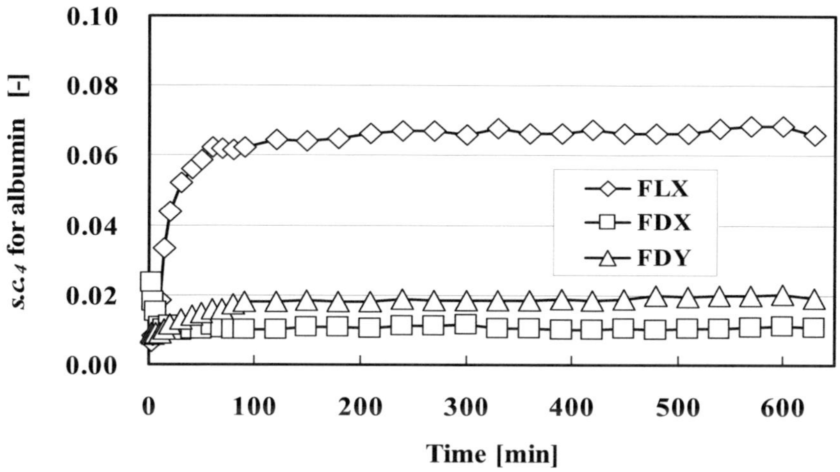

Figure 9. Time courses of the sieving coefficient for albumin under a fixed albumin concentration (3.64 mg/mL) in three PEPA membrane dialyzers Curves are different from the ones found with PSf membrane. Q_{Bi}=200 mL/min, Q_F=10 mL/min, Volume of test sol'n=2.0 L.

The time courses of $s.c._4$ for albumin of the latest version of PEPA dialyzers are depicted in Figure 10 for albumin concentration of 3.64 mg/mL. It should be noted that the peak values were found in new PEPA membranes that included increased amount of PVP at 6 minutes after starting the experiments. Moreover, time dependent pattern of these curves are different from the ones shown in Figure 9 and are similar to those found with PSf membrane in Figure 8. Then it may be concluded that the time course of $s.c._4$ for albumin is strongly dependent on the amount of PVP included in the membrane and not on the main material of the membrane.

Since the albumin concentrations of the test solutions were lower by the factor of 1/30-1/10 to the standard albumin concentration in human blood (3.6 – 4.0 g/dL), $s.c._4$ values for albumin shown above do not directly correspond to the clinical results. One should, however, need to consider that the membrane separation characteristics depend on the pore diameter, amount of hydrophilic agent as well as experimental conditions [11].

5.2. Clinical performance of super-high flux dialyzers/diafilters

According to the Japanese reimbursement system, all the commercial dialyzers are classified into five categories in accordance with the clearances for β2-microglobulin (β2-MG, MW 11800) under Q_B=200 mL/min, Q_D=500 mL/min for dialyzers with surface area of 1.5 m^2 (Table 3). Classes IV and V dialyzers, clearances for β2-MG greater or equal to 50 and 70 mL/min,

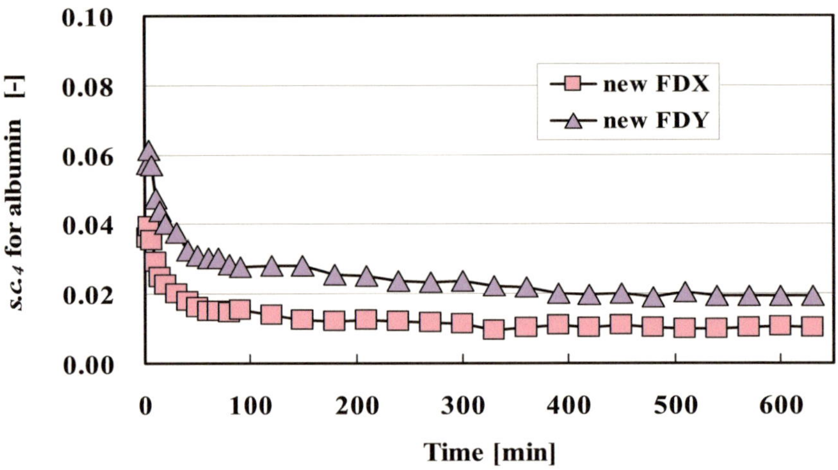

Figure 10. Time courses of the sieving coefficient for albumin under a fixed albumin concentration (3.64 mg/mL) in two new PEPA membrane dialyzers Curves are similar to the ones found with PSf membrane. Q_{Bi}=200 mL/min, Q_F=10 mL/min, Volume of test sol'n=2.0 L.

respectively, are the "super-high flux" models and more than 95 % of Japanese dialysis patients are treated with dialyzers of this kind [12]. These dialyzers had been used also for on-line hemodiafiltration (HDF) with considerable amount of albumin removal (> 3 g/treatment) until 2010 before on-line HDF has been officially announced to be included in the reimbursement system.

Class	β_2-MG clearance [mL/min]	Reimbursement
I	< 10	low
II	>=10～< 30	↓
III	>=30～< 50	↓
IV	>=50～< 70	↓
V	>= 70	high

1. Flow conditions: Q_B=200 mL/min, Q_D=500 mL/min, Q_F=10 mL/min/m^2.

2. A_0=1.5 m^2

3. *If* A_0 is NOT1.5 m^2, use of the closest model is recommended. Clearance for β_2-MG under A_0=1.5 m^2 may be estimated by using the performance evaluation equations with K_oA as a constant.

Table 3. Classification of dialyzers in Japanese reimbursement system

Although 99 uremic toxins are compiled by Vanholder [13], clinicians and researchers have different opinions on which solutes to be removed or up to how much albumin may be leaked out. Figure 11 shows the relationship between the reduction rate of β2-MG and albumin loss taken with various dialyzers in different modalities. Only a limited increase in β2-MG reduction was found with the increase of albumin removal. Therefore β2-MG removal may not be directly related to convection transport when super-high flux dialyzers are used. In other words, super high-flux dialyzers are the ones in which β2-MG removal does not correlate with the amount of albumin loss or the convection transport.

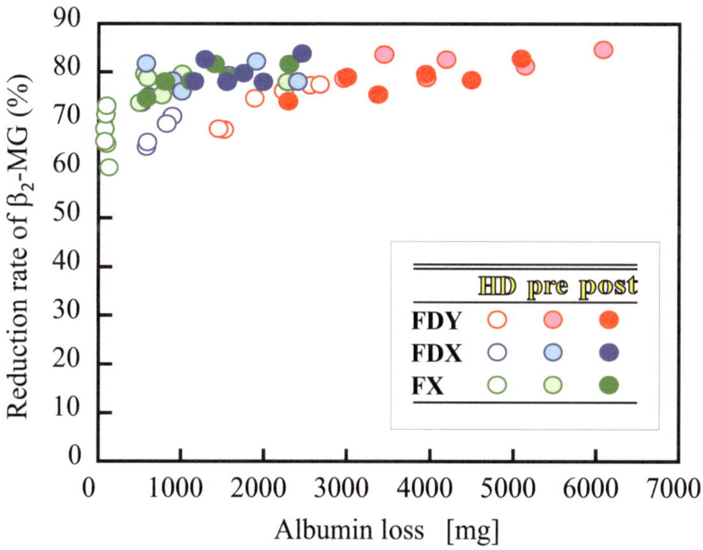

Figure 11. Relationship between the reduction rate of β2-microglobulin (MW: 11,800) and albumin loss.

Figure 12 shows the same relationship between the reduction rate of α_1-microglobulin (α_1-MG, MW 33,000) and albumin loss. Up to albumin loss of 3 g/session, almost linear relationship was observed, meaning that it may not be possible to remove α_1-MG without removing albumin, although the molecular weight of albumin is twice as large as that of α_1-MG. There is no such article that reports α_1-MG is toxic; moreover, α_1-MG is not even included in Vanholder's list [13]. We, however, experienced fairly good number of patients who have become better with albumin loss of 3 g or more for bone pain, shoulder pain, and improvement of fingertip power, and 5 g or more for finger numbness, restless legs syndrome. Therefore α_1-MG may be a possible surrogate marker of HDF treatment for those who have symptoms with normal HD therapy. Relief of clinical symptoms with various treatment modalities is summarized in Figure 13.

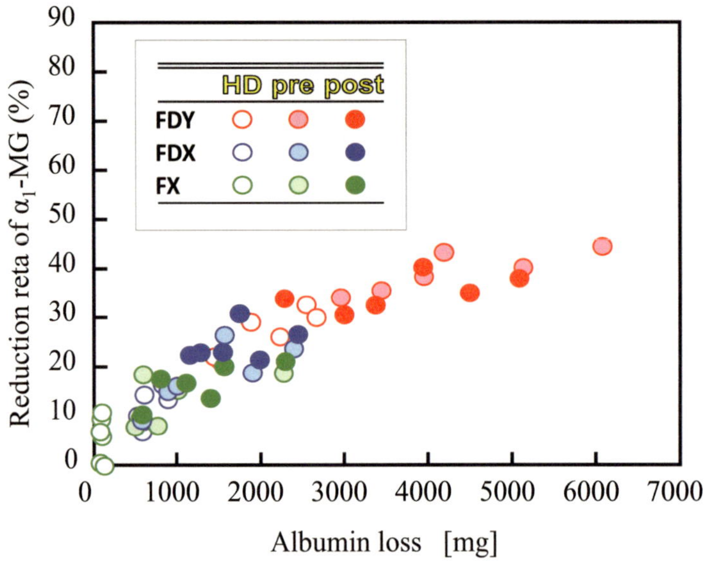

Figure 12. Relationship between the reduction rate of α1-microglobulin (MW: 33,000) and albumin loss.

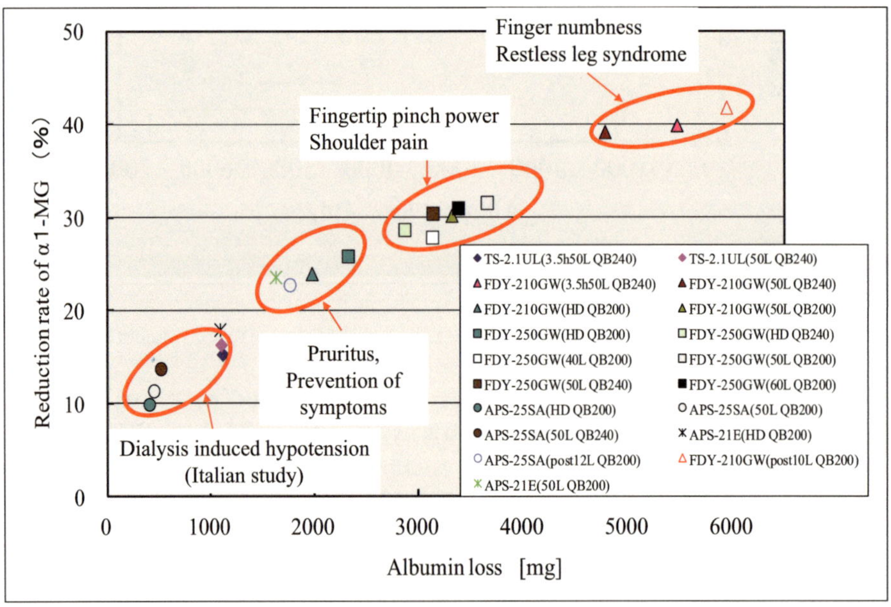

Figure 13. Relief of clinical symptoms by employing various protein-losing treatment modes.

5.3. Consideration of on-line HDF

On-line HDF is mostly performed in post-dilution mode with high Q_B (400 mL/min) in European countries, whereas that is mostly performed in pre-dilution mode with limited Q_B (250 mL/min) in Japan. Diafilters preferred in post-dilution and pre-dilution HDF must be designed under different concepts. Membrane for the post-dilution HDF requires a limited permeability for albumin, otherwise unexpected large amount of albumin may be leaked out. Therefore relatively large surface area is preferred for achieving large amount of fluid exchange (20 L/session). Since usually higher clearances are expected with post-dilution HDF, membrane for the pre-dilution HDF prefers higher solute permeability that may allow much albumin to penetrate across the membrane. Amount of albumin loss, however, may be relatively easily controlled by changing the amount of ultrafiltration that is usually around 60 L/session. In the recent market, since diafilters specifically designed for either post-dilution or pre-dilution are available, choice of diafilters must be paid much attention not only for effective treatment but also for safety. Moreover, a proposal of technical specifications for the future diafilters is also reported [14].

Many randomized control studies have been done in order to verify superiority or better outcomes of on-line HDF [15-[19]; however, we have not yet come into a conclusion that states on-line HDF is better than other treatment modalities. These studies showed that on-line HDF was at least better than low-flux HD; however, the difference between on-line HDF and high-flux HD was ambiguous [18, 19], in terms of survival rate within a study period of three years or so. Post–hoc analyses and sub-analyses of those studies showed superiority of on-line HDF with large amount of fluid exchange (at least > 15 L) to other treatment modalities in terms of dialysis-induced hypotension, reaction to ESR medications, as well as survival rate. Among them, the ESHOL study [20] greatly encouraged patients on dialysis as well as medical staffs in which on-line HDF showed better clinical outcomes in all the end points than high-flux HD. Many debates, however, still continues also elsewhere including in Japan where the number of patients on on-line HDF is rapidly growing and exceeded 10 % of the total patients [21].

6. Biological consideration of dialysis membrane

Biological consideration of the dialysis membrane is often referred to biocompatibility. Since dialyzers are repeatedly used four hours a session, three times a week, even a small event that repeatedly would occur each time may cause undesired side effects such as chronic inflammation.

6.1. Improvement of biocompatibility of the regenerated cellulosic membrane

Up until 1970s, RC membrane dominated over the market, and it was gradually replaced by synthetic polymeric membranes. Transient leukopenia that is an abrupt decease of leukocytes occurs at 15 to 30 minutes after starting the treatment has been one of the best known bio-incompatible events [22]. Reprocessing dialyzers was common in 1970's and since bio-incompatible events were often found when a dialyzer was used for the first time, this was called the "first use syndrome" [23].

Craddock *et al.* reported that complement activation under the use of RC membrane induced transient accumulation of leukocytes in the blood vessels and in the lung [24]. As shown in section 2, RC has three hydroxyl groups in its backbone, and these hydroxyl groups have been realized to be closely related to undesired complement activation. Then acetate groups was introduced to the one, two, or all three of hydroxyl group(s) to produce cellulose acetate (CA), cellulose diacetate (CDA), and cellulose triacetate (CTA), respectively. Since these semi-synthesized cellulosic membranes have not only better biocompatibility but also higher permeabilities for solutes and water transport, they are still on the market.

6.2. Improvement of biocompatibility of synthetic polymeric membrane

It is well known that the Glomerular basement membrane (GBM) in human kidney is negatively charged. Although AN-69® is also a negatively charged membrane, one must pay much attention for the use of this membrane because it may cause anaphylaxy shock soon after starting the treatment [25]. Strong negative charge (-70 mV) would activate Hageman (XII) factor to XIIa that eventually produces bradykinin from kininogen as a substrate. Under normal situation bradykinin may be deactivated by kininase II; however, if the patient takes angiotensin-converting enzyme (ACE) inhibitor, it deactivates kininase II. This would induce the cascade reaction with bradykinin, including NO generation, increased vascular permeability, expansion of blood vessels, suppressing blood pressure, and ending up with shock during the treatment. This is often called "negative charge syndrome" (NCS, Figure 14). Although all dialysis membranes are negatively charged, it is usually a contraindication to prescribe ACE inhibitor to a patient under the use of AN69®.

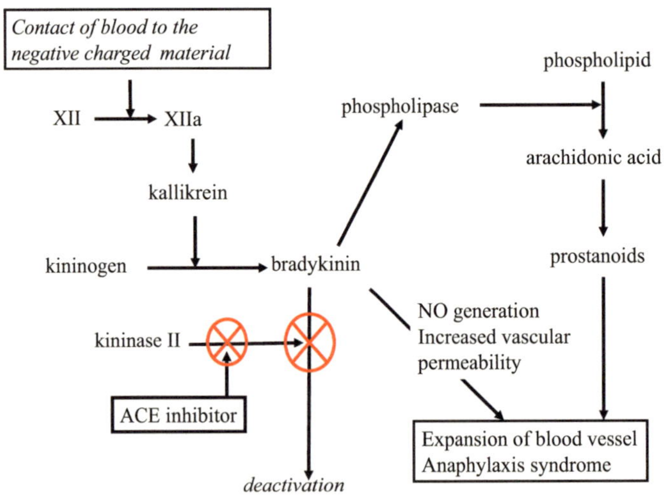

Figure 14. Mechanisms of negative charge syndrome (NCS).

6.3. Surface improvement technique

Hemophan® was developed by introducing a positively charged substance, diethylaminoethyl (DEAE), to RC membrane in order to improve its surface character (Membrana, Germany). Although only a limited amount of DEAE was introduced relative to entire amount of cellulose, complement activation was greatly suppressed. Hemophan®, however, adsorbed heparin, which induced blood coagulation. Because of this fact, the production of this membrane was ceased. Another trial was made by coating the membrane surface with vitamin E in order to make the RC membrane antioxydative (Terumo, Tokyo, Japan). Later, this technique was applied to PSf membrane and the commercial model is still available (Asahi Kasei Medical Co., Tokyo, Japan).

6.4. Membranes with polyvinylpyrrolidone

PSf and the ones whose chemical structures are similar to PSf have the highest market share among all dialysis membranes. They usually include polyvinylpyrrolidone (PVP) as a hydrophilic agent since they are hydrophobic in nature. PVP was once used as a supplement of plasma in medicine. Anaphylaxy shock, however, was reported, the cause of which was strongly doubted to be the PVP included in the membrane. Then we performed the following clinical investigation by using dialyzers with PSf and the ones with PEPA membrane with different amount of PVP [11].

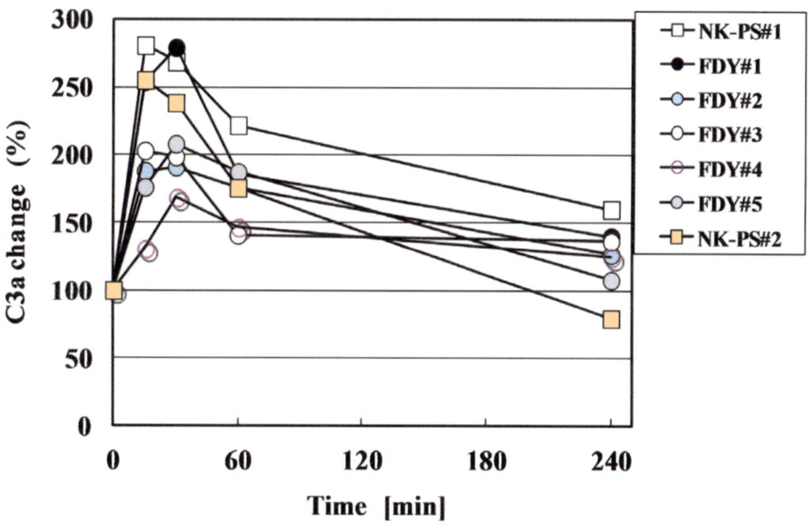

Figure 15. Time course of C3a change during four hr treatment. The same PSf dialyzers with PVP(+++) were used in the 1-st and last (7-th) weeks. The same FDY dialyzers with PVP(+) were used from the 2nd to the 6th weeks.

The time course of C3a concentration profile in clinical study is shown in Figure 15. PSf with PVP(+++) showed three times higher concentration 15 minutes after the start of treatment. The C3a elevation was slightly lower at the first use of PEPA with PVP(+) and the peak concentrations were approximately halved or even less from the second to the fifth week. The peak concentration, however, returned back to three folds in the first use of PSf after five-week use of PEPA with PVP(+).

According to another clinical data shown in Figure 16, PSf with PVP(+++) showed highest C3a elevation, followed by PEPA with PVP(++), PVP(+), and PVP(-). The degree of C3a elevation was a function of amount of PVP included in the membrane regardless of the main material of the membrane.

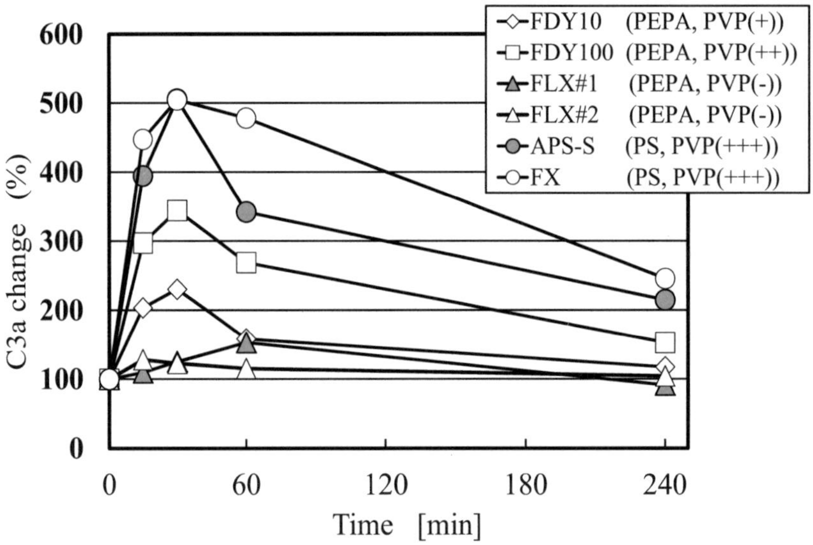

Figure 16. Time course of C3a change during four hr treatment in 1 patient. Symbols are arranged in the chronological order from the top to the bottom.

From these results, we learned that PVP may not be the best choice as a hydrophilic agent in terms of blood compatibility.

7. Future perspectives of dialysis membrane

With above mentioned technique, we will be able to expect an even better dialysis membrane to come into the market. Several futuristic functions desired for dialysis membrane is also introduced, expecting a new era to come. Followings are the problems to be solved in the future perspectives of dialysis membrane.

7.1. Solute removal performance

Since on-line HDF has been gaining popularity in European countries as well as in Japan, HDF with much larger amount of fluid exchange has to be more easily performed for the further success of this modality. Standard on-line HDF in European countries is performed in post-dilution system with Q_B=400 mL/min, Q_D=700 mL/min, Q_F=90 mL/min, Q_S=80 mL/min=19.2 L/4hr in single patient dialysis machine (SPDM) system, whereas that in Japan is performed in pre-dilution system with Q_B=250 mL/min, Q_D=500 mL/min, Q_F=260 mL/min, Q_S=250 mL/min=60 L/4hr in central dialysis fluid delivery system (CDDS) [26] (Figure 17). In terms of solute removal, the difference between these two methods is the largest target solute to be removed, i.e., "European HDF" is targeted to remove β2-MG (MW 11,800) with little loss of albumin (some ten mg/treatment), whereas "Japanese HDF" is targeted to remove α 1-MG (MW 33,000) or even greater ones with albumin "removal" less than 4 g/treatment because enough removal of α1-MG cannot be possible without removing considerable amount of albumin (Figure 13). Although ultra-"super-high flux" dialyzers are commercially available in Japan, termed class V in Japanese reimbursement system, which remove α1-MG to achieve clinically effective reduction rate (> 30 %) [26], they also remove considerable amount of albumin (> 5 g/treatment) as well as amino acids, important small solutes from the nutritional point of view. Therefore when more precise prescriptions are necessary, on-line pre-dilution HDF is preferred because it removes α1-MG more than 30 % with albumin loss of 4 g/treatment or less and with considerably reduced clearance for small solutes, including amino acids, due to reduced net dialysis fluid flow rate (net Q_D=500-250=250 mL/min).

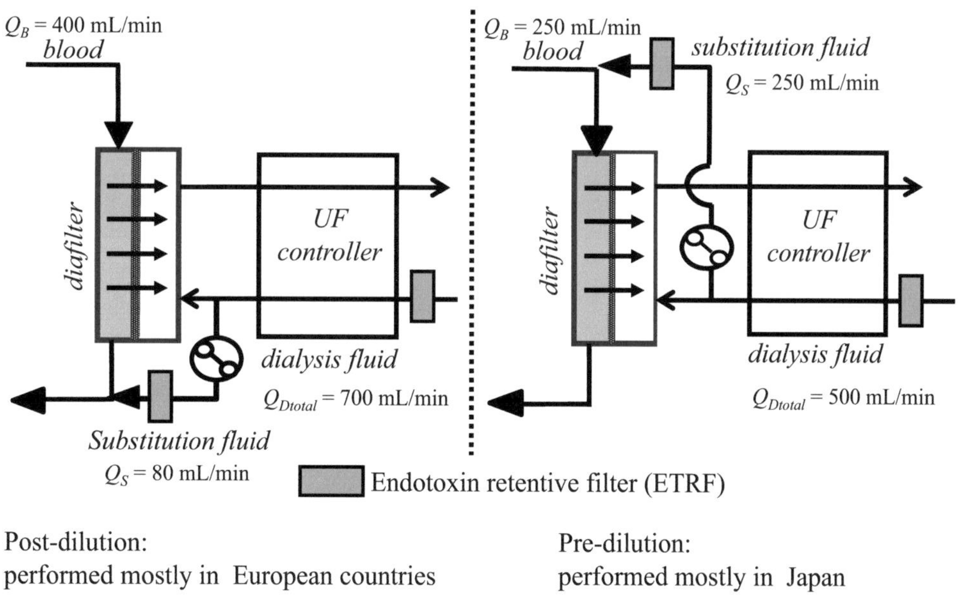

Figure 17. Comparison of post-dilution and pre-dilution on-line HDF with typical European and Japanese flow rates, respectively.

According to the Italian study [17], on-line HDF/HF is a useful tool for treating patients with dialysis induced hypotension. Then diafilters with higher hydraulic permeability with little albumin loss that do not aim to achieve higher solute removal may be useful for those patients. Not to mention, design specifications of dialyzer/diafilter is as important as the membrane permeability in terms of solute removal under given therapeutic conditions.

7.2. Biocompatibility

Many classic problems with biocompatibility in the past such as transient leukopenia, complement activation, negative charge syndrome, etc., have already been dissolved by modifying physical and chemical structures of the dialysis membrane. Most currently available synthetic polymeric membranes, however, employ PVP as a hydrophilic agent as well as a pore-forming agent. Study shows that many symptoms including abrupt decrease of blood pressure or shock right after starting treatments could be induced most probably due to PVP included in the membrane, and it is sometimes called "PVP intolerance". Novel hydrophilic agents may be studied for the purpose of replacing PVP. Alternately, novel casting technique in which no hydrophilic agent is necessary has to be studied, knowing that PMMA, EVAL, and PEPA are cast with no additives although they are also originated from petroleum.

7.3. Surface modification and adsorption

Surface modification with the third substances is another way to obtain membranes with preferred permeability as well as biocompatibility. For example, PSf membrane coated with vitamin E showed a great success for reducing reactive oxygen species (ROS) as well as free radicals that also showed preferable clinical results (Terumo, Asahi-Kasei). Toray introduced a novel technique with NV polymer to their PSf membrane to reduce adsorption of cells as well as protein molecules on the membrane. Although both two membranes work well clinically, they still utilize PVP in the same amount as previously included before. Then it should be noted since surface modification is closely related to solute transport as well as biocompatibility, biomimicry situations under dialysis must be further taken into consideration.

8. Conclusions

Since hemodialysis experiments with canines were first reported, many membranes, either natural or synthetic polymeric ones, have been developed and the latter have been the main stream due to higher solute and hydraulic permeabilities as well as better biocompatibility. The mass transport mechanism across the membrane can be expressed by the Fick's 1-st law of diffusion; however, not only the membrane permeability but also the design specifications are important for assembling dialyzers with better performances.

The chemical structure of the dialysis membrane determines the hydrophilicity and hydrophobicity of the membrane. Since all synthetic polymeric membranes are made from petroleum, they are hydrophobic in nature. Most of these membranes include a hydrophilic agent such as PVP for anti-thrombosis purpose. According to the in vitro experiments and clinical observations, it was proved that PVP was closely related to the sieving coefficient for albumin and had big influence on the complement activation. Then we must pay much attention on additives in addition to the main material(s) of the membrane.

Physical structure of the dialysis membrane can be discussed in two ways, i.e., direct observations by taking microscopic views (SEM) and the theoretical analysis by using a mathematical model. There are two kind of dialysis membranes, "homogeneous" and "asymmetry", among which the latter is gaining popularity because of the much smaller thickness that contributes to the resistance of solute and water transport. The pore theory is a useful tool for analyzing mass and water transport across the membrane and for designing a physical structure of the membrane.

Since the number of on-line hemodiafiltration (HDF) is growing these days not only from the solute removal point of view but also from the improvement of dialysis-induced hypotension during the treatment, membranes specifically designed for performing HDF has to be more extensively studied both clinically and fundamentally. Importance of biocompatibility of the membrane should be more carefully taken into account for selecting a device, considering membrane characteristic such as adsorption, especially in the field of acute kidney injury (AKI).

Author details

Akihiro C. Yamashita[1*] and Kenji Sakurai[2*]

*Address all correspondence to: yama@hosei.ac.jp

1 Department of Chemical Science and Technology, Faculty of Bioscience and Applied Chemistry, Hosei University, Kajino-cho, Koganei, Tokyo, Japan

2 Hashimoto Clinic, Hashimoto, Midori-ku, Sagamihara, Kanagawa, Japan

References

[1] Abel JJ, Rowntree, LG, Turner BB: On the removal of dissosible substances from the circulation blood of living animals by dialysis. *J Pharmcol Exp Ther* 1914; 5: 275-316.

[2] Kolff W J, Watschinger B: Further development of a coil kidney: disposable artificial kidney. *J Lab and Clin Med* 1956; 47: 969–77.

[3] Lipps BJ, Stewart RD, Perkins HA, Holmes GW, McLain EA, Rolfs MR, Oja PD: The hollow fiber artificial kidney, *Trans ASAIO* 1967; 13: 200-7.

[4] Sakai Y, Tsukamoto H, Fujii Y, Tanzawa H: Formation of poly(methyl methacrylate) membranes utilizing stereocomplex phenomenon. New York: Plenum Press: Ultrafiltration Membranes and Applications Plenum; 99–107, 1980.

[5] Hayama M, Yamamoto K, Kohori F, Sakai K: How polysulfone dialysis membranes containing polyvinylpyrrolidone achieve excellent biocompatibility?, *J Membrane Sci* 2004; 234: 41–9.

[6] Pappenheimer JR, Renkin EM, Borrero, LM: Filtration, diffusion and molecular sieving through peripheral capillary membranes – a contribution to the pore theory of capillary permeability, *Am J Physiol* 1951; 167: 166.

[7] Verniory A, Dubois R, Decoodt P, Gassee JP, Lambert PP: Measurement of the permeability of biological membranes – Application to the glomerular wall, *J Gen Physiol* 1973; 62: 489-507.

[8] Sakai K: Technical determination of optimal dimensions of hollow fiber membranes for clinical dialysis, *Nephrol Dial Transplant* 1989; 4 (Suppl): 79.

[9] Yamashita AC, Sakiyama R, Hamada H, Tojo K: Two new definitive equations of the sieving coefficient, *Kidney and Dialysis* (*JIN TO TOSEKI*) 1998; 45: S36-8. (in Japanese)

[10] Yamashita AC: New dialysis membrane for removal of middle molecule uremic toxins, *Amer J Kid Dis* 2001; 38 suppl.1: S217-9,.

[11] Yamashita AC, Tomisawa N, Takezawa A, Sakurai K, Sakai T: Blood compatibility and filtration: characteristics of newly developed polyester polymer alloy membrane, Hemodial Int 2004; 8: 99 – 100.

[12] Japanese Society for Dialysis Therapy (JSDT): An overview of regular dialysis treatment in Japan, Table 1913, as of Dec. 31, 2012, JSDT, 2012.

[13] Vanholder R, De Smet R, Glorieux G, *et al.*, European Uremic Toxin Work Group (EUTox): Review on uremic toxins: classification, concentration, and interindividual variability, *Kidney Int* 2003; 63: 1934-43.

[14] Yamashita AC: Diafilters for predilution and postdillution on-line hemodiafiltration, *Blood Purif* 2013; 35 (suppl 1): 29-33.

[15] Panichi V, Rizza GM, Paoletti S, *et al.* (RISCAVID Study Group): Chronic inflammation and mortality in haemodialysis: effect of different renal replacement therapies. Results from the RISCAVID study, *Nephrol Dial Transplant* 2008; 23: 2337-43.

[16] Canaud B, Bragg-Gresham JL, Marshall MR, *et al.*: Mortality risk for patients receiving hemodiafiltration versus hemodialysis: European results from the DOPPS, *Kidney Int* 2006; 69: 2087-93.

[17] Locatelli F, Altieri P, Andrulli S, *et al.*: Hemofiltration and Hemodiafiltration Reduce Intradialytic Hypotension in ESRD, *J Am Soc Nephrol* 2010; 21: 1798–807.

http://dx.doi.org/10.5772/59430

[18] Penne EL, Blankestijn PJ, Bots ML, *et al.* (the CONTRAST study group): Effect of increased convective clearance by on-line hemodiafiltration on all cause and cardiovascular mortality in chronic hemodialysis patients-the Dutch CONvective TRAnsport STudy (CONTRAST): rationale and design of a randomised controlled trial, *Curr Control Trials Cardiovasc Med* 2005; 6: 8.

[19] Ok E, Asci G, Toz H, et al. (Turkish Online Haemodiafiltration Study): Mortality and cardiovascular events in online haemodiafiltration (OL-HDF) compared with high-flux dialysis: results from the Turkish OL-HDF Study, *Nephrol Dial Transplant* 2013; 28: 192-202.

[20] Maduell F, Moreso F, Pons M, et al. (ESHOL Study Group): High-efficiency postdilution online hemodiafiltration reduces all-cause mortality in hemodialysis patients, *J Am Soc Nephrol* 2013; 24: 487-97.

[21] Japanese Society for Dialysis Therapy (JSDT): An overview of regular dialysis treatment in Japan, Table 34, P.38, as of Dec. 31, 2013, JSDT, 2014.

[22] Kaplow LS, Goffiret JA: Profound neutropenia during the early phase of hemodialysis, *JAMA* 1968; 203: 1135-7.

[23] Villarroel F: First-use syndrome in patients treated with hollow-fiber dialyzers, *Blood Purif* 1987; 5: 112-4.

[24] Craddock PR, Fehr J, Dalmasso AP *et al.*: Hemodialysis leukopenia. Pulmonary vascular leukostasis resulting from complement activation by dialyzer cellophane membranes, *J Clin Inves* 1977; 59: 879-88.

[25] Tielemans C, Madhoun P, Lenaers M, *et al.*: Anaphylactoid reactions during hemodialysis on AN69 membranes in patients receiving ACE inhibitors, *Kidney Int* 1990; 38; 982-4.

[26] Yamashita AC, Sato T: Central online hemodiafiltration in Japan: Management of water quality and practice, *Blood Purif* 2009; 27 (suppl 1): 50-5.

Chapter 11

The Role of the Dialysate Flow Rate in Haemodialysis

Peter Ahrenholz, Roland E. Winkler and
Diego Zendeh-Zartochti

Additional information is available at the end of the chapter

http://dx.doi.org/10.5772/58878

1. Introduction

Modern dialysis devices such as the Fresenius FMC 5008 allow the relationship between the flow rates of blood Q_B and dialysate Q_D to be fixed at a set ratio (e.g. Q_D=1.2 Q_B oder Q_D=1.5 Q_B). The FMC-Genius®-Therapy System, which uses a double-sided peristaltic pump for both the patient's blood and the dialysis fluid (50…350 ml/min), even allows a ratio of Q_B=Q_D.

The relationship between the effectiveness of haemodialysis on the one hand, and the flows of blood and dialysate on the other, is guided by physical principles. These principles have been known for some time and have been widely discussed in the literature [1]. However, the fact that dialysis machines are completely automated makes it easy to neglect the underlying principles, so much so that knowledge of these may at times be lacking. There are also financial pressures that result in a desire to economise on water and dialysate concentrate, and a desire to work with as low a dialysate flow rate as possible.

The following sections will provide a brief summary of the theory behind the principles involved. In vitro and in vivo testing results from some of the more commonly available dialysers are used to provide a clearer picture of the theoretical principles involved. These measurements show that in spite of modern dialysis membranes and structural changes, it is not in fact possible to reduce the dialysate flow rate without also reducing the dialysis dose.

2. Theoretical principles

The connection between the dialyser's technical parameters and the flow rates involved (QB, QD in the counter current flow) is based on the following relationship [1]:

$$K_O A = \frac{Q_B}{(1 - Q_B / Q_D)} \ln \left[\frac{1 - K / Q_D}{1 - K / Q_B} \right] \quad a$$
$$K_O A = \frac{K}{(1 - K / Q_B)} \quad b \qquad (1)$$

For $Q_B = Q_D$ the following applies: $K_O A = \frac{K}{1 - K / Q_B}$

where *Ko* is the "overall mass transfer coefficient" and *A* is the dialyser membrane surface area.

In dialysis log sheets, the *KoA*-value is usually recorded for urea, thus allowing the calculation of urea-clearance in relation to blood and dialysate flow rates.

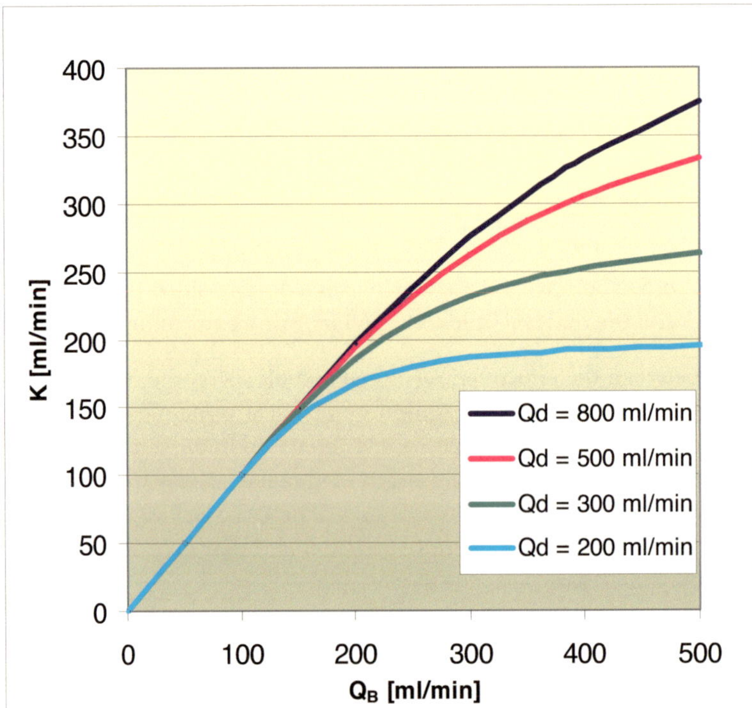

Figure 1. Dependence of clearance K on the flow rates of blood Q_B and dialysate Q_D (KoA=1000 ml/min)

Fig. 1 shows how clearance rate K, derived from the KoA value for a low molecular substance (urea), changes in relation to blood flow rates, with the relationship demonstrated at different dialysate flow rates, and for a high-flux dialyser. At low dialysate flow rates, the dialysate compartment soon becomes saturated, leading to a large reduction in the concentration gradient. This in turn means that an increase in blood flow will no longer produce a substantial improvement in the rate of clearance. It is only when the dialysate flow rate is high enough for the substance in question to be removed quickly from the dialysate chamber that a higher blood flow rate can produce substantial improvements in the rate of clearance. This is effectively only ever the case when the dialysate flow rate Q_D is at least 1.5…2.0 times as high as the blood flow rate, Q_B.

This theoretical relationship requires the KoA value to be constant for all dialysate and blood flow rates. This does of course not apply in practice in cases where the total surface area of the dialyser's fibre bundle is not completely bathed in dialysate. This may happen when low dialysate flow rates lead to preferential channels being formed (please also refer to Sections 3 and 4). In the presence of relatively low dialysate flow rates, therefore, clearance values which may seem possible in theory are in fact unachievable in practice.

It must be emphasised, however, that these observations only apply to transport by diffusion, the most important transport mechanism for low molecular weight substances such as urea, creatinine and phosphate. As far as larger molecules are concerned, it is convective solute transport that becomes increasingly important as the molecular weight of the solute increases. With regard to the manner in which the overall clearance K_T depends on both of these mechanisms, only an incomplete explanation can be provided. Werynski's equation [2] offers a reasonable approach:

$$K_T = K_{diff} + TrQ_F \text{ where } Tr = S(1 - K_{diff} / Q_{Bi}) \tag{2}$$

Tr: transmittance coefficient; S: sieving coefficient; Q_F: ultrafiltration rate

As the value for clearance by diffusion, K_{diff} in relation to blood flow rate, Q_B, decreases, the transmittance coefficient approaches the sieving coefficient, and the overall clearance K_T is effectively determined by the ultrafiltration rate Q_F. It follows that the dialysate flow rate Q_D has less significance with regard to larger molecules than it does with regard to smaller ones.

3. Structural changes to allow optimisation of the dialysate compartment

Fig. 2 shows an enhanced ultrasound image depicting an unfortunate case of channelling observed in a test dialyser during the inflow of dialysate.

In order to avoid, or at least reduce, this channelling phenomenon, different structural alterations are commonly applied:

- Flat sheet arrangement of hollow fibres
- Wave-shaped hollow fibres (Moiré structure)
- Spacer yarns
- Pinnacle structure in the dialysate inflow and outflow areas.

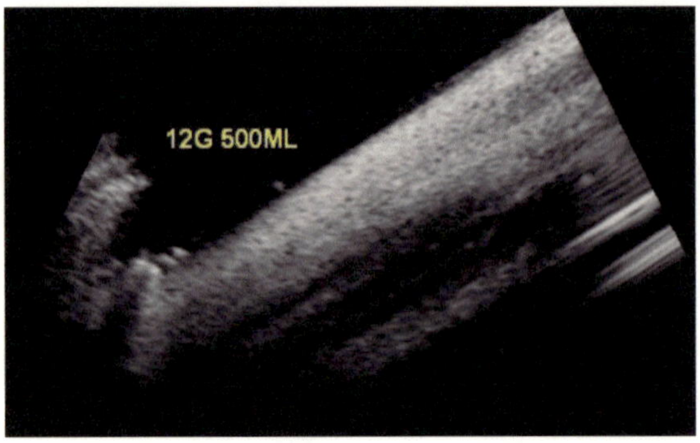

Figure 2. Enhanced ultrasound image of inflowing dialysate at Q_D=500 ml/min (Dialyser Altair 12G, US-machine Logic 7, GE Medical Systems, contrast agent: Optison®)

Although a number of manufacturers at one point utilised flat-plate arrangements of interweaved hollow fibres in their dialysers (e.g. HFD 1.0 by MLW), this method has since been abandoned-probably due to cost reasons. Almost all manufacturers prefer the Moiré structure of fibres in order to obtain adequate spacing. In some instances-and sometimes in addition to the Moiré structure-spacing filaments (spacer yarns) are added (e.g. Asahi PAN650SF, MTP VitaPES). Although these measures ensure improved dialysate flow distribution within the cross-sectional area of the dialyser, in vitro testing using CT imaging has revealed that some preferential channelling through peripheral areas of the dialysate compartment remains [3, 4, 5]. With its FX series, Fresenius Medical Care followed a different path. Via a pinnacle structure in the inflow and outflow tracts, the dialysate is forced into even distribution across the entire surface area [6]. In the early days, dialyser technology included a number of devices whose inlet and outlet headers were fitted diagonally to improve the distribution of dialysate across the fibre bundle (e.g. EMC TriEx). For reasons unknown, this very simple solution did not prevail.

4. In vitro analyses examining dialysate flow dependence of solute clearance

A dialysis machine (FMC 4008) was used to perform in vitro measurements of clearance rates in accordance with standard ISO 8637. A batch of 7.0 L stirred and thermostatically warmed dialysis liquid served as "blood" with dissolved urea and vitamin B12 as test substances. Measurements were carried out at different dialysate and blood flow rates, with each dialysate flow rate (Q_D=300, 500, 800 ml/min) being measured at blood flow rate settings of Q_B=100, 200, 300, 400 ml/min. These measurements were repeated for the 3 different types of dialysers.

Clearance data were obtained for one small molecule (urea, relative molecular weight=60) and one larger molecule (vitamin B12, relative molecular weight=1357). KoA values were then calculated according to GI. 1a, b and compared with the values provided by the manufacturers.

http://dx.doi.org/10.5772/58878

Dialyser	Membrane	Manufacturer	KoA urea [ml/min]
FDY-150 GW	PEPA®	Nikkiso	874
FX 60	Helixone®	FMC	967
VitaPES 150HF	Purema®	MTP Pirna	1167

Table 1. List of dialysers used for in vitro testing

Fig. 3 shows that the measured characteristics generally followed the theoretical model (refer to Fig. 1). However, the clearance rates calculated using the catalogue KOA values were not achieved at low dialysate flow rates. It was not until Q_D=800 ml/min that the values obtained managed to improve slightly on the ones provided. Similar curves were obtained for the other types of dialysers. The KoA values calculated from clearance, Q_B and Q_D were dependent upon both blood flow rate of blood and dialysate flow rate. In an ideal scenario, this kind of relationship should not exist. The overall mass transfer coefficient, Ko, is a physical characteristic of the fibre bundle and does not vary with the flow rates that might exist on the blood-side or the dialysate-side. Different KoA values in the presence of different flow rates can be easily explained provided if the effective surface area A, which is involved in solute transport, fails to remain constant. Values that may be theoretically possible will of course not be achieved in situations where a low dialysate flow rate results in sections of the fibre bundle not being immersed in dialysate. Fig. 4 shows that the KoA value calculated for the dialyser FDY150GW depends upon the dialysate flow rate.

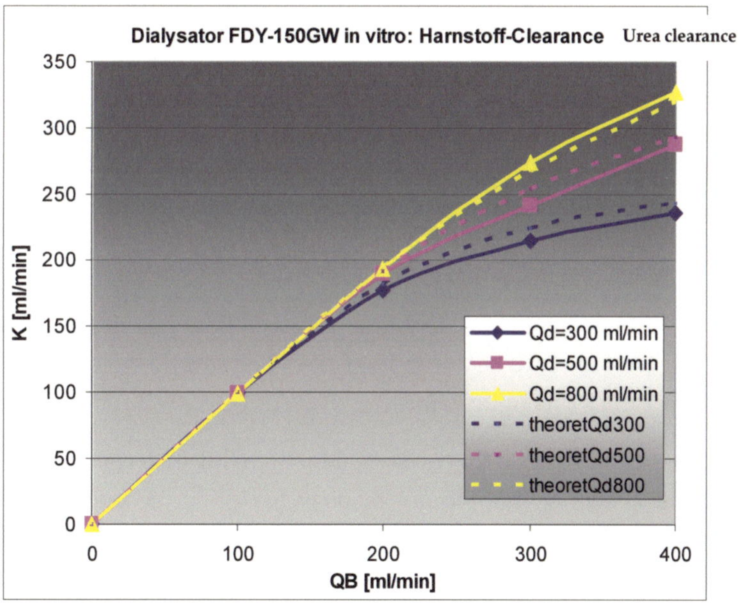

Figure 3. Comparison of measured urea clearance values and urea clearance values derived from KoA data provided by the manufacturers.

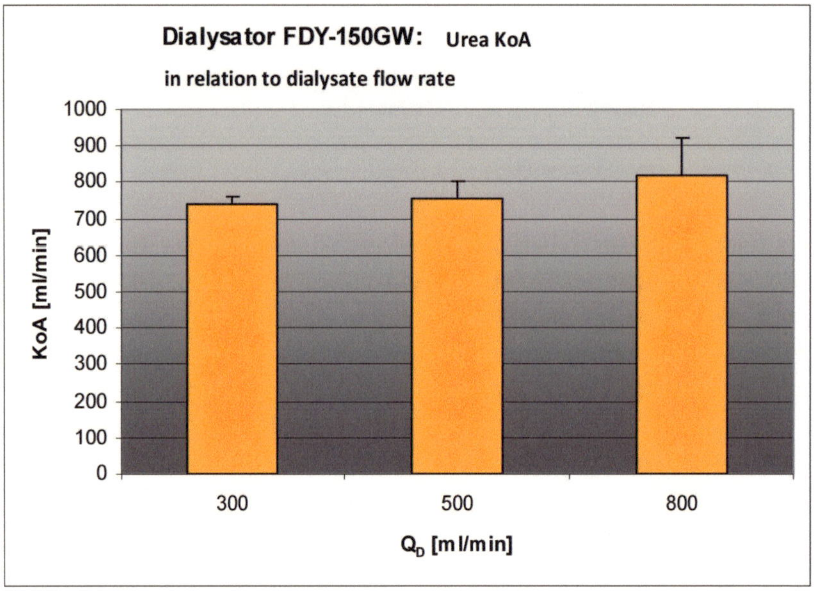

Figure 4. KoA values calculated based on clearance, Q_D and Q_B, using the dialyser FDY150GW as an example

Q_D/dialyser type	*FDY150GW*	*FX60*	*VitaPES150HF*
Q_D = 300 ml/min	740 ± 21	728 ± 26	792 ± 64
Q_D = 500 ml/min	753 ± 49	751 ± 42	936 ± 34
Q_D = 800 ml/min	817 ± 104	756 ± 70	1063 ± 106
Catalogue value	874	937	1167

Table 2. In vitro KoA values [ml/min] for urea at different dialysate flow rates Q_D (mean values for different blood flow rates Q_B)

The dialyser FX60 showed the lowest degree of dialysate flow rate dependence of the KoA value. Although this was likely to be due to improved dialysate flow, the device still failed to achieve the manufacturer's catalogue value.

In summary, it has to be concluded that even modern high flux dialysers providing structural changes to optimise dialysate flow do not manage to negate the underlying relationship between the flow rates of blood and dialysate. Furthermore, full use of the fibre bundle's effective surface area A can only be guaranteed at high dialysate flow rates of around 800ml/min. Whilst this mirrors the results obtained by Leypolt [7], it contradicts the assumptions made by Golper and Ward, who concluded that structural improvements have made high dialysate flow rates unnecessary.

5. In vivo analyses examining the dialysate flow rate dependence of solute clearance

Naturally, in vitro investigations involving dialysers have to be treated with caution, with results not directly transferable to the clinical dialysis setting. Due to its viscosity and non-Newtonian flow properties, blood is a much more complex substance than an aqueous test solution. Also, unlike dialyser clearance rates, in vivo clearance rates depend upon physiological factors such as compartmentalisation of the blood and the uraemic toxins contained therein, fistula recirculation, cardiopulmonary recirculation, individual differences in haematocrit, as well as differences in protein and lipid concentrations. In spite of this, when looking at a sufficiently large number of patients and dialyses treatments, the basic principles discussed above should be mirrored in the clinical dialysis setting.

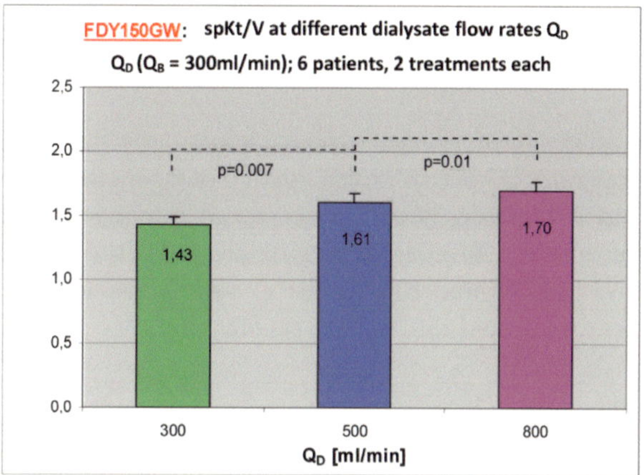

(a)

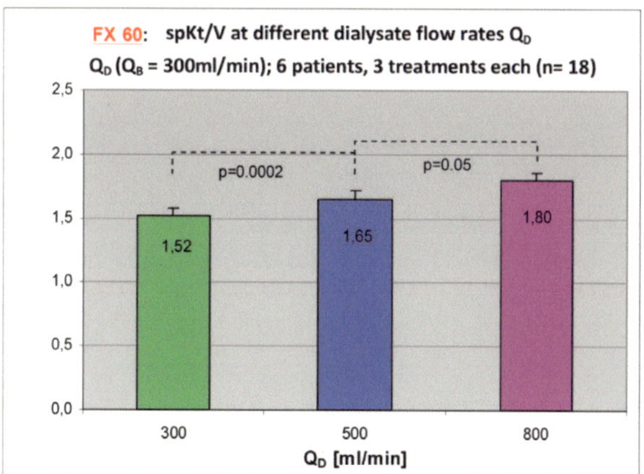

(b)

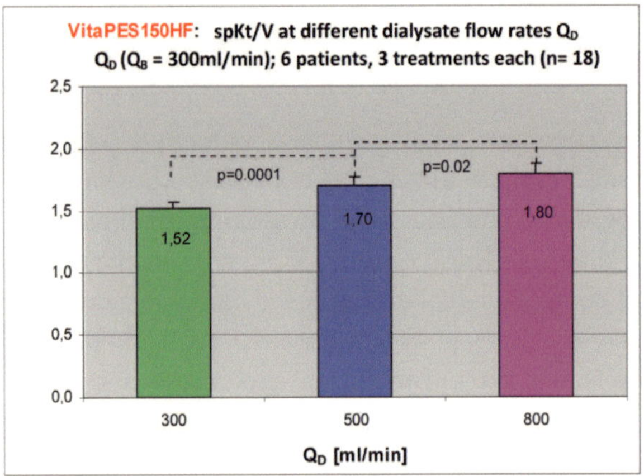

(c)

Figure 5. (a): Dialysate flow rate dependence of the spKt/V value in dialyser FDY150GW (b): Dialysate flow rate dependence of the spKt/V value in dialyser FX60 (c): Dialysate flow rate dependence of the spKt/V value in dialyser VitaPES150HF

At a constant blood flow rate (Q_B=300 ml/min), a group of 6 patients received three treatments each at Q_D=300, 500 und 800 ml/min, with each set repeated for each of the 3 types of dialysers tested in vitro. In order to assess the effectiveness of treatment, the urea reduction ratio, single pool Kt/V (spKt/V) and equilibrated Kt/V (eqKt/V) were obtained (Daugirdas formula). In addition, OCM data were obtained for the dialysis machine FMC 5008 (Eff.Kt, Eff.Kt/V).

The figures show (as do the urea reduction ratios and eqKt/V results) that each step increase in dialysate flow can significantly improve the effectiveness of haemodialysis.

The interesting question for dialysis patients is of course the exact impact this may have on treatment time. A sample calculation using results from the FX60 dialyser will demonstrate this (see Table 3).

Patient	BW_{opt}	V_{calc}	K_{300}	K_{500}	K_{800}	KtV_{300}	t_{300}	$t_{calc500}$	$t_{calc800}$	t_{300}-t_{500}	t_{300}-t_{800}
No.	*kg*	*L*	*ml/min*	*ml/min*	*ml/min*		*min*	*min*	*min*	*min*	*min*
1	75.0	37.1	186	199	209	1.18	240	220	209	**20**	**31**
2	60.0	26.9	181	197	207	1.57	240	215	204	**25**	**36**
3	66.0	23.0	158	190	202	1.35	180	163	154	**17**	**26**
4	75.5	33.6	184	202	216	1.71	300	285	267	**15**	**33**
5	69.0	31.8	173	199	207	1.36	240	217	208	**23**	**32**
6	69.5	27.9	178	188	201	1.93	300	287	268	**13**	**32**

(Vcalc from OCM EffKt and measured Kt/V; tcalc=Kt/V(QD300)*V/K)

Table 3. Time saved by using a dialysate flow rate of $Q_{D=}$500 ml/min or Q_D=800 ml/min instead of a dialysate flow rate of $Q_{D=}$300 ml/min

The same Kt/V value achieved at a dialysate flow rate Q_D=300 ml/min can be achieved at a dialysate flow rate of Q_D=500 ml/min, whilst treatment time can be reduced by between 13 and 25 minutes, depending on the individual patient's body mass and clearance. If a dialysate flow rate of Q_D=800 ml/min is used, treatment time will be reduced accordingly, namely by 26-36 min. Treatment time reduction of this order is certainly of interest to patients and should be able to outweigh the slight increase in costs incurred by higher dialysate flow rates. Naturally, if treatment time remains unchanged, a higher dialysate flow rate can also be used to improve the Kt/V value-as depicted in Fig. 5.

6. Summary

In vitro measurements obtained from a number of different modern high flux dialysers show that the characteristics "Clearance (Q_B, Q_D)" manage to closely match theoretical scenarios of expected interdependence. However, in spite of a number of different structural improvements, the KoA value remains dependent upon the dialysate flow rate. A higher dialysate flow rate of around 800 ml/min ensures that the fibre bundle is bathed more evenly in dialysate, thus improving the effectiveness of dialysis.

In vivo investigations confirm that increases in dialysate flow rates are likely to produce significantly improved Kt/V values.

Author details

Peter Ahrenholz[1], Roland E. Winkler[1*] and Diego Zendeh-Zartochti[2]

*Address all correspondence to: roland.winkler@praxisverbund-rostock.de

1 BioArtProducts GmbH Rostock, Rostock, Germany

2 Praxisverbund Dialyse und Apherese Rostock, Rostock, Germany

References

[1] Klein E, Autian J, Bower JD, Buffaloe G, Centella LJ, Colton CK, Darby TD, Farrell PC, Holland FF, Kennedy RS, et al.: Evaluation of hemodialyzers and dialysis membranes. Report of a study for the artificial kidney-chronic uremia program NIAMDD-1977. Artif Organs. 1978 Aug; 2(3):284-92.

[2] Weryński A: Evaluation of the impact of ultrafiltration on dialyzer clearance. Artif Organs. 1979 May;3(2):140-2.

[3] Ronco C, Bredolan A, Crepaldi C, Rodighiero M, Scabardi M: Blood and dialysate flow distributions in hollow-fiber hemodialyzers analyzed by computerized helical scanning technique. J Am Soc Nephrol 13: S53-S61, 2002

[4] Gastaldon F, Brendolan A, Crepaldi C, Frisone P, Zamboni S, d'Intini V, Poulin S, Hector R, Granziero A, Martins K, Gellert R, Inguaggiato P, Ronco C: Effects of novel manufacturing technology on blood and dialysate flow distribution in a new low flux "alpha Polysulfone" hemodialyzer. Int J Artif Organs. 2003 Feb;26(2):105-112

[5] Kim JC, Kim JH, Kim HC, Kim KG, Lee JC, Kang E, Kim HC, Min BG, Ronco C: Three-dimensional dialysate flow analysis in a hollow-fiber dialyzer by perfusion computed tomography. Int J Artif Organs. 2008 Jun;31(6):553-60.

[6] Külz M, Nederlof B, Schneider H: In vitro and in vivo evaluation of a new dialyzer. Nephrol Dial Transplant (2002) 17: 1475-1479

[7] Leypoldt JK, Cheung AK, Agodoa LY, Daugirdas JT, Greene T, Keshaviah PR: Hemodialyzer mass transfer-area coefficients for urea increase at high dialysate flow rates. The Hemodialysis (HEMO) Study. Kidney Int. 1997 Jun;51(6):2013-7.

[8] Golper TA, Ward RA: Dialysate... Ho-hum! Clin J Am Soc Nephrol. 2009 Sep;4(9): 1403-4. Epub 2009 Aug 20.

Chapter 12

Principles and Practices of Haemodiafiltration

Eric T. Chou, Ross S. Francis, David W. Mudge,
Carmel M. Hawley and David W. Johnson

Additional information is available at the end of the chapter

http://dx.doi.org/10.5772/59470

1. Introduction

Options for renal replacement therapy (RRT) for patients with end-stage kidney disease (ESKD) include haemodialysis, peritoneal dialysis and renal transplantation. Although renal transplantation offers the best outcomes in terms of quality and quantity of life, most patients with ESKD will be treated with dialysis, either because they are ineligible for transplantation due to their burden of comorbid medical conditions, or because they commonly have to wait several years on dialysis before they are able to receive a kidney transplant. Survival of patients on dialysis remains poor, with reported annual mortality rates ranging from 12.7% in Australia and 14.6% for New Zealand [1] to 17.9% in Europe [2] to 25% in the United States of America [3]. Alternative ways of delivering dialysis that will materially improve patient outcomes are therefore required.

Emerging data suggest that haemodiafiltration (HDF), a form of haemodialysis that combines both diffusive and convective solute removal, may offer clinical benefits when compared to standard high-flux haemodialysis (HD). Despite these findings, the global uptake of haemodiafiltration is variable and generally low, ranging from minimal use in the United States, 3.1% in the United Kingdom to 6% in Australia and 28.8% in Belgium [2]. This chapter will provide an overview of the principles and technical aspects of haemodiafiltration, as well as review the clinical evidence comparing HDF outcomes with those of HD.

2. Diffusive versus convective therapy

Physical removal of solutes across a dialysis membrane occurs via diffusion (passive movement down a concentration gradient) and/or convection (obligatory "dragging" of solutes by fluid removal across the dialysis membrane, i.e. solvent drag) [4]. Some solutes, especially proteins, may also be removed to a limited extent by adsorption to the dialysis membrane.

In conventional low-flux haemodialysis, solute clearance predominantly occurs via diffusion across the dialysis membrane in a counter-current set up whereby blood flows in one direction and the dialysate flows in the other (Figure 1). Solutes move across the semi-permeable dialysis membrane down a concentration gradient. The factors that lead to a higher rate of diffusive exchange are 1) larger concentration gradient; 2) larger membrane pore size; 3) smaller solute molecular size; 4) larger exchange surface area; 5) higher blood flow rate; and, 6) higher dialysate flow rate. Diffusion represents the main mechanism for removal of low molecular weight molecules (<500 Daltons), such as urea (60 Da) and creatinine (113 Da), but is relatively inefficient at removing middle molecules (500 – 60,000 Daltons) [5], such as β2-microglobulin (11,500 Da), and does not appreciably remove large molecules (>60,000 Da), such as albumin (66,500 Da). This limitation can be overcome to a certain extent by the use of high-flux dialysis membranes with a larger pore size. High-flux dialysers permit increased blood water transfer across the membrane at the proximal end of the dialyser, compensated by the phenomenon of backfiltration, in which dialysate flows across the membrane at the distal end of the dialyser under a hydrostatic pressure gradient. Concentration of plasma proteins in the blood compartment will also exert osmotic pull, further contributing to backfiltration [6]. This process results in "internal" convection of up to 5-10L per dialysis treatment, and improves clearance of middle molecules compared to low-flux dialysis.

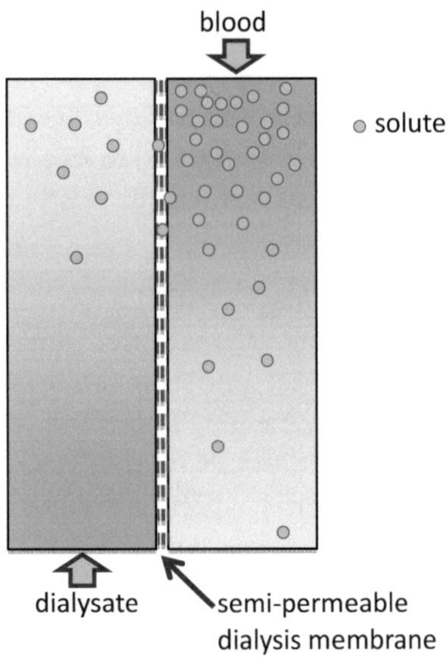

Figure 1. Conventional haemodialysis. A solute, shown dissolved in blood, moves across the semi-permeable dialysis membrane by diffusion, into the dialysate, with blood and dialysate flowing in opposite directions (countercurrent). The rate of diffusion is dependent on the initial concentration in the blood, the blood flow rate, the permeability of the membrane for the solute, and the dialysate flow rate. Removal of water (ultrafiltration) is determined largely but the pressure across the membrane.

http://dx.doi.org/10.5772/59470

In contrast to haemodialysis, haemofiltration clears solutes primarily via convection, allowing water and solutes up to 20 kDa to cross the membrane and achieving more efficient removal of middle and large molecular weight solutes (Figure 2). The factors that lead to a higher rate of convective removal of solute are 1) volume of ultrafiltration, 2) a higher sieving coefficient (solute concentration in the ultrafiltrate divided by plasma concentration) and 3) a higher transmembrane pressure (which leads to a higher ultrafiltration rate) [7]. Given that haemofiltration is dependent upon large volume ultrafiltration, replacement fluid needs to be infused back into the patient to prevent excessive fluid removal. However, although haemofiltration provides efficient clearance of middle and large molecular weight molecules, it is less efficient at removing small molecular weight solutes than conventional haemodialysis.

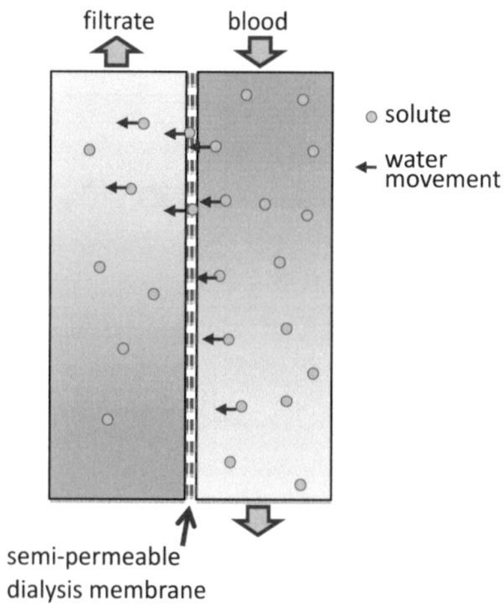

Figure 2. Haemofiltration (convection). Movement of water across the more water-permeable membrane 'drags' solute across, and leads to production of a filtrate which contains the solute. Solute removal is largely dependent on the ultrafiltration rate, but is limited by haemoconcentration and so 'pure' haemofiltration is not practical without replacement of fluid.

The distinct and separate advantages of haemofiltration (efficient middle and large molecule clearance) and haemodialysis (efficient small solute clearance) are combined by the technique of HDF, which provides both diffusive and convective clearances (Figure 3). This theoretically offers better overall clearance of small, middle and large molecular weight substances. HDF can produce convective volumes of greater than 20L per session, and this can be achieved by several different means:

1. "Internal" HDF: Achieved through the process of backfiltration in high flux haemodialysis. As mentioned above, this results in smaller convective volumes compared to dedicated HDF modality.

2. Classical HDF: Characterised by the use of an external substitution fluid in the form of sterile solution stored in plastic bags. Logistic and cost issues limit the use of this modality.

3. Online HDF: A form of HDF whereby substitution fluid is produced by the dialysis machine, creating ultrapure dialysate that is sterile, non-pyrogenic, continuous and unlimited while the machine is in operation [4].

As discussed later in the chapter, convective volume, and therefore enhanced removal of larger uraemic toxins, has emerged as an important parameter in outcomes relating to convective therapies. Convective dose is defined as the total ultrafiltered volume, which equates to the sum of volume gained/lost and substitution fluid given [7]. Convective dose has been proposed as the key quantifier of online-HDF by the European Dialysis (EUDIAL) group [8].

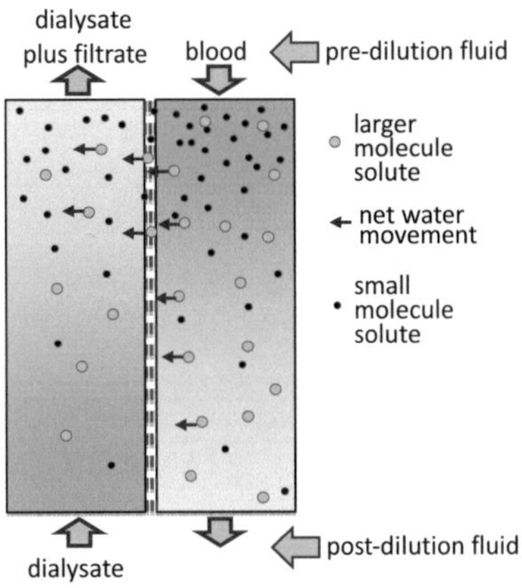

Figure 3. Haemodiafiltration (HDF). HDF combines dialysis and filtration across a semi-permeable membrane but uses much larger volumes of dialysate. Extra ultrapure water can be added either pre-dilution or post-dilution to replace the filtrate. Small solutes are removed largely by diffusion whereas larger solutes (middle molecules) are removed by convection. Water removal (ultrafiltration) is regulated by varying the volume of replacement fluid.

3. Important considerations for haemodiafiltration

3.1. Membrane

Haemodialysis and haemodiafiltration utilise filter membranes composed of cellulose, substituted cellulose or synthetic material. The ideal membrane will provide both solute removal capability as well as biocompatibility [9]. Contact of blood with dialysis membranes elicits inflammatory response, including activation of complement system, polymorphonuclear cells and mononuclear cells [10]. A biocompatible membrane is one that elicits the least amount of inflammatory response in patients exposed to it [11]. Membranes can be described in terms of their efficiency (rate of removal of small solutes) and flux (rate of removal of middle molecules).

High-flux membranes can remove molecules as large as 20kDa, which is better than a traditional low-flux membrane, but still inferior to glomeruli, which can clear molecules up to

http://dx.doi.org/10.5772/59470

65kDa [12]. 'Super high-flux' or 'high cut-off' membranes have been developed to remove larger molecules of up to 50-60kDa, in an attempt to remove larger uraemic toxins and inflammatory mediators [12, 13]. Early data using these membranes have indicated enhanced clearance of free light chains and myoglobin, in patients with myeloma and rhabdomyolysis respectively, although larger clinical trials are required to demonstrate their impact on important clinical outcomes. Loss of important serum proteins such as albumin is significant, and represents a potential disadvantage of using 'high cut-off' membranes, because of the risk of protein malnutrition [12].

3.2. Ultrapure dialysate

Convective therapies result in infusion of substantial quantities of dialysate and substitution fluid, and a major challenge in HDF is the generation of ultrapure dialysate that is sterile and non-pyrogenic. This is because dialysate contaminants can enter the blood via convection or by direct infusion as substitution fluid [14]. The European Best Practice Guidelines (ERPG), American National Standards Institute / Association for Advancement of Medical Instrumentation (ANSI/AAMI) and International Organization for Standardisation (ISO) all mandate that ultrapure fluid contains no more bacteria than 0.1 colony forming units (CFU)/mL, and endotoxins no more than 0.03 endotoxin unit (EU)/mL [14]. Previous studies indicate that ultrapure dialysate improves inflammation-related parameters such as C-reactive protein [14], albumin and haemoglobin [14-17], although endpoints such as mortality and cardiovascular events have not been adequately demonstrated in high quality trials to date.

3.3. Site of fluid replacement

In HDF, ultrafiltration for convective solute clearance necessitates that replacement fluid is administered to maintain appropriate fluid balance. The site at which the replacement fluid is infused has an important impact on several dialysis variables.

In post-dilution mode, replacement fluid is added to the venous side of the circuit, distal to the filter. The convective clearance is the same as the volume of filtrate. This is the most efficient form of HDF, with respect to solute clearance, however this modality is complicated by the effects of haemoconcentration. At high ultrafiltration rates the haematocrit rises within the dialyser, increasing the risk of the filter clotting as well as membrane pore occlusion caused by adherence of plasma proteins [8]. Haemoconcentration is proportional to the filtration fraction, typically defined as the ratio of ultrafiltration rate to blood flow rate, which is usually limited to $<25\%$ in post-dilution HDF, and necessitates a high blood flow rate [6].

In pre-dilution mode, replacement fluid is given to the arterial side of the circuit, diluting blood before it is filtered. This mitigates the effect of ultrafiltration on haemoconcentration, but at the cost of reducing the efficiency of both diffusive and convective solute clearance. As a result, to achieve equivalent clearances, the ultrafiltration rate is typically set two-fold higher when performing pre-dilution HDF compared to post-dilution HDF. While many centres use post-dilution HDF, dialysis centres in Japan have more experience employing pre-dilution HDF [18,

19]. From their experience, pre-dilution has comparable effects on removal of uraemic toxins, reduces shear stress and results in stable blood pressures during treatment [18].

Recently, mid-dilution HDF has been made possible with the development of specialised dialysis circuits that permit infusion of replacement fluid between an initial post-dilution and subsequent pre-dilution stage. The advantage of this design is the ability to allow higher reinfusion rates, and early studies show better clearance of urea, β2-microglobulin and phosphate compared with high-flux HD [20, 21].

Finally, mixed dilution combining pre-and post-dilution has been developed with the aim of providing the most safe and efficient clearance of solutes. A small study of ten patients suggested that mixed dilution may provide superior clearances compared to mid-dilution, citing high transmembrane pressures in the mid-dilution dialyser potentially compromising membrane permeability and therefore infusion rate [22]. While different modes of fluid replacement in HDF have demonstrated advantages and disadvantages in small pilot studies, more data from larger studies are required to convincingly demonstrate the relative efficacy and safety of each method. For now, regional availability and experience tend to dictate the method utilised.

3.4. Cost effectiveness

One important consideration when deciding whether to adopt HDF is that of cost and cost-effectiveness. One French centre estimated that for each session, additional consumables (-€2.55 to+€3.35), microbiological analysis (€1.10) and water consumption (€0.15 to €0.23, based on 50.8 to 74.8 L), resulted in a cost of €-1.29 to €+4.58 per session for HDF over conventional HD [23]. Another cost analysis conducted in the United Kingdom over a 12 month period comparing HDF and high-flux HD found variable consumables costs (-£0.78 to+£1.16, depending on type of line used), similar erythropoiesis stimulating usage and less phosphate binder use (£3.8 and £5.0 weekly) in the HDF group [24].

A cost analysis of HDF versus haemodialysis was performed based on data from the CONTRAST study (mentioned later in the chapter) comparing low-flux HD and HDF. It was found that the annual costs for HDF and HD were €88,722 ± 19,272 and €86,086 ± 15,945, respectively, in 2009 in Europe [25]. However, when cost-utility analysis was applied to assess difference in quality of life, the incremental cost per quality-adjusted year (QALY) of HDF over HD was €287,769. Based on this analysis, the authors concluded that HDF was not cost effective, as concurred by McBrien, et al [26].

3.5. Potential role in home haemodialysis

To date, little data has been published regarding HDF utlisation in the home setting. This is not surprising, given that it is yet to be established as the predominant method of haemodialysis. If applied in the home setting, an extra filter used to produce ultrapure dialysate may provide benefits relating to inflammatory parameters, as mentioned above.

http://dx.doi.org/10.5772/59470

4. Clinical benefits of HDF compared with HD

4.1. Mortality

The first large randomised trial performed to compare different doses and flux of dialyser was published in 2002. The Effect of Dialysis Dose and Membrane Flux in Maintenance Hemodialysis (HEMO) study [27] was a two-by-two factorial design randomised controlled trial which enrolled 1846 patients between 1995 and 2000, and assigned them to receive standard dose (Kt/V urea of 1.05) or high dose (Kt/V urea of 1.45) dialysis, and to a low-flux or high-flux dialyser. Flux was estimated based on β2-microglobulin clearance, with the low-flux group achieving 3±7mL/min and the high-flux group achieving 34±11mL/min. The primary outcome measured was death from any cause, with mean follow up of 2.84 years. The study found 0.166 deaths per patient-year, and that the rate of mortality did not vary significantly across the groups [27].

However, potential survival benefit from convective therapy was suggested by subsequent clinical data, such as the Dialysis Outcomes and Practice Pattern Study (DOPPS) – Mortality risk for patients receiving haemodiafiltration versus haemodialysis: European results from the DOPPS [28]. In this prospective cohort study involving 2165 patients recruited between 1998 and 2001, patients were stratified into four groups: low-or high-flux HD, low-or high-efficiency HDF. The usage of HDF varied greatly between countries, with 1.8% in Spain and up to 20.1% in Italy [28]. Adjusted mortality rate showed high-efficiency HDF patients had a 35% lower mortality risk than those receiving low-flux HD (p=0.01) [28], suggesting that high convective clearance lowers risk of death, independent of dialysis dose. However, this needs to be considered in the context of the observational nature of the study and possible selection bias with residual confounding.

In a Cochrane review in 2009, published evidence on HDF, HF and HD were compared, including 20 randomised trials. There was no significant difference in mortality or hospitalisations [29] between the 3 treatment modalities. However, given the relatively small number of patients in the studies and their heterogeneous nature, the conclusion of this review suggested that larger studies would be needed to prove the benefit of convective therapies.

Recently, three large, randomised controlled trials have compared haemodiafiltration with haemodialysis. While their designs were slightly different, they all measured important patient-level outcomes such as mortality, cardiovascular events, and hospitalisations, amongst others. These three trials were, respectively, the Convective Transport Study (CONTRAST) [30], Comparison of Post-dilution Online Haemodiafiltration and Haemodialysis (Turkish OL-HDF study) [31] and Online Haemodiafiltration Survival Study (ESHOL: *Estudio de Supervivencia de Haemodiafiltracion*) [32]. These three trials will be described in further detail.

In the CONTRAST study, 714 patients across the Netherlands, Canada and Norway, recruited between 2004 and 2009, were enrolled and randomised to post-dilution online HDF (n=358) or low-flux HD (n=356) [30]. One of the remarkable feats of this study was the achievement of 100% follow up. The mean follow up was 3.04 years. No significant difference was observed between the treatment groups with respect to the primary outcome measure of all-cause mortality (HR 0.95, 95% CI 0.75-1.20), even after adjustment for potential confounders. However, a subsequent *post hoc* analysis, indicated that patients who achieved a higher convective volume (>21.95 L per session), experienced a 38% risk reduction for mortality compared to the low-flux HD group (p=0.012). A potential limitation is that the pre-defined target convection of 6 L per hour (based on modelling calculations) was not reached: the mean convection volume was 20.7 L, and one third of patients received 18 L or less, mainly caused by inadequate vascular access [33].

In the Turkish OL-HDF study, 782 ESKD patients recruited between 2007 and 2008 were randomised to receive high-flux HD (n=391) or post-dilution online HDF (n=391) over a mean follow-up period of 22.7 months [31]. The primary outcome was a composite of all-cause mortality and non-fatal cardiovascular events. The investigators did not find a significant difference in event free survival (HD group 74.8% versus OL-HDF 77.6%, p=0.28). However, on *post hoc* analysis, it was again demonstrated that OL-HDF patients who received higher convective volumes (> 17.4 L per session) experienced a 46% lower risk of mortality (p=0.02) after adjustment for other potential risk factors [31]. Patients recruited in this study had spent considerably longer time on dialysis (average 57.9 months), and therefore mortality rate was likely affected by survival selection bias. The average age of patients selected was also far younger at 56.5 years.

The ESHOL study was an open-label, randomised controlled trial conducted in Catalonia, Spain [32]. 906 patients recruited between 2007 and 2008 who were already on haemodialysis were randomised to receive high-flux haemodialysis (n=450) or post-dilution online HDF (n=456). Unlike CONTRAST and the Turkish OL-HDF study, the ESHOL study specifically targeted high convective volumes in the HDF group. The median follow up was 2.08 years and the primary outcome measured was all-cause mortality. At 3 years, the detected mortality rate was 27.1% in the HD group compared to 18.6% in OL-HDF group (30% risk reduction, hazard ratio 0.53-0.92, p=0.01), in contrast with the two above studies. They also detected a lower risk of stroke (HR 0.39, p=0.03) and lower rate of hospitalisations (HR 0.78, p=0.001)

It is interesting that the three trials, conducted at similar times, produced different outcome results for all-cause mortality. Based on the *post-hoc* analyses of CONTRAST and the Turkish OL-HDF suggesting a mortality benefit in patients achieving higher convective volumes, a possible explanation for the difference is the higher convective volume achieved in the ESHOL trial (mean of 22.9 – 23.9 L per session, compared with 20.7L per session in CONTRAST and 17.2L per session in the Turkish OL-HDF). Furthermore, there was a difference in time already on dialysis at the point of randomisation, which may have contributed to lead-time bias. Different practices in various regions may also have led to centre-effect bias.

A meta-analysis undertaken in early 2014 (Wang A, et al) analysed 16 randomised controlled trials published thus far comparing HD and HF/HDF in terms of cardiovascular outcomes and mortality [34]. Of these, 11 included HDF, 4 incorporated HF, and one included either modality. The three recently published randomised trials contribute to the majority of the data analysis, due to their large patient numbers. The authors did not find significant reduction associated with convective therapies in terms of cardiovascular events (RR 0.85, 95% CI 0.66 – 1.10) or all-cause mortality (RR 0.83, 95% CI 0.65 – 1.05). There was reduction in symptomatic

http://dx.doi.org/10.5772/59470

hypotension (RR 0.49, 95% CI 0.30 – 0.81) and improved β2-microglobulin levels (-5.95mg/L, 95% CI-10.27 to – 1.64mg/L) [34].

	CONTRAST [30]	Turkish OL-HDF [31]	ESHOL [32]
Total patient number	714	782	906
Control group	Low-flux HD (n = 356)	High-flux HD (n = 391)	High-flux HD (n = 450)
HDF group	Post-dilution HDF (n = 358)	Post-dilution HDF (n = 391)	Post-dilution HDF (n = 456)
Average patient age	64.1 years	56.5 ± 13.9 years	65.4 ± 14.4 years
Prior time on dialysis	34.8 ± 33.6 months	57.9 ± 44.6 months	28.0 (12 – 59) months
Mean follow up	3.04 yrs, range 0.4-6.6	22.7 ± 10.9 months	1.91 ± 1.10 years
Primary outcomes measured	All-cause mortality	All-cause mortality Non-fatal CV events	All-cause mortality
Secondary outcomes measured	Fatal & non-fatal CV events	CV mortality Intradialytic complications Hospitalisation rate Laboratory parameters	CV mortality Hospitalisation Treatment tolerability Laboratory parameters
Ultrapure dialysate used for both groups	Yes	Not specified	Yes
Convective volume on HDF	20.7 L / session	17.2 ± 1.3 L / session	22.9 – 23.9 L / session
β2 microglobulin reduction	HDF: 4.3 mg/L HD: -3.1 mg/L (p < 0.001)	HDF: 0.67 ± 9.57 mg/L HD: -0.59 ± 9.02 mg/L	Not specified
Primary outcome result	Incidence HDF 121 vs HD 127 per 1000 person-yrs (95% CI 0.75-1.20) **Post hoc*: HDF with convective volume > 21.95L/ session 38% RR for mortality, p = 0.012	Event free survival HDF 77.6%, HD 74.8%, p = 0.28 **Post hoc*: HDF with convective volume > 17.4L/ session 46% RR for mortality, p = 0.02	3 year mortality rate HDF 18.6% vs HD 27.1% (p = 0.01)

*HD=haemodialysis, *HDF=haemodiafiltration, *CV=cardiovascular, *CI=confidence interval

Table 1. Comparison of recent randomised controlled trials

Another review performed by Mostovoya, et al. focused on six published randomised controlled trials only, namely The Italian Cooperative Dialysis Study Group [35], Hemofiltration and haemodiafiltration reduce intradialytic hypotension in ESRF [36], Efficacy of haemodiafiltration [37], alongside CONTRAST, Turkish OL-HDF and ESHOL. In this meta-analysis, HDF was found to have a decreased risk of mortality (RR 0.84, 95% CI 0.73-0.96) and cardiovascular death (RR 0.73, 95% 0.57-0.92) [38]. Data interpretation needs to be taken with caution given the heterogeneous mix of pre-, mid-and post-dilution modes used, as well as different convective volumes achieved.

While these two systematic reviews drew different conclusions based on different trials included in their analyses, there did appear to be a signal suggesting possibly reduced mortality and cardiovascular events when higher convective volumes were achieved. Indeed, in the CONTRAST study [30], convective volumes exceeding 21.95L were associated with a 38% risk reduction. Similarly, in the Turkish OL-HDF trial [31], convective volumes exceeding 17.4 L per session were associated with a 46% risk reduction in mortality. The ESHOL trial showed a difference in mortality, but it achieved higher convective volumes (22.9 – 23.9 L per session) [32] than the CONTRAST and Turkish OL-HDF trials.

4.2. Intradialytic hypotension

In meta-analyses, symptomatic hypotension was reduced by HDF compared to HD, with RR of 0.49 [34]. The ESHOL trial reported significant difference in occurrence, with 769.2 episodes per 100 patient-years in the HDF group compared with 937.7 episodes ($P<0.001$) [32].

4.3. Blood pressure and fluid control

Post-dialysis systolic blood pressure was not significantly affected by treatment modality [34]. The CONTRAST study reported insignificantly different pre-dialysis systolic blood pressure of 146 mmHg for HDF compared to 145 with low-flux HD, and intradialytic weight gain of 1.9 vs 1.85kg [30]. There was also no significant difference in systolic blood pressure in the Turkish study, however a difference in interdialytic weight gain was detected: 3.19% of body mass in the HD group, 3.87% in the low-efficiency HDF group and 3.29% in the high-efficiency group [31]. The ESHOL trial reported no difference in blood pressure levels [32].

4.4. Left ventricular mass

Higher left ventricular mass (LVM) has been associated with cardiovascular and overall mortality in patients on dialysis [39, 40]. A subset of 327 patients from the CONTRAST study was assessed in terms of their LVM at baseline with echocardiography [41]. These patients were stratified into tertiles, and those in the highest tertile (LVM > 260grams) had the highest risk of mortality, cardiovascular death and sudden death. So far one small trial involving 22 patients utilising HDF has demonstrated improvement in left ventricular mass index (131.9 to 116.5 g/m^2) at 1 year [42]. This surrogate marker will need to be more extensively studied to convincingly demonstrate potential long term clinical effect.

4.5. Dialysis related β2-microglobulin amyloidosis

Dialysis related amyloidosis is a syndrome of pain and loss of function due to deposition of amyloid composed of β2-microglobulin in the musculoskeletal system. While β2-microglobulin can be removed on dialysis, pre-dialysis levels often remain elevated [43]. The CONTRAST study demonstrated lower β2-microglobulin level in the HDF group (26.4 mg/L) compared to the HD group (35.4 mg/L), as well as a greater reduction in its level post treatment (4.3 mg/L) [30]. On the other hand, patients in the Turkish study had very similar levels, and achieved a much smaller reduction of 0.67 mg/L [31]. While advancements in renal replacement therapy have allowed manipulation in β2-microglobulin levels, enhanced clearance has not yet translated to clinical difference in dialysis related amyloidosis, particularly given the long periods required for the syndrome to manifest.

http://dx.doi.org/10.5772/59470

4.6. Inflammatory markers

Inflammation in chronic kidney disease has been associated with a range of negative outcomes, including cardiovascular mortality [44], atherosclerosis, protein energy wasting, hypo-responsiveness to erythropoiesis stimulating agents (ESAs), platelet dysfunction and endocrine dysfunction [45]. Chronic inflammation is caused by both cytokine dysregulation in chronic kidney disease [46], and the dialysis process itself [47]. A subset of patients from the CONTRAST study was screened for markers of inflammation, including C-reactive protein (CRP) and interleukin-6 (IL-6) [48]. 201 patients from the HDF arm and 204 patients from the HD arm were selected for this study. Baseline CRP levels were 3.0 mg/L in the HD group and 4.1 mg/L in the HDF group. After 3 years, there was a significant steady rise in CRP level in the HD group (~20% per year) whereas it remained stable in the HDF group. Similarly, IL-6 levels increased in the HD group but not for HDF patients. Both of these figures were adjusted for confounders including age, sex and residual renal function, and still remained significant [48]. Given that ultrapure dialysate were used for both groups, the different measurements appear to have arisen from different modalities of dialysis.

4.7. ESA hypo-responsiveness

Another clinical outcome examined by the CONTRAST investigators was whether use of HD or HDF resulted in a difference in resistance to erythropoiesis stimulating agents. This was done given the proposed concept that better clearance of middle molecular weight uraemic toxins would reduce inflammation, and therefore improve responsiveness to ESAs [49]. Starting at statistically similar haemoglobin levels (11.9 g/dL in HDF, 11.8 g/dL in HD), with iron replete, they measured ESA index (weekly weight adjusted ESA dose divided by haematocrit) as a measure of ESA resistance. After 12 months, there was no significant difference found [50]. This finding is in keeping with an earlier randomised controlled study involving 146 patients where allocation to low flux HD or HF/HDF did not improve haemoglobin levels or ESA resistance [51].

4.8. Quality of life measurement

Assessment quality of life is difficult, due to the subjective nature of outcomes as well as different assessment of tools used. One study reported lower physical wellbeing scores while on HD[52], however meta-analyses have shown inconsistent and insignificant differences in quality of life, particularly when measured with Kidney Disease Quality of Life Questionnaire [34, 53].

5. Further trials

As of September 2014, there are several proposed trials currently underway to further elucidate potential clinical benefits of haemodiafiltration, as registered on *ClinicalTrials.gov* [54]:

- Mid-dilution Hemodiafiltration International Randomised Prospective on Incident Patients Focused on Outcome (MILESTONE) [55]
    - Trial identifier: NCT01693354
    - Purpose: "to determine whether mid-dilution haemodiafiltration is effective in the reduction of the crude mortality risk in patients who have been undergoing renal replacement treatment for less than 1 year. Patients will be randomized since the beginning of the study in two groups: standard HF dialysis and mid-dilution HDF"
    - Study type: interventional
    - Estimated enrolment: 800
    - Arms: HF dialysis vs. mid-dilution HDF
    - Primary outcome: crude, all-cause mortality at 5 years
- Tolerance of "On Line" Hemodiafiltration and Impact on Mortality and Cardiovascular Risk Factor in Chronic Renal Failure Patients [56]
    - Trial identifier: NCT01327391
    - Purpose: "to appreciate the tolerance of "on line" hemodiafiltration and its impact on morbidity and cardiovascular risk factors in chronic renal failure patient."
    - Study type: interventional
    - Estimated enrolment: 600
    - Arms: on line hemodiafiltration vs high flux hemodialysis
    - Primary outcome: tolerance of online HDF in terms of adverse events occurring during dialysis sessions
- Randomised Study of High-flux Haemodialysis and Haemodiafiltration [57]
    - Trial identifier: NCT01862679
    - Purpose: to answer the following three main questions in regards to HDF and high-flux HF
        - Does HDF make patients feel better?
        - Is blood pressure more stable on HDF in comparison with HF-HD?
        - Are Phosphate levels and other blood parameters better controlled with HDF than HF-HD?
    - Study type: interventional
    - Estimated enrolment: 100
    - Arms: HF-HF and HDF, crossover at 8 weeks

http://dx.doi.org/10.5772/59470

  - Primary outcome: change in the average time taken to fully recover post dialysis
- The Effects of Haemodiafiltration vs Conventional Haemodialysis on Growth and Cardiovascular Markers in Children – 3H (HDF, Hearts and Height) Study [58]
  - Trial identifier: NCT02063776
  - Purpose: to monitor growth, heart and blood vessel scans, blood markers and quality of life in children
  - Study type: Observational case control
  - Estimated enrolment: 150
  - Arms: children on HDF, children on conventional HD
  - Primary outcome: change in carotid intimate thickness standard deviation score, change in height standard deviation score

6. Conclusion

Haemodiafiltration, utilising convection via high-flux dialysers and ultrapure dialysate, has been shown to exhibit certain advantages over conventional haemodialysis, such as a reduction of intradialytic hypotension, reduction of left ventricular mass and lower β2-microglobulin levels. However, when it comes to important patient-level outcomes such as mortality and cardiovascular events, HDF has not been shown conclusively to be of benefit, although studies to date have been limited by inadequate statistical power and suboptimal methodological quality. It may be that a minimum amount of convective volume needs to be achieved to demonstrate mortality benefits, and that this volume may be in the order between 17.4 and 23.9L per session, given the heterogeneous cut-offs in trials that have suggested a difference in mortality. A large, well-designed, multi-centre, multi-national randomised controlled trial examining this issue is indicated given the suggestive findings of a potential benefit with high volume HDF to date.

Author details

Eric T. Chou[1], Ross S. Francis[1,2], David W. Mudge[1,2], Carmel M. Hawley[1,2] and David W. Johnson[1,2*]

*Address all correspondence to: david.johnson2@health.qld.gov.au

1 Department of Nephrology, Princess Alexandra Hospital, Brisbane, Australia

2 School of Medicine, The University of Queensland, Brisbane, Australia

References

[1] McDonald S. ANZDATA Registry Report 2012. Chapter 3. Deaths. Australia and New Zealand Dialysis and Transplant Registry. 2013:3.1-3.9.

[2] ERA-EDTA Registry. ERA-EDTA Registry Annual Report 2012. Academic Medical Center, Department of Medical Informatics, Amsterdam, The Netherlands. 2014.

[3] US Renal Data System. USRDS 2013 Annual Data Report: Atlas of Chronic Kidney Disease and End-Stage Renal Disease in the United States. National Institutes of Health, National Institute of Diabetes and Digestive and Kidney Diseases. 2013.

[4] Fischbach M, Fothergill H, Zaloszyc A, Seuge L. Hemodiafiltration: the addition of convective flow to hemodialysis. Pediatric nephrology. 2012;27(3):351-6.

[5] Clark WR, Winchester JF. Middle molecules and small-molecular-weight proteins in ESRD: properties and strategies for their removal. Advances in renal replacement therapy. 2003;10(4):270-8.

[6] Petrie J, Ng T, Hawley C. Is it time to embrace haemodiafiltration for centre based haemodialysis? Nephrology. 2008;13:269-77.

[7] Bowry SK, Canaud B. Achieving high convective volumes in on-line hemodiafiltration. Blood purification. 2013;35 Suppl 1:23-8.

[8] Tattersall JE, Ward RA, group E. Online haemodiafiltration: definition, dose quantification and safety revisited. Nephrology, dialysis, transplantation : official publication of the European Dialysis and Transplant Association-European Renal Association. 2013;28(3):542-50.

[9] Sanaka T, Koremoto M. Selection guidelines for high-performance membrane. Contrib Nephrol. 2011;173(30-5).

[10] Grooteman MP, Nube MJ. Impact of the type of dialyser on the clinical outcome in chronic haemodialysis patients: does it really matter? Nephrology, dialysis, transplantation : official publication of the European Dialysis and Transplant Association-European Renal Association. 2004;19(12):2965-70.

[11] Hakim RM. Clinical implications of hemodialysis membrane biocompatibility. Kidney international. 1993;44(3):484-94.

[12] Gondouin B, Hutchison CA. High cut-off dialysis membranes: current uses and future potential. Advances in chronic kidney disease. 2011;18(3):180-7.

[13] Naka T, Haase M, Bellomo R. 'Super high-flux' or 'high cut-off' hemofiltration and hemodialysis. Contrib Nephrol. 2010;166:181-9.

[14] Glorieux G, Neirynck N, Veys N, Vanholder R. Dialysis water and fluid purity: more than endotoxin. Nephrology, dialysis, transplantation : official publication of the Eu-

ropean Dialysis and Transplant Association-European Renal Association. 2012;27:4010-21.

[15] Arizono K, Nomura K, Motoyama T, Matsushita Y, Matsuoka K, Miyazu R, et al. Use of ultrapure dialysate in reduction of chronic inflammation during hemodialysis. Blood purification. 2004;22 Suppl 2:26-9.

[16] Izuhara Y, Miyata T, Saito K, Ishikawa N, Kakuta T, Nangaku M, et al. Ultrapure dialysate decreases plasma pentosidine, a marker of "carbonyl stress". American journal of kidney diseases : the official journal of the National Kidney Foundation. 2004;43(6):1024-9.

[17] Rahmati MA, Homel P, Hoenich NA, Levin R, Kaysen GA, Levin NW. The role of improved water quality on inflammatory markers in patients undergoing regular dialysis. The International journal of artificial organs. 2004;27(8):723-7.

[18] Tsuchida K, Minakuchi J. Clinical benefits of predilution on-line hemodiafiltration. Blood purification. 2013;35 Suppl 1:18-22.

[19] Masakane I, Esashi S, Igarashi H. Biocompatibility of predilution on-line hemodiafiltration. Blood purification. 2013;35 Suppl 1:34-8.

[20] Santoro A, Conz PA, De Cristofaro V, Acquistapace I, Gaggi R, Ferramosca E, et al. Mid-dilution: the perfect balance between convection and diffusion. Contrib Nephrol. 2005;149:107-14.

[21] Krieter DH, Falkenhain S, Chalabi L, Collins G, Lemke HD, Canaud B. Clinical crossover comparison of mid-dilution hemodiafiltration using a novel dialyzer concept and post-dilution hemodiafiltration. Kidney international. 2005;67(1):349-56.

[22] Feliciani A, Riva MA, Zerbi S, Ruggiero P, Plati AR, Cozzi G, et al. New strategies in haemodiafiltration (HDF): prospective comparative analysis between on-line mixed HDF and mid-dilution HDF. Nephrology, dialysis, transplantation : official publication of the European Dialysis and Transplant Association-European Renal Association. 2007;22(6):1672-9.

[23] Lebourg L, Amato S, Toledano D, Petitclerc T, Creput C. Online hemodiafiltration: is it really more expensive? Nephrologie & therapeutique. 2013;9(4):209-14.

[24] Oates T, Cross J, Davenport A. Cost comparison of online haemodiafiltration with high-flux haemodialysis. Journal of nephrology. 2012;25(2):192-7.

[25] Mazairac A, Blankestijn P, Penne E, van der Weerd N, den Hoedt C, Buskens E, et al. The cost-utility of haemodiafiltration versus haemodialysis in the convective transpot study. Nephrology, dialysis, transplantation : official publication of the European Dialysis and Transplant Association-European Renal Association. 2013;28:1865-73.

[26] McBrien K, B M. Haemodiafiltration: not effective or cost-effective compared with haemodialysis. Nephrology, dialysis, transplantation : official publication of the Eu-

ropean Dialysis and Transplant Association-European Renal Association. 2013;28:1630-3.

[27] Eknoyan G BG, Cheung A, Daugirdas J, Greene T, Kusek J. Effect of dialysis dose and membrane flux in maintenance hemodialysis. N Eng J Med. 2002;347(25): 2010-19.

[28] Canaud B, Bragg-Gresham JL, Marshall MR, Desmeules S, Gillespie BW, Depner T, et al. Mortality risk for patients receiving hemodiafiltration versus hemodialysis: European results from the DOPPS. Kidney international. 2006;69(11):2087-93.

[29] Rabindranath KS SG, Roderick PJ, Wallace SA, MacLeod AM. Haemodiafiltration, haemofiltration and haemodialysis for end-stage renal disease (review). The Cochrane Collaboration. 2006.

[30] Grooteman MP, van den Dorpel MA, Bots ML, Penne EL, van der Weerd NC, Mazairac AH, et al. Effect of online hemodiafiltration on all-cause mortality and cardiovascular outcomes. Journal of the American Society of Nephrology : JASN. 2012;23(6):1087-96.

[31] Ok E, Asci G, Toz H, Ok ES, Kircelli F, Yilmaz M, et al. Mortality and cardiovascular events in online haemodiafiltration (OL-HDF) compared with high-flux dialysis: results from the Turkish OL-HDF Study. Nephrology, dialysis, transplantation : official publication of the European Dialysis and Transplant Association-European Renal Association. 2013;28(1):192-202.

[32] Maduell F, Moreso F, Pons M, Ramos R, Mora-Macia J, Carreras J, et al. High-efficiency postdilution online hemodiafiltration reduces all-cause mortality in hemodialysis patients. Journal of the American Society of Nephrology : JASN. 2013;24(3): 487-97.

[33] Kuhlmann MK. On-line hemodiafiltration: not a self-fulfilling prophecy. Journal of the American Society of Nephrology : JASN. 2012;23(6):974-5.

[34] Wang AY, Ninomiya T, Al-Kahwa A, Perkovic V, Gallagher MP, Hawley C, et al. Effect of hemodiafiltration or hemofiltration compared with hemodialysis on mortality and cardiovascular disease in chronic kidney failure: a systematic review and meta-analysis of randomized trials. American journal of kidney diseases : the official journal of the National Kidney Foundation. 2014;63(6):968-78.

[35] Locatelli F, Mastrangelo F, Redaelli B, Ronco C, Marcelli D, La GG, et al. Effects of different membranes and dialysis technologies on patient treatment tolerance and nutritional parameters. The Italian Cooperative Dialysis Study Group. Kidney international. 1996;50(4):1293-302.

[36] Locatelli F, Altieri P, Andrulli S, Bolaco P, Sau G, Pedrini LA, et al. Hemofiltration and hemodiafiltration reduce intradialytic hypotension in ESRD. Journal of the American Society of Nephrology : JASN. 2010;21(10):1798-807.

[37] Wizemann V, Kulz M, Techert F, Nederlof B. Efficacy of haemodiafiltration. Nephrology, dialysis, transplantation : official publication of the European Dialysis and Transplant Association-European Renal Association. 2001;16(Suppl 4):27-30.

[38] Mostovaya IM, Blankestijn PJ, Bots ML, Covic A, Davenport A, Grooteman MPC, et al. Clinical Evidence on Hemodiafiltration: A Systematic Review and a Meta-analysis. Seminars in Dialysis. 2014;27(2):119-27.

[39] Zoccali C, Benedetto FA, Mallamaci F, Tripepi G, Giacone G, Stancanelli B, et al. Left ventricular mass monitoring in the follow-up of dialysis patients: prognostic value of left ventricular hypertrophy progression. Kidney international. 2004;65(4):1492-8.

[40] London GM, Pannier B, Guerin AP, Blacher J, Marchais SJ, Darne B, et al. Alterations of left ventricular hypertrophy in and survival of patients receiving hemodialysis: follow-up of an interventional study. Journal of the American Society of Nephrology : JASN. 2001;12(12):2759-67.

[41] Mostovaya IM, Bots ML, van den Dorpel MA, Goldschmeding R, den Hoedt CH, Kamp O, et al. Left ventricular mass in dialysis patients, determinants and relation with outcome. Results from the COnvective TRansport STudy (CONTRAST). PloS one. 2014;9(2):e84587.

[42] Ohtake T, Oka M, Ishioka K, Honda K, Mochida Y, Maesato K, et al. Cardiovascular protective effects of on-line hemodiafiltration: comparison with conventional hemodialysis. Therapeutic apheresis and dialysis : official peer-reviewed journal of the International Society for Apheresis, the Japanese Society for Apheresis, the Japanese Society for Dialysis Therapy. 2012;16(2):181-8.

[43] Drueke TB, Massy ZA. Beta2-microglobulin. Semin Dial. 2009;22(4):378-80.

[44] Herzog CA, Asinger RW, Berger AK, Charytan DM, Diez J, Hart RG, et al. Cardiovascular disease in chronic kidney disease. A clinical update from Kidney Disease: Improving Global Outcomes (KDIGO). Kidney international. 2011;80(6):572-86.

[45] Leurs P, Lindholm B, Stenvinkel P. Effects of hemodiafiltration on uremic inflammation. Blood purification. 2013;35 Suppl 1:11-7.

[46] Carrero JJ, Yilmaz MI, Lindholm B, Stenvinkel P. Cytokine dysregulation in chronic kidney disease: how can we treat it? Blood purification. 2008;26(3):291-9.

[47] Schindler R. Inflammation and dialysate quality. Hemodialysis international International Symposium on Home Hemodialysis. 2006;10 Suppl 1:S56-9.

[48] den Hoedt CH, Bots ML, Grooteman MP, van der Weerd NC, Mazairac AH, Penne EL, et al. Online hemodiafiltration reduces systemic inflammation compared to low-flux hemodialysis. Kidney international. 2014;86(2):423-32.

[49] van der Weerd NC, Den Hoedt CH, Blankestijn PJ, Bots ML, van den Dorpel MA, Levesque R, et al. Resistance to erythropoiesis stimulating agents in patients treated

with online hemodiafiltration and ultrapure low-flux hemodialysis: results from a randomized controlled trial (CONTRAST). PloS one. 2014;9(4):e94434.

[50] van der Weerd N, Den Hoedt C, Blankestijn P, Bots M, van der Dorpel M, Levesque R, et al. Resistance to erythropoiesis stimulating agents in patients treated with on-line hemodiafiltration and ultrapure low-flux hemodialysis: results from a randomized controlled trial (CONTRAST). PloS one. 2014;9(4):e94434.

[51] Locatelli F, Alteiri P, Andrulli S, Sau G, Bolasco P, Pedrini L, et al. Predictors of haemoglobin levels and resistance to erythropoiesis-stimulating agents in patients treated with low-flux haemodialysis, haemofiltration and haemodiafiltration: results of a multicentre randomized and controlled trial. Nephrology, dialysis, transplantation : official publication of the European Dialysis and Transplant Association-European Renal Association. 2012;27:3594-600.

[52] Ward RA, Schmidt B, Hullin J, Hillebrand GF, Samtleben W. A comparison of on-line hemodiafiltration and high-flux hemodialysis: a prospective clinical study. Journal of the American Society of Nephrology : JASN. 2000;11(12):2344-50.

[53] Nistor I, Palmer SC, Craig JC, Saglimbene V, Vecchio M, Covic A, et al. Convective versus diffusive dialysis therapies for chronic kidney failure: an updated systematic review of randomized controlled trials. American journal of kidney diseases : the official journal of the National Kidney Foundation. 2014;63(6):954-67.

[54] ClinicalTrials.gov. Search of hemodiafiltration 2014 [cited 2014 Sep 11]. Available from: http://clinicaltrials.gov/ct2/results?term=hemodiafiltration.

[55] Maduell F, Panichi V, Alijama P, Jadoul M, Brunet P, A S. Mid-HDF Randomized Controlled Study on Outcome (MILESTONE): ClinicalTrials.gov; 2014 [cited 2014 Sep 11]. Available from: http://clinicaltrials.gov/ct2/show/NCT01693354?term=hemodiafiltration&rank=37.

[56] Canaud B, al e. Tolerance of "on Line" Hemodiafiltration in Chronic Renal Failure Patients (on-line-HDF): ClinicalTrials.gov; 2014 [cited 2014 Sep 11]. Available from: http://clinicaltrials.gov/ct2/show/NCT01327391?term=hemodiafiltration&rank=2.

[57] MacTier R. Randomised Study of High-flux Haemodialysis and Haemodiafiltration: ClinicalTrials.gov; 2014 [cited 2014 Sep 11]. Available from: http://clinicaltrials.gov/ct2/show/NCT01862679?term=hemodiafiltration&rank=14.

[58] Shroff R. Haemodiafiltration vs Conventional Haemodialysis in Children (3H) Great Ormond Street Hospital for Children NHS Foundation Trust: ClinicalTrials.gov; 2014 [Sep 11]. Available from: http://clinicaltrials.gov/ct2/show/NCT02063776?term=hemodiafiltration&rank=17.

Chapter 13

Water Treatment for Centre and Home-Based Haemodialysis

Shyam Dheda, Carolyn Van Eps, Carmel Hawley and David W. Johnson

Additional information is available at the end of the chapter

http://dx.doi.org/10.5772/59380

1. Introduction

The process of haemodialysis is mirrored on the physiological principles of the kidney. Specifically the process of diffusion, where blood is made to flow in a counter current to the direction of dialysis fluid and ultrafiltration, where fluid is pressured across a semi permeable membrane using a convective force.

A large quantity of high purity dialysis water is required to safely perform a dialysis treatment. A single 4-hour dialysis treatment can require up to 150L of dialysis quality "ultra pure" water. Producing this high quality water is a multi step filtration process requiring several levels of processing before it is of a sufficient quality to be presented to the dialyser membrane and the patient's blood. Depending on the quality of the source water, the production of this 150L of dialysis quality water, can require the processing of up to 1000L of drinking quality water. This results in between 60 – 90% of source water being rejected to waste.

Ideally pure water used for dialysis should contain no contaminants eg. particles, trace elements, chemicals, organic matter, bacteria or bacterial fragments. Since this water is in direct contact with the blood stream any impurities in the dialysis water has the potential to pass to the patient. Published accepted standards of water quality do exist and specify the minimum concentrations of contaminants that are allowed, bearing in mind that absolute purity is impossible and is often limited by testing thresholds.

Several contamination incidents, some fatal have been described in the literature where patients have inadvertently been exposed to contaminants due to a breakdown in the water purification process. Historical examples include fatal haemolysis from chlorine exposure, bone disease and dementia from aluminium exposure and fatal bacterial contamination resulting in liver failure [1-3]. There is also evidence that bacteria and bacterial fragments especially gram-negative lipopolysaccharide can induce an inflammatory state contributing to erythropoietin resistance, hypotension and a poor nutritional status [4].

Ultrapure water has more stringent microbiological criteria than standard dialysis water and has become the standard in most dialysis units. This is particularly relevant when considering the increasing use of on-line haemodiafiltration, which necessitates large volumes of ultrapure replacement fluid to be infused directly into the patient bloodstream, without the traditional barrier protection of the dialyser membrane. In addition the use of high flux dialyser membranes, theoretically may also allow bacterial fragments to cross into the blood compartment hence further necessitating the need for stringent water standards. Use of ultrapure water is associated with improvement in inflammatory and nutritional markers as well as anaemia and can be produced safely [4-6].

In the home setting much training, education and preparation is necessary prior to a patient safely performing dialysis at home and in turn this is also important with regards to water quality. Patient factors such as dexterity, visual acuity, hygiene, desire to be independent and ability to follow protocols are important. Importantly in the home setting, patients must correctly perform their own chlorine testing, equipment maintenance and WRO disinfection.

This chapter will discuss the various components of the water purification process required for haemodialysis both in the home and in dialysis units. We will also discuss the components of water quality testing and international standards. Finally, with the increasing constraints on water supply, there is a growing awareness of the need for, so called 'green dialysis units', where water conservation practices are utilised.

2. Water source

The quality of the feedwater must be appreciated when setting up a purification system for dialysis, either in a home or an in-centre setting. On a basic level, the lower the concentrations of contaminants the less elaborate the purification system. For instance, the size, number and types of filters necessary for a water purification installation in an inner city suburb with good quality piped water would be different from those for a rural setting with borehole water. Even within the same city and despite similar purification steps there is a considerable difference in the organic and inorganic substances in municipal water due to the difference in the origin of the water. This can be due to geology in the area of the source water (e.g. high iron or clay content), and local industry or farming practice (e.g. pesticide use or heavy metal contamination) in the area.

Rainwater collection tanks are commonly in use in many rural and remote Australian areas. However, this water can also have both microbiological and inorganic contaminants present, due to the roofing materials used and wildlife that have access to the roof (e.g. birds and possums). In one study of 27 households in Brisbane using rainwater tanks, 63% of tank water samples tested positive for E Coli and 78% tested positive for enterococci. [7]

http://dx.doi.org/10.5772/59380

Municipal water is primarily sourced from 2 areas, surface water and groundwater. Groundwater includes wells, aquifers and springs. They have less organic materials but higher inorganic ions eg. metals. Surface water, incudes lakes, ponds and rivers and have more organic matter, microbes and contaminants (eg pesticide, sewerage)

There are several processes involved in converting source water to drinking water standard. These include:

- **Sedimentation**, by which large particles are allowed to settle
- **Flocculation** where particles that remain suspended are removed by adding a coagulant (e.g. aluminium or iron sulphates) to form larger complexes called flocs, which are then removed, through a process of filtration and adsorption
- **Softening**: where calcium and magnesium salts are removed
- **Oxidation and disinfection**: is most commonly achieved with the addition of chlorine.
- **Carbon filtration**: the water is finally passed through a carbon filter to remove any remaining chemicals.

Type:	Ground water	Surface water	Rainwater
Example:	Wells, springs	Lakes, ponds, rivers	Rooftop
Inorganic ions eg metals	High	Normal	Variable (dependent of roof construction)
Organic material eg bacteria, pesticides	Less	High	Present, variable

Table 1. Types of source water

Several instances in the literature highlight the unfortunate morbidity experienced by patients due to a failure to recognize the importance of knowing the source and nature of feed water used for dialysis. One such incident occurred in Brazil in 1996 where 26 patients died from acute liver failure following failure to recognize that the water supply was not being chlorinated. This led to poisoning by bacterial cyanotoxins, which are highly hepatotoxic. [8]

3. Components of the water system

Improving water quality to a standard required for safe haemodialysis utilises a step wise, water filtration process. Each component is specially designed to remove certain contaminants and is arranged in a manner so as to protect and increase the efficiency of the downstream components (Figure 1). For example, carbon filters efficiently remove chlorine, which is not removed by water reverse osmosis (WRO) and can damage WRO membranes, thereby reducing their efficiency.

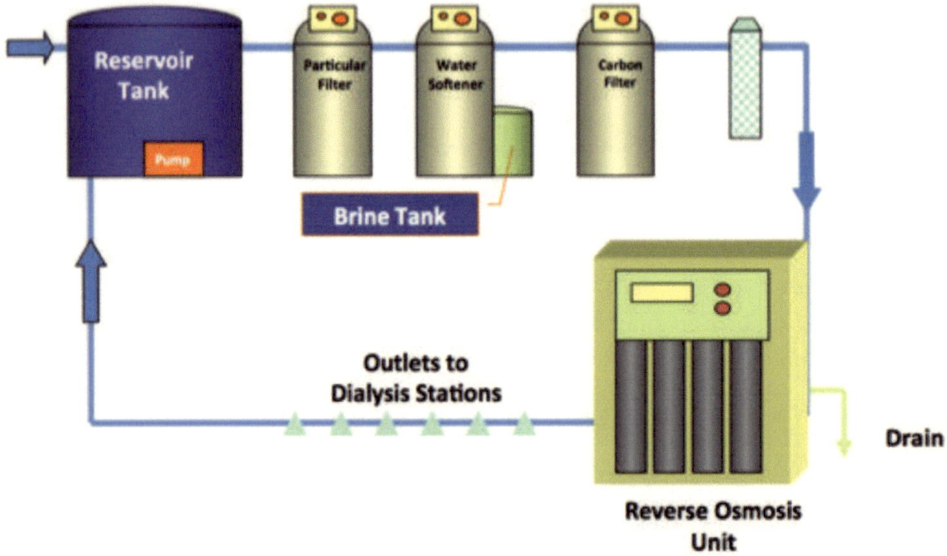

Figure courtesy of Fresenius Medical Care © Australia Pty Ltd. A typical dialysis water treatment setup consists of a reservoir tank, particle filters (multimedia, micron, bag filters), a water softener and 2 carbon tanks in series.

Figure 1. Schematic representation of a typical dialysis water treatment circuit

In centre dialysis units supplying multiple dialysis machines, which are used up to thrice a day, require large amounts of dialysis water and hence more involved filtration systems. However, even though home haemodialysis setups supply only one machine, they also are used in different feedwater settings, which may require minor changes in the type and size of filters (Figure 2).

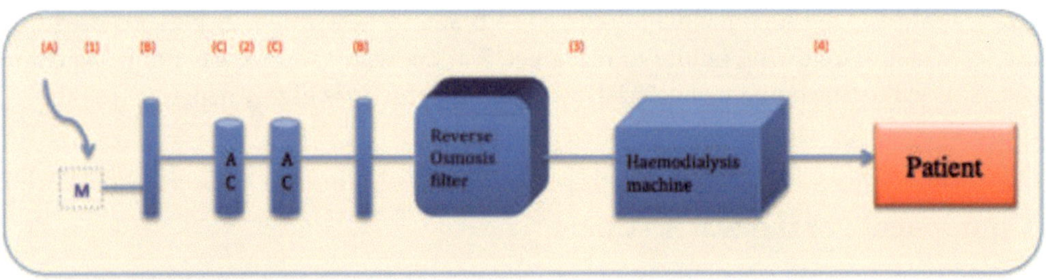

1. *M – Merlin reverse osmosis filter*
2. *AC – activated carbon*

(A) The Cartridge unit is an easily changed, optional unit sometimes used to "pre treat" the source water. (B) micron particle filters, usually either 5u and 1u size, (C) activated carbon tanks

Figure 2. Schematic of home water treatment setup

http://dx.doi.org/10.5772/59380

3.1. Micron filters

Water contains particulate matter, which may include sand, clay, silt, or colloidal matter. This particle load can be quantified by calculating the silt density index, which measures the time taken for a 0.45μm filter to experience a reduction in flow. These filters function to exclude particles on the basis of size and prevent fouling of the RO membrane (Figure 3). They are located both pre and post carbon filters. In addition the post carbon filter also traps any carbon flecks that may pass out of the carbon tanks.

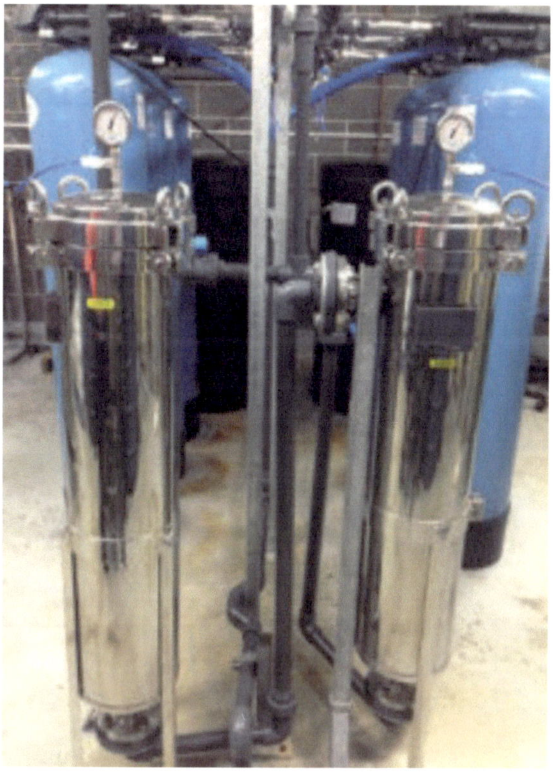

These micron filters are of a woven bag structure. Water passes through the filters in series, the 1st a 25u and the second 10u. They are changed every 4 weeks. Note the pressure gauges. The pressure differential between the 1st filter (inlet) and the gauge on the softener (outlet, not Figured here) is closely monitored. The pressure differential slowly rises as the filter integrity drops.

Figure 3. Micron particle filters (bag filters)

For **home dialysis,** typically, a 10-inch 1μm filter would be used but larger capacity e.g. 20 inch may be necessary in some areas with significant particle load such as areas with high clay concentrations. The International Organization for Standardization (ISO) recommends changing these according to the manufacturers specifications or using a change in pressure test, across the filter to check its integrity [9]. Common practice is to change these on schedule every two to four weeks.

3.2. Softener and multimedia filter

Dissolved salts within in the water contribute to the hardness of water, which can cause 'hard deposits' and can foul the downstream WRO filter. Softeners function to reduce this hardness by removing the salts, commonly calcium and magnesium, by passing water through a resin, exchanging them for sodium (Figure 4). The ISO guidelines recommend a softener be used where feed water has hardness in excess of 10 GPG (grains/gallon) [9]. The softener is 'regenerated' by backwashing it with a high salt solution from the brine tank, effectively stripping the resin of bound calcium and magnesium salts. This can be set to a required time or volume schedule. Typically the softener is replaced every 3 – 5 yrs. Multimedia filters are composed of multiple layers of media, typically coal, sand and garnet, which are of differing sizes. As water passes through the filter, particles up to 10μm, suspended in the water are removed. Some units do not use multi-media filter, opting rather for the micron filters, which are cheaper and easier to replace.

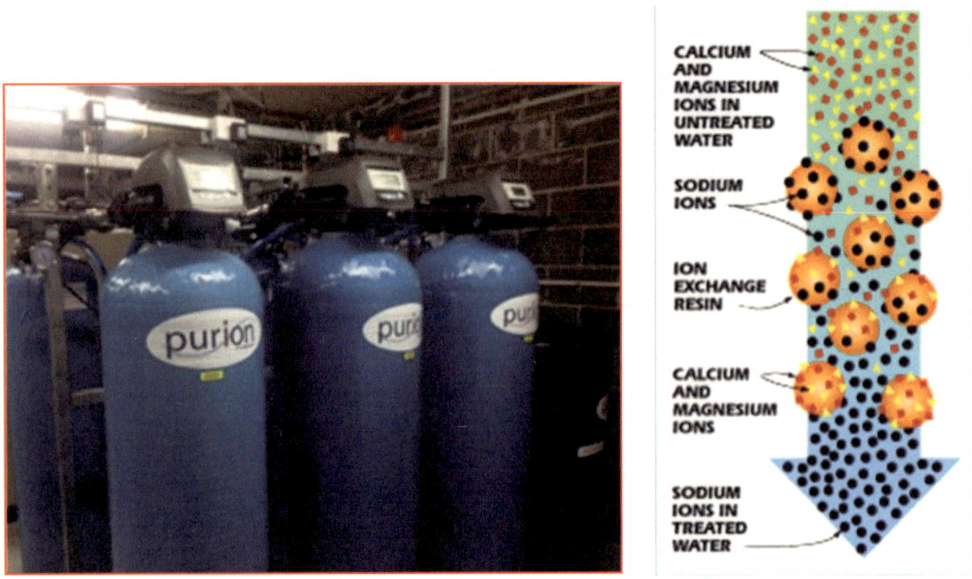

(A) 2 carbon filters, 1 softener tank and a brine tank in series.

(B) Mechanism of softener function, illustrating ion exchange

Figure 4. Softeners and mechanism of action.

Large amounts of particulate matter and salts have the potential to affect the efficiency of the carbon and WRO filters. In **home dialysis** installations, our local experience has been that multimedia filters and softeners do not affect the water quality standards. We do not routinely use these filters in our home water setup. Our RO membranes are routinely changed approximately every 5 years and the absence of the multimedia filter and softeners has not led to early failure of the WRO. Once again this will be dependent on the quality of the feed water.

http://dx.doi.org/10.5772/59380

3.3. Activated carbon

Activated carbon is a highly porous carbon material that is created by adding heat and steam to carbon containing products such as coal and wood. The carbon is then acid washed to clean and increase its porosity. The primary purpose of the carbon filter is to remove chlorine and its related compounds, including chloramines and halogenated organic material, like trihalomethanes (Figure 5). With regular use the carbon becomes spent with no further binding available along its large surface area.

Chloramines are derived from chlorine and ammonium and is added to drinking water, as a disinfectant as it is more stable, does not dissipate as rapidly as free chlorine and reduces the formation of chlorinated organic compounds such as trihalomethanes [10] (see section on water testing). It is important to note that the RO filter does not remove chlorine. Activated carbon is the best method of removing chloramines and is achieved by physical adsorption and chemical catalysis to its parent compounds. The adsorptive capacity of the carbon filter is determined by the contact time of the carbon with water, known as empty bed contact time (EBCT) and the Iodine number of the carbon. The iodine number of a carbon is calculated by its ability to absorb iodine per gram of carbon. The EBCT is directly proportional to the volume of carbon in the carbon tank and inversely proportional to the flow and can be exactly calculated using a formula. The larger the carbon tanks, the higher the EBCT provided the flow rate is constant.

The tanks are connected in series with the first tank providing most of the chlorine removal; hence it is usually referred to as the 'worker' tank and the second called the 'polisher'. With regular use, the absorptive sites on the carbon particles become exhausted and their efficiency declines. Conditions within the carbon tanks, especially the polisher, are ideal for bacterial proliferation in that it is chlorine deplete and contains organic matter. To increase the efficiency and prolong its lifespan, the carbons are backwashed ie 'fluffing the carbons'. This is usually performed weekly and the tanks are changed every 12 months.

Both in the home and in-centre setting, patients and staff, respectively, test the dialysis water daily prior to treatment. If chlorine is detected, dialysis is not initiated and an immediate carbon change is effected. Our center, also tests for trihalomethanes (THMs) (*see section on water testing*), in both the home and in centre setting. The carbons effectively remove THM's. In our experience, elevated THM levels often precede a chlorine breakthrough and are also a marker of the organic load in the water. The ISO guidelines recommend an EBCT of at least 10 minutes and a Iodine number >900. It also recommends that carbon be acid washed by the manufacturer and that regenerated carbon not be used [9].

3.4. UV

The ultra violet (UV) light emitters function to deactivate microorganisms. Exposure to UV results in damage to the nucleic acids of the cell. The ISO recommends that a minimum radiant energy dose should be 16 milliwatt-s/cm^2 and that unit replacement and maintenance should occur annually [11-13].

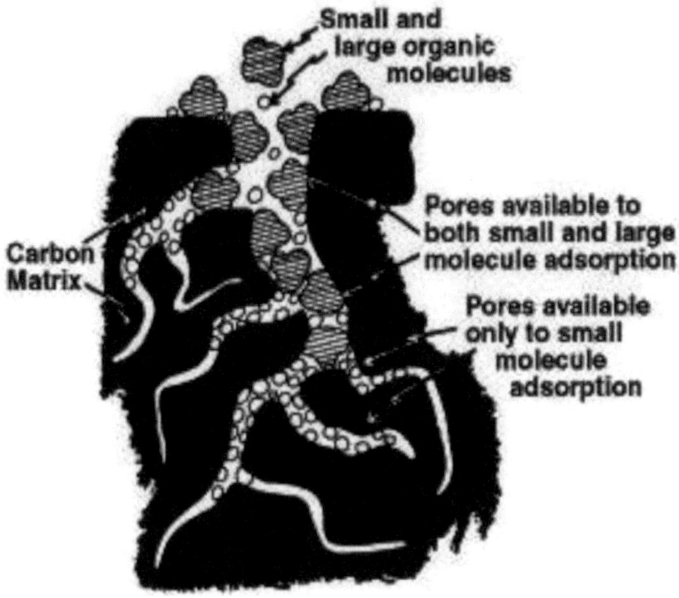

Adapted from Culp, G.L., and R.L. Culp. 1974. New Concepts in Water Purification. Van Nostrand Reinhold Co., New York.

Figure 5. Activated carbon particle

3.5. De-ioniser

Deionisers work on the principle of ion exchange to remove organic or inorganic ions from the water. Typically a mixed bed, anion and cation exchange resin would be used. These have largely been replaced by the use of reverse osmosis technology.

3.6. Reverse osmosis

Water reverse osmosis (WRO) units operate by pumping water, at pressure, across a semi permeable membrane, using a cross flow, membrane filtration system (Figure 6). Here a single stream of water is presented to the membrane, at which point it can either pass across the membrane as pure permeate or be "rejected" by the membrane and flow to waste. The WRO will remove metals (e.g. manganese, iron and fluoride), as well as organic molecules (e.g. bacteria). Effective and efficient operation of the WRO is proportional to the quality of feedwater; hence making the pre-treatment process obligatory to maximise the longevity of the membrane.

There are various WROs available on the market, differing in membrane type (e.g. cellulose, synthetic, composite) and membrane configuration. Typically, a polyamide, thin film composite in a spiral configuration is used in haemodialysis.. Water pH ideally should be between 5 and 8.5. A higher pH will cause the carbon filters chloramine absorption to be less effective and also reduce the efficiency of the RO membrane.

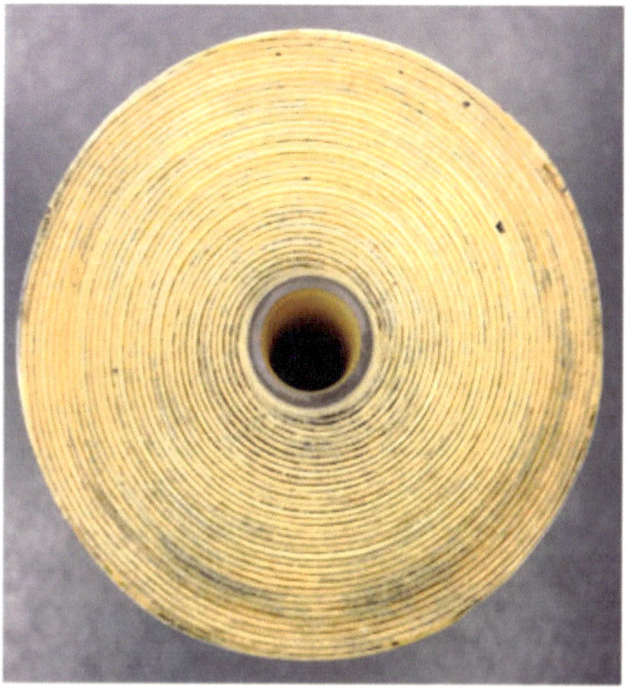

Figure 6. Used RO membrane from a home dialysis WRO machine

The WRO unit has an internal conductivity sensor and uses this to monitor the efficiency of the WRO membrane by measuring the conductivity both pre-and post-filtration and then calculating a percentage efficiency. Post membrane water usually has a conductivity of between 2 – 10 μSm/cm. The machine has programmable alarm limits, which can be adjusted by the technicians. Although our unit routinely sets the initial alarm at 50μSm/cm, our technicians usually intervene if the post RO water conductivity exceeds 20μSm/cm. The machine is programmed to shut down if this exceeds 150μSm/cm. Measurements of RO conductivity efficiency is only a guide and not an absolute measure of suitability for dialysis, which can only be ascertained by performing a detailed water analysis.

In the home setting, portable WROs are disinfected, by the user, either using heat, weekly or chemically, twice a week. Chemical disinfection is performed using agents, such as Dialox® solution (peracetic acid 0.35%, hydrogen peroxide 6.6%). Some units use a weekly or even fortnightly disinfection schedule. The use of chemicals reduces the longevity of the RO membrane. Newer WRO's use only heat to disinfect by heating water up to 90°C. This has the advantage of not needing to store and transport chemicals and also prevents the rare but real danger of mistakenly using the dialysis machine bleach in the WRO. Using heat disinfection WRO's also offers the unique advantage of integrated disinfection. Here the heated solution is not limited to the WRO but extends simultaneously to the HD machine, thus disinfecting the piping in between and resulting in fewer breaches in water quality. In the in-centre setting, the loop delivery piping connecting the WRO and the dialysis machines, is heat disinfected daily, using water heated to 85°C with the WRO membranes being disinfected weekly.

As the WRO is used over time, several different processes start to affect its efficiency. These 3 processes include:

- fouling – the entrapment of particles in the membrane,
- scaling – deposition of eg calcium salts and
- membrane degradation.

Hence, WROs do need to be serviced regularly. This involves calibrating the conductivity sensors, checking the pump flows, descaling, checking for leaks and sterilising the machine (see Figure 8). In the home setting, the machines first undergo a high pH, sodium hydroxide, flush followed by a low pH acidic solution (e.g. a citrate based solution.) Specific practices will be dependent on whether or not softeners have been used, the quality of the feed water and manufacturer specific guidelines for servicing. The WRO membranes are usually replaced every 3 – 5 years.

The ISO recommends daily monitoring of the WRO unit's instrumentation panel. This usually includes, a constant readout of the product water conductivity and percentage efficiency [9]. The purpose is to monitor and log trends and confirm that the machine is operating within the manufacturer's specifications. It also recommends repeating a laboratory water analysis when significant seasonal changes in water quality are suspected or if rejection rates change by more than 10%.

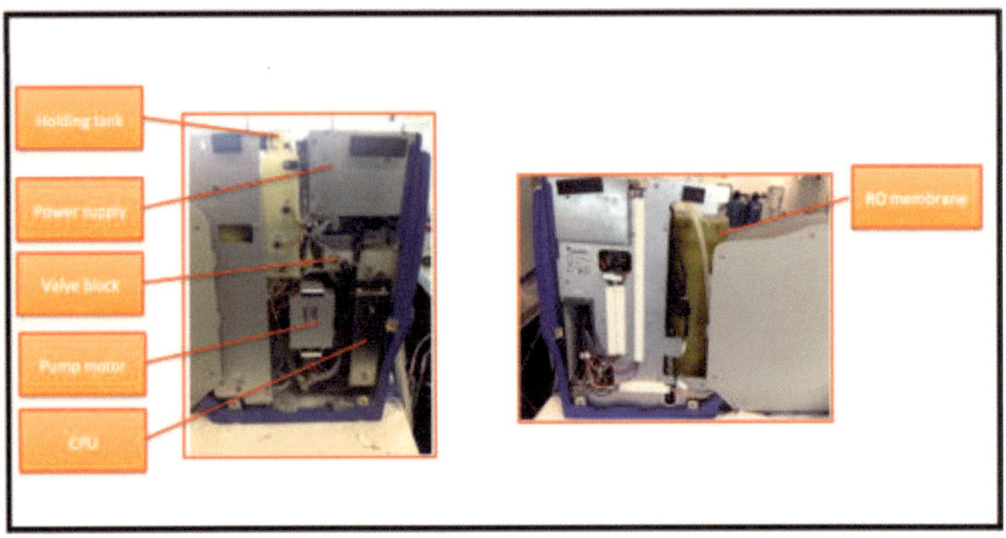

Figure 7. Portable WRO with casing removed

http://dx.doi.org/10.5772/59380

3.7. Ultra filters or endotoxin retentive filters

Ultra filters, also known as endotoxin retentive filters, are cartridge type filters that are installed onto the dialysis machine (Figure 9). They are composed of a polysulfone material used to achieve "ultra pure" water by removing bacteria and endotoxin. This is by a process of adsorption and exclusion by particle size. Flow through the filter cartridge can be either in a "dead end" or "cross flow" configuration. In 'cross flow' mode, water flows parallel to the membrane surface with impurities "washed away" in the reject stream. In 'dead end' mode, water flows perpendicular to the membrane surface.

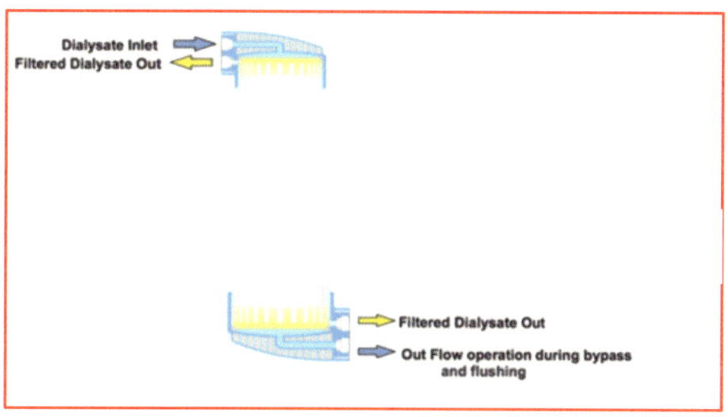

(A) Ultrafilter

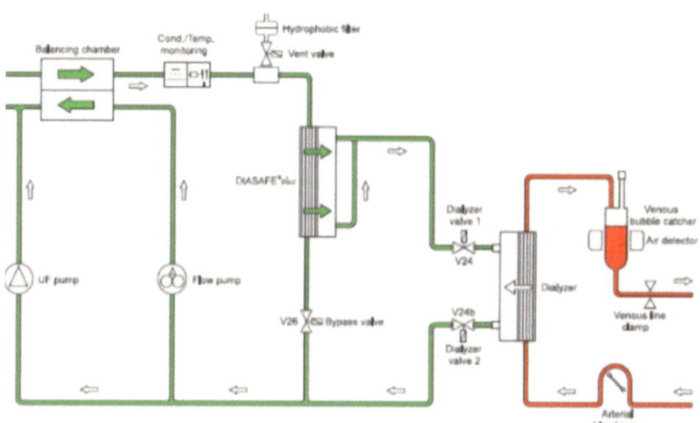

(B) Schematic of flow and creation of ultra pure water. Dialysis water is mixed with solute to create the mixed dialysis fluid that is then presented to the ultrafilter. During flushing, the bypass valve is opened whilst the dialyser valves are closed.

Figure 8. Example of an ultrafilter showing dialysate flow

These filters are usually operated in dead end mode as a cost saving measure. Any "fouling" of the membrane is limited by regular flushing to a drain valve. In addition, these filters are included in the dialysis machine disinfection cycle further limiting bacterial contamination. Prior to each treatment, the dialysis machine conducts a pressure integrity check (ΔP) to ensure the membrane is functioning adequately.

Patients on haemodiafiltration (HDF) require a high quality "substitution fluid' to be infused directly in to the circulation. Hence, a second ultrafilter is used, which greatly minimises the possibility of contamination.

3.8. Plumbing

Only qualified plumbers registered with the local water board and with prior experience in water systems are used to plumb new installations. The main components are the filters and the piping in between. Plumbing installations including those for haemodialysis must comply with the *Plumbing and drainage standard* of that country.

3.8.1. Backflow device and stop valve

This prevents treated water, containing disinfectants, from back flowing into municipal water supply. The device cannot be tested and so are changed routinely every two years according to the manufacturer's specification.

3.8.2. Piping, couplings, micro fittings and sealants

The 2009 ISO guidelines recommend that piping should not contribute any chemicals eg copper, lead, zinc or chemicals. [9]. Common practice is the use of PVC (polyvinyl chloride) piping as it is non corrodible, is able to withstand high temperatures achieved during disinfection and has a smooth inner surface to prevent biofilm.

Much controversy surrounds the potential leaching of plasticizer compounds from the dialysis tubing, including the dialyser membrane and their effects on health. Two compounds in particular, Bisphenol A and phthalate diesters are known to act as 'oestrogenic disrupting chemicals' which have been shown in rodent models, to cause liver, pancreatic, thyroid and developmental abnormalities [28, 29]. Their role in human disease remains unclear. Copper piping is used only for reject water and not for the piping that supplies the WRO and the dialysis machine, as copper can leach from the piping and result in copper toxicity to the patient [14]. Brass fittings may be minimally used for certain fixtures due to the risk of leaks and blowout with plastic couplings. Particular care needs to be taken to prevent use of and contamination from adhesives, epoxy resins or bonding cements.

3.9. Water disposal and saving – Green dialysis

There are two grades of wastewater created from the water filtration process. The first is reject water from the WRO, which has not come into contact with the patient and second, post dialysis effluent, which is produced during the actual dialysis process. Safe disposal of dialysis effluent water poses two issues. **Firstly**, because dialysis fluid is in contact with blood, it is a biological waste product and theoretically may contain bacterial or viral particles from the patient. There is however no evidence that this poses a definite infective risk. In one study dialysis wastewater was analysed and compared to municipal, industry, Food and Agriculture Organization of the United Nations (FAO) and World Health Organization (WHO) standards for wastewater use for agricultural applications. Apart from an expected higher conductivity, the dialysis wastewater did not exceed FAO standards for biochemical oxygen demand or bacteria [15]. **Secondly**, dialysis wastewater in the home setting is diverted to sewerage, which poses a practical dilemma for patients in the rural setting, where septic tanks are used. With the large volumes of dialysis wastewater created per treatment, this could quickly overflow

http://dx.doi.org/10.5772/59380

these tanks and hence there is a need to be able to accommodate this volume. **Thirdly**, addition of chemicals used in the disinfection process would damage the bio flora essential in the normal function of the septic system used by some patients. For these situations, the current practice is to construct an independent water disposal pit for chemically tainted water during the disinfection process whilst all other effluent water is diverted to sewerage.

There is a high percentage of reject water (approximately 65 – 90%) created by the WRO. This water, created from drinking standard feed water, has already passed through, in most cases, particle *filters*, carbon filters, softeners or multimedia filters. Although "reject" by dialysis purity standards, it is "pre patient" and is still drinkable in some cases [16]. Although not traditional standard practice, experts in the field, especially in water shortage areas in Australia, advocate the use of water conserving practice. This entails storing and using the 'reject' water for "grey water' purposes (e.g. gardening, cleaning etc.) [16, 17]. As a rough estimate, a dialysis unit in a tertiary hospital, servicing approximately 20 dialysis beds, can reject almost 3,000,000 litres of water annually! Secondly, reject water (RW) can be recycled back into the dialysis filtration system [18]. Here the RW is pumped into a separate storage tank, which is then re-presented to the filtration system for reuse and reprocessing. This can result in up to an 80% water saving [18]. Thirdly, water saving WRO's that internally reuse RW can also result in water saving. For example, there would typically be a 3 way valve that would redirect reject water flow away from waste and back into the supply pipe. This valve would operate in short eg. 20-second cycles, alternating between waste and the supply pipe. The recirculation rate can be varied on the machines. Commonly home dialysis and in-centre WRO units use a recirculation rate of between 10% and 65%.

However recirculating reject water or using the water saving feature, will increase the feed water concentration of contaminants, which will reduce the efficiency of the WRO membrane and likely reduce its lifespan. The average water conductivity in an urban area is usually <500mSm/cm and it is sensible in such areas to trial a higher water recirculation percentage eg 30%-50%. Areas where feed water quality is poor with high conductivity > 1000mSm/cm should probably not use the water saving feature to better protect the RO membrane. Ultimately, the cost and safety concerns involved in balancing water saving against membrane longevity and water quality need to be monitored. Without trialing the water saving feature, it is impossible to know where this balance lies.

4. Additional and optional equipment

4.1. Cartridge filter with basic RO membrane

These are small, under-counter-size WRO units. In remote areas where patients are supplied by borehole water, the feedwater can have high amounts of particulate matter, dissolved salts and metals (e.g. arsenic). A cheap pre-filtering system is required to return water to near drinking water standard to protect the more expensive downstream components of the filtration system. Water from rainwater and borehole supplied tanks requires a pump that provides pressures between 300 – 500Kpa as these filters operate on line pressure. The filter typically has a 3 stage system that involves a carbon prefilter cartridge leading into a RO cartridge. Typically the cartridges are changed every 6 months, although this is variable depending on the feedwater quality. When the reject rate of water starts to increase (i.e. less water per minute of treated water is produced), then the cartridges are changed sooner. Typically patients will notice that the storage tank takes longer to fill alerting them that an earlier change is necessary.

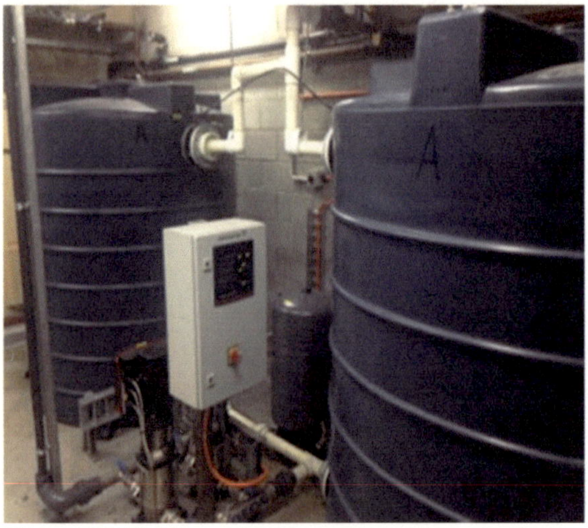

A) Two 3000L holding tanks to provide an uninterrupted water supply in case of emergency. Note also the booster pumps in the centre. These ensure an inlet pressure of at least 550Kpa

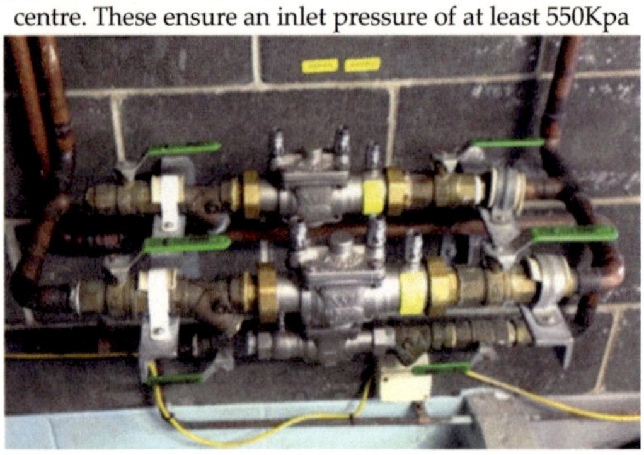

(B) A backflow device.

Figure 9. Holding tanks with booster pumps and back flow preventor

4.2. Water temperature regulators

As blood is passed through a dialysis circuit, heat is radiated to the cooler ambient temperature and then is brought into contact with dialysis water. The temperature of this water may have significant seasonal or diurnal variation. Dialysis machines are capable of heating but not

http://dx.doi.org/10.5772/59380

cooling dialysis water to the required temperature. Feed water less than 10 degrees Celsius and greater than 30 degrees would require temperature adjustment. Feed water temperature also affects the integrity of the RO and particle filters, which have a maximum operating temperature set by the manufacturer, usually less than 35 degrees Celsius. In most units the temperature of dialysis water is typically 35ºC. A high dialysate temperature can result in haemolysis [19]. If feed water temperature is outside the recommended range then water temperature will need to be adjusted. This is usually not required in more temperate climates.

4.3. Booster pumps

When feedwater originates from rainwater or borehole, it is stored in a tank. A booster pump is necessary to pump water to the filtration system (Figure 11). Some homes especially older ones may have low mains water pressure. This may be due to low supply pressure from the municipality, corrosion or faulty pressure restrictors. If not correctable then such homes may also require a booster pump. This must be sufficient to meet the minimum pressure requirements of the RO filter, which is typically between 1 to 8 bars.

4.4. Iron removal units

In some circumstances high iron content in the feedwater may necessitate an independent iron removal system. A dedicated iron filter (e.g. BIRM® Clack Corporation, Wisconsin 53598-0500 USA) is available. The ISO does not specify a level for iron in dialysis water but does recognise that it may foul downstream filters [9].

5. Water quality testing

The water purification system is a multiple layer system designed to progressively purify water at each step. The resulting dialysis water needs to meet minimum criteria for chemical and microbiological characteristics. These criteria form the basis of the definition for standard quality and ultrapure quality dialysis water. There are several available guidelines specifying the minimum allowable standards for water quality. (eg U.S. Association for the Advancement of Medical Instrumentation (AAMI) and the European best practice guidelines (EBPG). The ISO (international organisation for standardisation) is an international collaboration of national standard bodies (ISO member bodies). Minimum water testing parameters from the ISO are summarised below. The ISO recommends at least annual testing for chemical contaminants and quarterly testing for microbiological contaminants (Table 2) [9]. Ultimately a schedule of water testing must achieve two goals. Firstly, testing must ensure that a high quality of dialysis water is being delivered at the end of the filtration process. Perturbations in feed water quality and breakthrough in upstream filters do not usually result in fouling of the dialysis water, as there is a fair degree of redundancy built into each filter. Hence, even if, for example, a post-WRO sample reveals an elevated bacterial load, a well maintained further downstream ultrafilter should still prevent this exposure to the patient. Secondly, testing at different points in the circuit enables troubleshooting and localization of the problem area. As in the example above, the problem would be proximal to the WRO testing port and hence the carbon filters would be backwashed and the RO disinfected. A suggested schedule for water testing frequency in the home environment in outlined below. *(see Table 3).*

There are 4 main points of water testing. (see table 3 and Figure 2). Water samples are best sent to an experienced testing facility for all water analyses.

	Drinking water standards: mg/l [10]	**Standard dialysis water mg/l** [11, 12]	**Ultrapure dialysis fluid**	**Symptoms and disease associations:**
Contaminant:				
Aluminium	0.1	0.01		Anaemia, neuropathy, bone disease
Total chlorine	5	0.1		Haemolysis
Chloramine [13]	3	0.1		Haemolysis
Copper	2	0.1		Haemolysis
Fluoride	1.5	0.2		Bone disease
Lead	0.01	0.005		Haemolysis, neuropathy, gout [14]
Nitrate	50 - 100	2		Hypotension, Haemolysis
Sulphate	250	100		Acidosis
Zinc	3	0.1		Anaemia
Antimony	0.003	0.006		
Arsenic	0.01	0.005		Encephalopathy, cancer [15, 16]
Barium	2	0.1		
Beryllium	0.06	0.0004		
Cadmium	0.002	0.001		
Chromium	0.05	0.014		
Mercury	0.001	0.0002		
Selenium	0.01	0.09		
Silver	0.1	0.005		
Thallium	NS	0.002		
Copper	2			Anaemia
Calcium	200	2 (0.05)		Muscle weakness
Magnesium	TDS (600)	4 (0.15)		Muscle weakness
Sodium	180	70		
Potassium	TDS	8		
Microbiological criteria:				
Microbial count (CFU/ml) [11]	Individual bacterial levels, eg Ecoli	< 100 CFU/ml	<0.1 CFU/ml [(1)]	Hypotension, inflammation
Endotoxin Concentration EU/ml	NS	< 0.25 EU/ml	<0.03 EU/ml	Hypotension, inflammation

1. ISO 2009 standards for haemodialysis water recommend Ultra pure water for routine dialysis, defined as a microbial count < 0,1 cfu/ml and an endotoxin concentration <0.03EU/ml
2. Total dissolved solids (TDS) consist of inorganic salts and small amounts of organic matter that are dissolved in water. The palatability of drinking water has been rated according to TDS concentrations. High TDS values, apart from taste, may also be associated with excessive scaling in pipes, fittings and household appliances

Table 2. ISO recommendations for water quality in dialysis water [20]

http://dx.doi.org/10.5772/59380

Collection point	Bacteria and Endo[4] count	Pesticides[5]	THM	Heavy metals	Anions, cations, pH, conductivity:	Standard water analysis:[3]
1 – Feed water	Rural: 3 – 6 monthly & pre initial install	As requested[4]		As requested		6 – 12 monthly rural
2 – Inter carbon			3 monthly[2]			
3 - Post RO	3 monthly (monthly HDF until stable)	Annually (Rural 3 – 6 monthly)		Annually (Rural 3 – 6 monthly)	Annually (Rural 3 – 6 monthly)	
4 – HD machine	3 monthly (monthly HDF until stable)					

1. Nos 1 – 4 correspond to schematic representation of water circuit
2. Chlorine testing occurs routinely before each treatment using a dipstick-colour chart based system. 3 monthly, total chlorine testing is also performed by water testing staff
3. Standard water analysis includes pH, conductivity, turbidity (see below sample report)
4. Colony forming units and endotoxin count
5. Pesticide testing frequency is also dependent on area, eg farmlands and rural areas are tested more frequently compared to metropolitan areas. In addition seasonal variations are also considered. Generally 4/yr

Table 3. Schedule for water testing

[redacted]

HCF: [redacted]
WARD:
DOCTOR:

DOB: [redacted]
GENDER:
CONSULTANT:

UR No: [redacted] **DOB:** [redacted] **Patient:** [redacted]

Lab No : 55519-6136
Standard Water Analysis
SPECIMEN : Water Feed(Retic)

Collected : 08:00 21-May-13
Registered: 11:03 21-May-13
Ward of Collection HTHU~PAH

		Units	Ref. Range
Conductivity	665	uS/cm	
pH	7.80	Std pH Units	(6.50 - 8.50)
Total Hardness	124	mg/L CaCO3	(< 200)
Alkalinity	124	mg/L CaCO3	
Silica	16.5	mg/L	
Total Diss Solids	414	mg/L	(< 500)
True Colour	4	Hazen	(< 15)
Turbidity	<1	NTU	(< 5)

OTHER DISSOLVED ELEMENTS

		Units	Ref. Range
Iron Fe	<0.010	mg/L	(< 0.30)
Manganese Mn	<0.01	mg/L	(< 0.10)
Zinc Zn	0.04	mg/L	(< 3)
Aluminium Al	0.01	mg/L	(< 0.20)
Boron B	0.1	mg/L	(< 4.0)
Copper Cu	< 0.03	mg/L	(< 2.00)

CATIONS

		Units	Ref. Range
Sodium Na^+	55	mg/L	(< 180)
Potassium K^+	2.8	mg/L	
Calcium Ca^{++}	38.5	mg/L	
Magnesium Mg^{++}	22.2	mg/L	
Hydrogen H^+	0.0	mg/L	

ANIONS

		Units	Ref. Range
Bicarbonate HCO_3^-	150	mg/L	
Carbonate CO_3^{--}	0.5	mg/L	
Hydroxide OH^-	0.0	mg/L	
Chloride Cl^-	100	mg/L	(< 250)
Fluoride F^-	0.8	mg/L	(< 1.5)
Nitrate NO_3^-	3.8	mg/L	(< 50.0)
Sulphate SO_4^{--}	40	mg/L	(< 250)

Figure 10. Example of a standard water analysis report

5.1. Chemical testing

Chlorine is a strong oxidising agent used in the disinfection of municipality drinking water. Inadequately treated dialysis water can result in significant patient exposure to chlorine. Here ferrous iron (Fe^{2+}) in haemoglobin is converted ferric iron (Fe^{3+}) resulting in the formation of methaemoglobin, haemolysis and anaemia [21, 22]. Due to its toxic nature and abundance, testing for chlorine occurs twice daily in dialysis units. This is performed using indicator test strips or testing tablets, which cause a colour change in the presence of chlorine. Electronic chlorimeters are also used and these are serviced regularly. In the home setting, patients are trained to perform a chlorine check before any dialysis session is initiated. In addition, trained water technicians visiting the home for maintenance reasons, also check chlorine levels. Chlorine testing is not routinely performed in the lab, as the samples need to be tested within 4 hours of collection due to the instability of the chlorinated compounds.

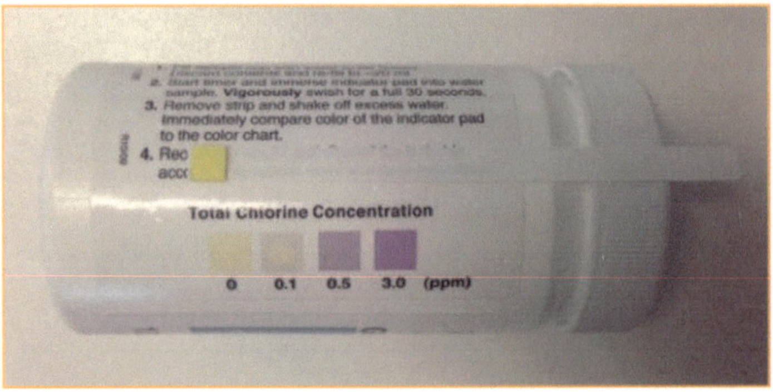

Figure 11. Colour based chlorine test strips

Aluminium has been associated with renal bone disease, anaemia and dementia [1). Although measurable, serum levels are not a good marker of organ concentration and proper water treatment is the only preventative measure possible. Other disease associations with contaminants are summarised in the table 3. Gas or liquid chromatography with mass spectrometry are powerful tools used in analytical chemistry to separate, identify and quantify compounds in a liquid and can also be used as a screening test to detect contaminants in water samples. It is important to realise that chemicals detected in ultrapure samples tested at the end of the circuit may have originated not only from the feed water but also the plumbing, membranes or heated plastics, within the circuit.

Trihalomethanes levels are not specified in the ISO guidelines but are part of routine testing at certain facilities. (also see carbon filters above). These are a group of organic chemicals that are formed by the water disinfection process, by the reaction of chlorine with organic matter eg decaying plant and vegetable matter. Exposure to trihalomethanes in drinking water has been associated with liver damage, carcinogenicity and adverse reproductive effects [10, 23, 24]. Our institution currently tests for THM's in our water circuit between carbon tanks. The Australian drinking water guideline specifies a maximum concentration of trihalomethanes not greater than 0.25g/l [250ppb) [25]. The EPA (Environmental protection agency) in the USA specifies a lower limit of 0.08g/l ie 80 parts per billion (ppb). There is no specification for THM levels in dialysis water. In Australia, dialysis facilities use a level of 1/10th of the EPA drinking water guideline. It is believed that the presence of THM's greater than 8ppb usually heralds the imminent breakthrough of chloramines and/or chlorine post carbon. Levels greater than 8ppb trigger an action protocol resulting in swapping out and rotation of the carbon tanks, which can be performed on a semi elective basis.

Standard quality dialysis water has minimum microbiological and contaminant concentrations, defined by the ISO [9]. (see table 3). **Ultrapure water** has more stringent microbiological criteria specifying a lower bacterial load and endotoxin concentration. Although ultrapure water can now be easily produced with the regular use of ultrafilters, the more stringent microbiological criteria make testing a more involved and lengthy process for instance longer culture times. Microbiological testing involves testing for bacteria and endotoxin and is discussed further below.

5.2. Microbiological testing

Microbiological analysis involves testing for bacteria and endotoxins. Endotoxins are the lipopolysaccharide layer of the gram-negative bacterial cell walls. However it is worth noting that bacterial culture and endotoxin testing do not exclude all possibility of bacterial contamination. For example, they do not detect gram-positive cell wall components e.g. peptidoglycan, or bacterial fragments, unculturable organisms or dead bacteria [26], all of which may still elicit an inflammatory response when introduced into the blood stream. The clinical relevance of this is unknown.

Various factors can affect the ability of bacteria to be cultured. These include the type of culture medium, length of incubation and temperature, all of which are specified in the ISO guideline [9]. The method of collection is also standardized by the ISO. Sampling ports are cleaned with alcohol, connectors soaked in ethanol to prevent contamination and water is allowed to run for the first 30 seconds. The [9) guidelines also recommend that samples be assayed within 4 hours of collection. The guideline recommends that this time can be extended by refrigeration, up to 24rs. However this is not easily achievable especially considering the remote location of many of the home dialysis patients.

Potential organisms that contaminate the water circuit are accustomed to a nutrient poor environment hence necessitating special consideration. These include using a nutrient poor culture medium (e.g. Reasoners agar [R2A]), the use of membrane filtration for low colony count detection, an incubation temperature of between 17 and 23 degrees Celsius and an incubation period of 7 days [27]. The concentration of contaminants at which action should be instituted is set at 50% of the maximum allowable level; that is intervention is required when 50% of the allowed maximum is reached.

Endotoxin testing is performed using the Limulus amoebocyte lysate (LAL) assay. Here serum (amebocytes) removed from the horseshoe crab (limulus) is exposed to endotoxin. This activates a proteolytic cascade in the crab serum resulting in the formation of a gel like substance. An artificial substrate added to the lysate is also proteolytically cleaved and the liberated protein can be measured by its ability to absorb light, which is the basis of the chromogenic test kits. The test can also be quantified by its ability to form a clot or produce turbidity. It is important to note that the LAL assay does not detect endotoxin < 8000 Da.

6. Unique environments eg rural home setup

Home dialysis has resulted in a multitude of benefits for patients. Most importantly with convenience, independence and improvement in biochemical and likely mortality figures. The availability of electricity and running water should not disparage patient's eligibility for dialysis. In Australia the possibility of solar powered dialysis has been shown to be a feasible option, if not completely then to significantly offset the power costs of dialysis [17]. Similarly the lack of running water should also not be a limiting factor. Illustrated below is an example of how home dialysis became a possibility for a patient living on a farm over 200km from the nearest major city.

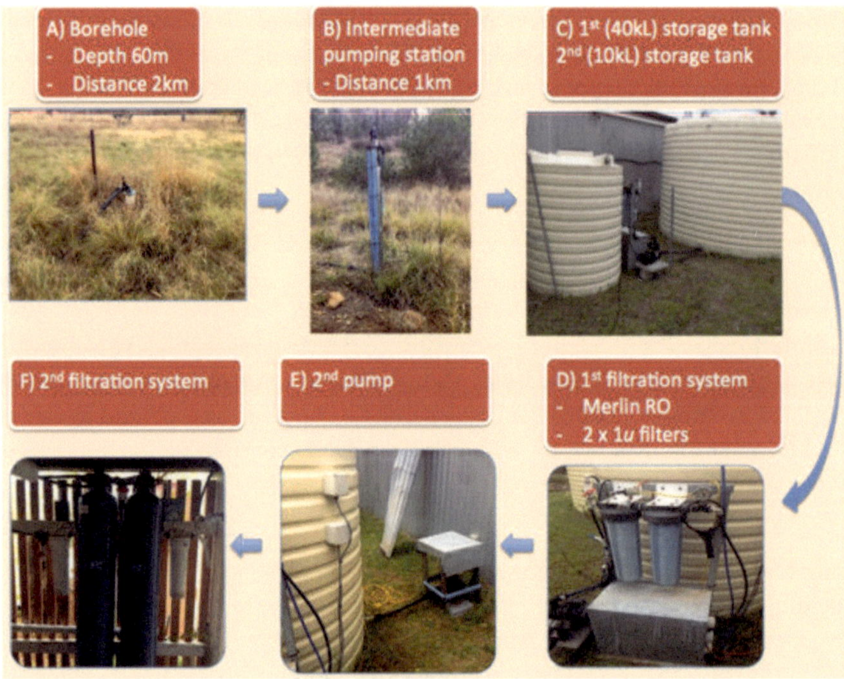
A) Borehole
- Depth 60m
- Distance 2km
B) Intermediate pumping station
- Distance 1km
C) 1st (40kL) storage tank
2nd (10kL) storage tank
F) 2nd filtration system
E) 2nd pump
D) 1st filtration system
- Merlin RO
- 2 x 1u filters

Figure 12. An Example of a rural home water treatment setup: (A) The borehole is approximately 2 km from the patient's residence and is determined by the geology of the area. (B) An intermediate pumping station operated using air pressure. (C) Storage tanks are continually replenished from the bore to ensure an uninterrupted water supply. (D) A basic pre filtration cartridge filter (located in the silver casing) and two micron filters pre treat the water (E) A second pump located approximately 100m from the patients residence (F) A second set of micron filters and carbon tanks. This is located underneath the patients home and feeds directly to dialysis machine inside the bedroom.

7. Special situations; floods and droughts

Floods are often devastating natural disasters that result in extensive disruption of transport, communication and power supply networks, as well as industrial, farming, business and personal property damage. Table 4 summarises some of the important implications for haemodialysis patients. Experience from previous natural disasters has highlighted the importance of dialysis units having a practiced disaster management plan to manage these situations. During the 2005 Hurricane Katrina disaster, 94 dialysis centres closed for at least one week affecting close to 6000 patients [30, 31]. The national kidney foundation provides a useful guide for disaster planning for people with chronic kidney disease. It includes useful information for patients such as fluid and dietary advice, including salt, potassium and water restriction, medical record management, dialysis rationing and medication supply [32].

Problem:	**Proposed Action:**
Water contamination:	
Increased particulate matter from surface run off	Increase capacity and schedule of micron filter change
Increased pesticides/herbicides/organic contaminants	Consider increasing EBCT, increasing capacity and schedule of carbon change
Increased chlorine load from municipality	As above and ensure regular chlorine testing
Increased ionic/dissolved solute load	Monitor WRO conductivity and reject rates. Consider increasing disinfection schedule
Variations in water supply and pressure	Liaise with local water authority and ensure appropriate capacity reservoir tanks
Power disruptions	Backup generators

EBCT: Empty bed contact time

Table 4. Problems associated with flooding

Water is clearly a precious resource. Unfortunately large volumes of reject water are created for the provision of dialysis. (See **Water disposal and saving-green dialysis**). Drought prone areas should consider water recycling, water saving WRO's and rainwater collection tanks to conserve water. Close liaison with the local water authority regarding supply rationing and trucked water is imperative.

8. Conclusion

High volumes of ultrapure water are required for safe and effective haemodialysis. A sequential and progressive water purification system ensures that this is delivered safely to the patient. With proper maintenance and monitoring of these systems many of the incidents of the past can be avoided. With the increased uptake of home dialysis therapies the need for similarly robust systems is necessary. Home dialysis differs in that home patients have longer dialysis hours and are exposed to more water. Water systems are also used in different areas with differing feed water quality and machines are left unused for periods of up to 48 hours. These factors increase the risk of exposure to chemical and microbial contaminants.

Important factors that need to be considered in the management of a dialysis water treatment system, both in the home and in-centre include: the quality of the feed water, including the abundance of its supply, reliable electricity, an adequate capacity to dispose of water and a validated water-testing program. A good working relationship and communication with the local council is important; particularly in providing prior warning regarding planned maintenance, expected fluctuations in feed water quality and assistance with water subsidy schemes. In the home setting, the patient, the ultimate end user, needs to be well trained not only to perform their dialysis properly but also regarding maintenance and testing of the water system. Failure to regularly backwash carbons, test for chlorine, change particle filters or perform scheduled disinfections will ultimately lead to failure of the water treatment system. However, the needs for maintenance routines has to be balanced against patient fatigue and ultimately poor compliance. Complex protocols and frequent changes should be avoided and any episodes of technique failure should be regarded as an indication to reinforce proper protocol.

A comprehensive water analysis is the only quantitative measure of water purity. Frequent testing would theoretically be more likely detect a breakthrough contaminant, however important considerations include cost of testing and false positives especially as a consequence of collection contamination. In addition there is a remarkable degree of redundancy built into the system. Upstream failure in the proximal part of the filtration system is extremely unlikely to breach both the RO and the ultra filters. Different institutions may vary the extent of their water treatment system, with additional or larger filters; use of deionisation, multimedia filters or duplicate ultra filters and automated systems. Ultimately this increases the cost of operation with diminishing returns in improvement of water quality.

Finally, we must retain the ability to adapt our methods and reflect on our practice. Changes in the environment, water quality standards, technology and patient needs will continue to evolve and will call in to question traditional practice, such as exhaustive and costly testing and prophylactic maintenance. Ultimately, patient safety and optimising treatment efficacy will remain a priority.

Abbreviations

WRO: Water reverse osmosis unit

HDF: Haemodiafiltration

HD: Haemodialysis

EU: Endotoxin units

RW: Reject water

http://dx.doi.org/10.5772/59380

Acknowledgements

Janine Jefferies, Sally Carpenter, John Poulton.

Author details

Shyam Dheda, Carolyn Van Eps, Carmel Hawley and David W. Johnson

*Address all correspondence to: shyam.dheda@gmail.com

Department of Nephrology, Princess Alexandra hospital, Brisbane, Australia

References

[1] Malluche HH. Aluminium and bone disease in chronic renal failure. Nephrology, dialysis, transplantation : official publication of the European Dialysis and Transplant Association-European Renal Association. 2002;17 Suppl 2:21-4.

[2] Berend K, van der Voet G, Boer WH. Acute aluminum encephalopathy in a dialysis center caused by a cement mortar water distribution pipe. Kidney international. 2001;59 (2):746-53.

[3] de Oliveira RM, de los Santos CA, Antonello I, d'Avila D. Warning: an anemia outbreak due to chloramine exposure in a clean hemodialysis unit--an issue to be revisited. Renal failure. 2009;31 (1):81-3.

[4] Susantitaphong P, Riella C, Jaber BL. Effect of ultrapure dialysate on markers of inflammation, oxidative stress, nutrition and anemia parameters: a meta-analysis. Nephrology, dialysis, transplantation : official publication of the European Dialysis and Transplant Association-European Renal Association. 2013;28 (2):438-46.

[5] Penne EL, Visser L, van den Dorpel MA, van der Weerd NC, Mazairac AH, van Jaarsveld BC, et al. Microbiological quality and quality control of purified water and ultrapure dialysis fluids for online hemodiafiltration in routine clinical practice. Kidney international. 2009;76 (6):665-72.

[6] Ouseph R, Ward RA. Ultrapure dialysate for home hemodialysis? Advances in chronic kidney disease. 2007;14 (3):256-62.

[7] Ahmed W, Huygens F, Goonetilleke A, Gardner T. Real-time PCR detection of pathogenic microorganisms in roof-harvested rainwater in Southeast Queensland, Australia. Applied and environmental microbiology. 2008;74 [17]:5490-6.

[8] Jochimsen EM, Carmichael WW, An JS, Cardo DM, Cookson ST, Holmes CE, et al. Liver failure and death after exposure to microcystins at a hemodialysis center in Brazil. The New England journal of medicine. 1998;338 [13]:873-8.

[9] ISO11663. Quality of dialysis fluid for haemodialysis and related therapies. 2009.

[10] Perez-Garcia R, Rodriguez-Benitez P. Chloramine, a sneaky contaminant of dialysate. Nephrology, dialysis, transplantation : official publication of the European Dialysis and Transplant Association-European Renal Association. 1999;14 [11]:2579-82.

[11] Hijnen WA, Beerendonk EF, Medema GJ. Inactivation credit of UV radiation for viruses, bacteria and protozoan (oo)cysts in water: a review. Water research. 2006;40 (1):3-22.

[12] ISO. ISO 13959 Water for haemodialysis and related therapies. 2009.

[13] Cutler TD, Zimmerman JJ. Ultraviolet irradiation and the mechanisms underlying its inactivation of infectious agents. Animal health research reviews / Conference of Research Workers in Animal Diseases. 2011;12 (1):15-23.

[14] Lyle WH, Payton JE, Hui M. Haemodialysis and copper fever. Lancet. 1976;1 [7973]: 1324-5.

[15] Tarrass F, Benjelloun M, Benjelloun O. Recycling wastewater after hemodialysis: an environmental analysis for alternative water sources in arid regions. American journal of kidney diseases : the official journal of the National Kidney Foundation. 2008;52 (1):154-8.

[16] Agar JW, Simmonds RE, Knight R, Somerville CA. Using water wisely: New, affordable, and essential water conservation practices for facility and home hemodialysis. Hemodialysis international International Symposium on Home Hemodialysis. 2009;13 (1):32-7.

[17] Agar JW. Conserving water in and applying solar power to haemodialysis: 'green dialysis' through wiser resource utilization. Nephrology (Carlton). 2010;15 (4):448-53.

[18] J Agar RS, JM Boddington, J Magoffin, R Hungerford, T Hinton. Water-wise home dialysis: re-using r/o reject water but with a high conductivity, revert-to-mains manual-alarming system. Nephrology (Carlton). 2007;12:1014.

[19] Jepson R, Alonso E. Overheated dialysate: a case study and review. Nephrology nursing journal : journal of the American Nephrology Nurses' Association. 2009;36 (5):551-3.

[20] ISO. International Organization for Standardization, Water for haemodialysis and related therapies, ISO 13959 :International Organization for Standardization, Geneva. 2002.

[21] Tipple MA, Bland LA, Favero MS, Jarvis WR. Investigation of hemolytic anemia after chloramine exposure in a dialysis center. ASAIO transactions / American Society for Artificial Internal Organs. 1988;34 (4):1060.

[22] Pyo HJ, Kwon YJ, Wee KS, Kwon SY, Lee CH, Kim S, et al. An outbreak of Heinz body positive hemolytic anemia in chronic hemodialysis patients. The Korean journal of internal medicine. 1993;8 (2):93-8.

[23] King WD, Marrett LD. Case-control study of bladder cancer and chlorination by-products in treated water (Ontario, Canada). Cancer causes & control : CCC. 1996;7 (6):596-604.

[24] Reif JS, Hatch MC, Bracken M, Holmes LB, Schwetz BA, Singer PC. Reproductive and developmental effects of disinfection by-products in drinking water. Environmental health perspectives. 1996;104 [10]:1056-61.

[25] NHMRC. NHMRC, NRMMC [2011] Australian Drinking Water Guidelines Paper 6 National Water Quality Management Strategy. National Health and Medical Research Council, National Resource Management Ministerial Council, Commonwealth of Australia, Canberra. 2011.

[26] Glorieux G, Neirynck N, Veys N, Vanholder R. Dialysis water and fluid purity: more than endotoxin. Nephrology, dialysis, transplantation : official publication of the European Dialysis and Transplant Association-European Renal Association. 2012;27 [11]:4010-21.

[27] van der Linde K, Lim BT, Rondeel JM, Antonissen LP, de Jong GM. Improved bacteriological surveillance of haemodialysis fluids: a comparison between Tryptic soy agar and Reasoner's 2A media. Nephrology, dialysis, transplantation : official publication of the European Dialysis and Transplant Association-European Renal Association. 1999;14 [10]:2433-7.

[28] Kanno Y, Okada H, Kobayashi T, Takenaka T, Suzuki H. Effects of endocrine disrupting substance on estrogen receptor gene transcription in dialysis patients. Therapeutic apheresis and dialysis : official peer-reviewed journal of the International Society for Apheresis, the Japanese Society for Apheresis, the Japanese Society for Dialysis Therapy. 2007;11 (4):262-5.

[29] Krieter DH, Canaud B, Lemke HD, Rodriguez A, Morgenroth A, von Appen K, et al. Bisphenol A in chronic kidney disease. Artificial organs. 2013;37 (3):283-90.

[30] Kopp JB, Ball LK, Cohen A, Kenney RJ, Lempert KD, Miller PE, et al. Kidney patient care in disasters: lessons from the hurricanes and earthquake of 2005. Clinical journal of the American Society of Nephrology : CJASN. 2007;2 (4):814-24.

[31] Johnson DW, Hayes B, Gray NA, Hawley C, Hole J, Mantha M. Renal services disaster planning: lessons learnt from the 2011 Queensland floods and North Queensland cyclone experiences. Nephrology (Carlton). 2013;18 (1):41-6.

[32] National Kidney Foundation. Planning for Emergencies: A Guide for People with Chronic Kidney Disease. 1995-2006.

Section 3

Vascular Access

Chapter 14

Vascular Access and New Trends

Eirini Grapsa and Konstantinos Pantelias

Additional information is available at the end of the chapter

http://dx.doi.org/10.5772/59464

1. Introduction

Patients suffering from end-stage renal disease (ESRD) treated with renal replacement therapy is a continuously growing population [1–3]. Hemodialysis is the most preferable modality among them [4], making a suitable permanent vascular access (VA) vital for their treatment. The ultimate purpose is the successful creation of a well-functioning, long-lasting VA, capable of delivering adequate dialysis to the patient with the minimum of complications under its appropriate management. In the last years in this field of nephrology, very few changes have taken place. Three types of permanent VA are in use, arteriovenous fistula (AVF), arteriovenous grafts (AVGs), and cuffed central venous catheters (CVCs). Long-lasting survival, adequate blood flow, and low complications rate are necessary characteristics of them. Native forearm AVF best fulfills this criteria and is the first choice of VA, the first native arteriovenous fistula (AVF) described in 1966 by Brescia and Chimino [5]. The second choice is upper arm AVF, followed by AVG and last one cuffed CVC [6–8]. Vascular access dysfunction is responsible for 20% of dialysis patients' hospitalizations in the USA [9], making it one of the most important causes of morbidity [10], while the annual cost of VA creation and maintenance is over 1 billion dollars yearly [11], with arteriovenous graft (AVG) cost be more than fivefold higher than AVF [12]. Thus, VA is called the "Achilles' heel" of hemodialysis [13].

2. History of vascular access

In 1924, Haas [14] carried out the first hemodialysis treatment in humans using glass needles in radial and cubital vein. In 1943, Kolff used venipuncture needles in the femoral artery and vein [15, 16]. Kolff's [17] twin-coil kidney made regular hemodialysis treatments possible in 1950s, making the need of a safe, reliable, long-lasting VA more imperative.

Aubaniac [18], in 1952, described the puncture of subclavian vein as a VA, while, in the 1960s, Dillard, Quinton, and Scribner [19], based on Alwall's experience, developed arteriovenous Teflon shunt inserted into radial artery and cephalic vein. Flexible silicon rubber replaced later Teflon. Based on Seldinger's technique, Shaldon inserted catheters into femoral artery and vein for dialysis sessions in 1961 [20, 21]. Vessels in different sites were used, over time, including the subclavian, jugular, and femoral vein.

Cimino and Brescia [22] described, in 1962, a "simple venipuncture for hemodialysis." Fogarty et al. [23] invented, in 1963, a special designed catheter for thrombectomy and embolectomy with an inflatable balloon at its distal tip. In 1965, the first AVF was created, and 14 more in 1966 when Brescia, Cimino, Appel, and Hurwich published their paper [24]. Sperling [25], in 1967, created an end-to-end anastomosis in the forearm, between radial artery and cephalic vein, in 15 patients, whereas Appell did side-to-side anastomosis. End-to-end anastomosis usually is not the first choice of AVF due to high risk of steal syndrome in aging, diabetic patients of dialysis, but it remains a useful option in revision procedures, although it is correlated with higher mortality risk from infections [26].

Nowadays, artery side-to-vein anastomosis seems to be a standard procedure [27], which began from Rohl et al. [28] in 1968. Girardet et al. [29] and Brittinger et al. [30] in 1970 described their experience with AVG between femoral vein and artery and subcutaneously fixed superficial femoral artery for chronic HD. Brittinger et al. [31] were the first to implant a plastic valve as a vascular access in an animal model, but unfortunately, their efforts did not proceed to a human one. In the early 1970s, Buselmeier et al. [32] developed a U-shaped silastic prosthetic AV shunt with either one or two Teflon plugged outlets, which communicated to the outside of the body. The U-shaped portion could be totally or partially implanted subcutaneously. Subsequently, pediatric hemodialysis patients were extremely favored by this procedure. In 1976, Baker [33] presented expanded PTFE grafts in 72 hemodialysis patients. In the subsequent years, several publications indicated the benefits and the shortcomings of the prosthetic material in question, remaining the primary choice of graft for hemodialysis VA to date. The same year, two authors, Mindich and Dardik, had worked with a new graft material: the human umbilical cord vein [34, 35]. Regrettably so, this material did not succeed in becoming a revolutionary graft material due to its inadequate resistance against the trauma of repeated cannulations and their complications (aneurysm and infection). After the subclavian route for hemodialysis access was firstly introduced by Shaldon in 1961, it was further processed in 1969 by Josef Erben, using the intraclavicular route [36]. In the next 20 years or so, the subclavian vein was the preferred access for temporary vascular access by central venous catheterization. Today, due to phlebographic studies revealing a 50% stenosis or occlusion rate at the cannulation site, subclavian route has been discarded. Subclavian stenosis and occlusion predispose to edema of the arm, especially after creation of an AV fistula [37].

The first angioplasty described by Dotter et al. [38], who introduced a type of balloon, was immensely conducive to the resolution of one of the most significant predicaments in vascular surgery and vascular access surgery.

In 1977, Gracz et al. [39] created the "proximal forearm fistula for maintenance hemodialysis," a variant of an AV anastomosis. An adjustment of this AVF became quite significant in the old,

http://dx.doi.org/10.5772/59464

hypertensive, and diabetic patients on the grounds that it allows a proximal anastomosis with a low risk of hyper circulation [40]. In 1979, Golding et al. [41] developed a "carbon transcutaneous hemodialysis access device" (CATD), commonly known as "button," as a blood access not requiring needle puncture. As a procedure of the third choice, these devices were expensive and never gained widespread acceptance. Shapiro et al. [42] described another type of "button," a device similar to that developed by Golding.

3. Classification of vascular access

Nowadays, and thanks to all above efforts, nephrologists have the ability to choose the most suitable VA for their patients depending on special needs of each one. Based on expected half-life, the first demarcation is of permanent and temporary VAs [43]. Long-term or permanent VAs are called the ones with an expected half-life of more than 3 years, and mainly include AVF [13] and PTFE AVG. VAs with expected half-life of less than 90 days are called temporary VAs and basically are noncuffed double lumen catheters and arteriovenous shunts. The VAs with half-life between the above categories (90 days to 3 years) are the mid-term VA containing tunneled cuffed catheters, port devices and external and internal shunts.

3.1. Acute hemodialysis vascular access

Acute hemodialysis is a lifesaving treatment, which needs a VA in order to be carried out. When a permanent VA is not available, the preferred and currently available VA for acute hemodialysis is cuffed tunneled and noncuffed nontunneled hemodialysis catheters (Figures 1–5). The reason is that they can be used immediately and placed relatively easily. For catheter insertion, a modified Seldinger guide wire technique is used, preferably with ultrasound guided assistance for minimizing acute placement complications [44, 45].

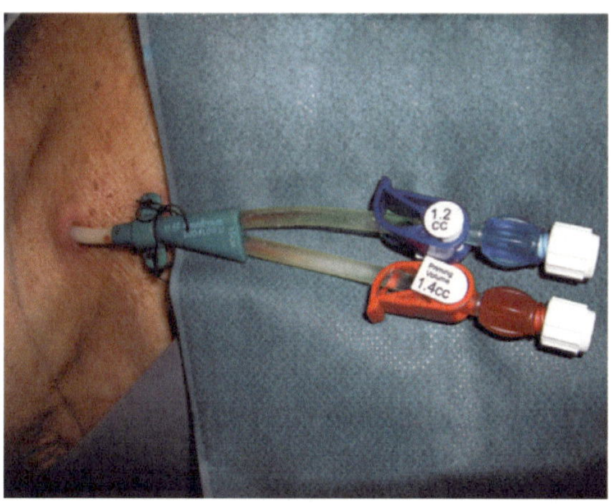

Figure 1. Noncuffed in jugular double lumen catheter.

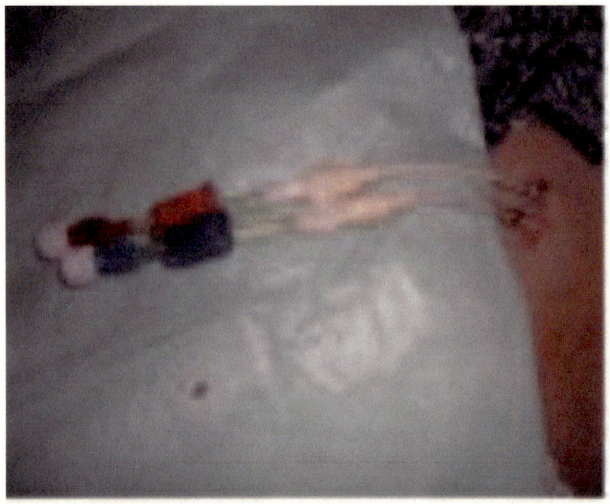

Figure 2. Cuffed tunneled in jugular double lumen catheter.

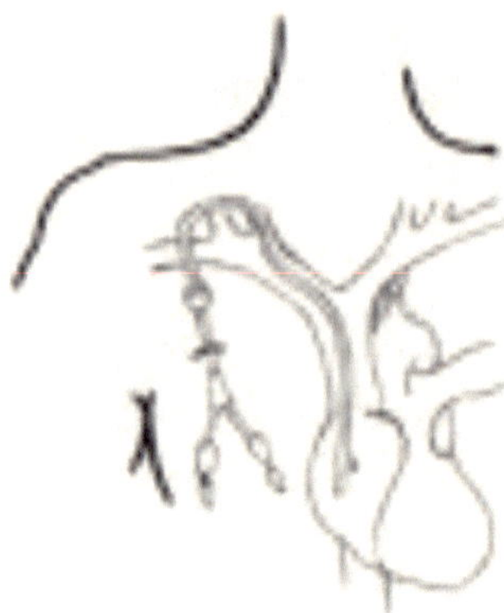

Figure 3. Permanent cuffed jugular catheter.

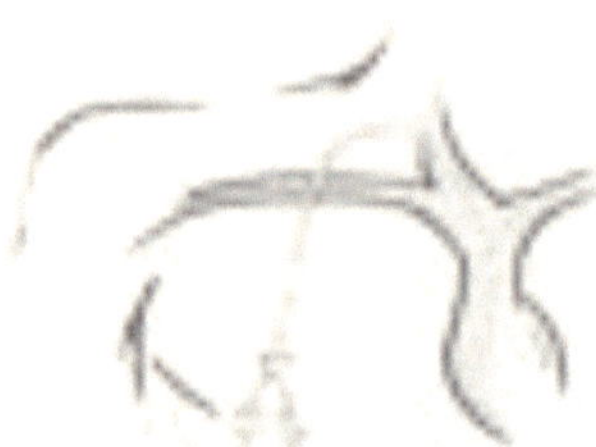

Figure 4. Acute noncuffed jugular catheter.

http://dx.doi.org/10.5772/59464

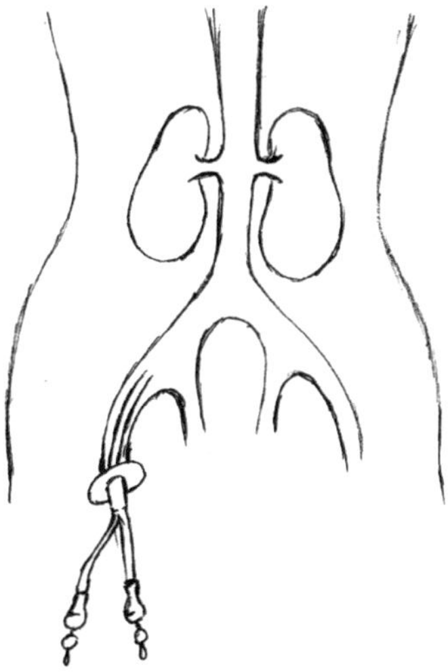

Figure 5. Femoral noncuffed catheter.

The most used and feasible are the noncuffed nontunneled catheters with easy insertion and availability for immediate use. They have some specific technical characteristics; they are made of polymers inelastic at room temperature, facilitating the insertion, but unstiffening at inner body temperature in order to be atraumatic for the vessels. The distance between the inflow and the outflow tip of the catheter must be at least 2 cm to lessen recirculation [46].

Central veins such as jugular or femoral can be used as insertion routes of these catheters [47]. Subclavian typically is an option, but due to its higher incidence of complications, such us lung injury, it is used when the others insertion sites are not feasible.

The National Kidney Foundation Dialysis Outcomes Quality Initiative (K/DOQI) 2006 guidelines recommend the radiographical identification of tip placement and any potential complications before catheter use or anticoagulation treatment [48]. Subclavian vein should be avoided for catheter insertion due to high frequency of stenosis and thrombosis.

There are restrictions concerning the use of these catheters such as the blood flow with a maximum pump speed of 300 ml/min, although actual blood flow tops at 250 ml/min, catheters for insertion in femoral vein should be no less of 18 to 25 cm long to minimize recirculation [49, 50]. Their insertion site determines their life use, with the ones in internal jugular vein be suitable for use for about 2 to 3 weeks, while in femoral vein are used for 3 to 7 days in bedridden patients and for a single treatment in ambulatory patients [51]. Nevertheless, according to KDOQI guidelines, the life use of noncuffed, nontunneled catheters must be of a week or less; when hemodialysis treatment will be required for a longer period, the placement of cuffed, tunneled catheters is suggested [48]. Especially in hospitalized patients, triple lumen catheters are placed, using the third lumen for intravenous drugs and fluid administration and for blood drawing. It seems that two and three lumen catheters have similar blood flow and inflections incidence [52]. The leader cause for catheter removal is infectious complications.

3.2. Permanent vascular access

Taking patient-dependent factors into consideration, such as life expectancy, comorbidities, the status of the venous and arterial vascular system, is very important in order to prescribe the appropriate access. Each type of access, such as arteriovenous fistula (AVF), arteriovenous graft (AVG) or TC, has a different effect on circulatory system, and this should be taken into consideration. Also, the duration of their functionality and the risk for infection and thrombosis are important factors to consider. Each type of surgical anastomosis has advantages and disadvantages [53]. Also, it seems that the advantages of an AVF attempt strategy lessened considerably among older patients, particularly women with diabetes, reflecting the effect of lower AVF success rate and lower life expectancy, suggesting that vascular access-related outcomes may be optimized by considering individual patient characteristics [54]. The American Association for Vascular Surgery and the Society for Vascular Surgery, in 2002, for better consultation and understanding between physicians and registration of VA set VA reporting standards in which three components should be listed, structure (autogenous, prosthetic), position and alignment (loop, direct, etc.) [55]. Risk factors such as female gender, age, diabetic nephropathy, dialysis initiation via CVC and inability of VA maturation before HD initiation are responsible for the majority of VA failure. Repetitive VA failures are risk factor for mortality [56]. It seems that early referral to nephrologist and patient's education leads to initiation of dialysis with permanent VA, better metabolic and clinical situation, lower long-term morbidity and higher 2-year survival [57–61]. It is of benefit to the patient to begin hemodialysis treatment via a functional AVF than with a TC [62–64]; however, grafts are a better alternative to TCs, when AVF is not feasible [65]. Patients with bilateral central vein stenosis often require more than one vascular access modality to achieve a "personal access solution." Native long saphenous vein loops provided the best long-term patency. Expedited renal transplantation with priority local allocation of cadaveric organs to patients with precarious vascular access provides a potential solution [66]. Patients who received either femoral AVG or HeRO VA device experience poor access patency. ESRD patients who receive either of these procedures appear to be at the end stage of available access options [67].

3.2.1. Arteriovenous fistula

The first choice of VA is AVF, for its longevity and low morbidity and mortality rates [68, 69], low complication incidence for infection (one-tenth of AVGs) and thrombosis (one-sixth of AVGs) [70, 71]. AVFs' primary patency rates at 1 year vary considerably between USA and Europe, with reports from the USA that include diabetic patients be as low as 40–43% [72, 73]. From the study of 748 AVFs in diabetic patients over 5 years, Konner et al. showed a primary patency rate of 69–81% [74], while Chemla et al. had a rate of 80% at 22 months in 552 radio-cephalic AVFs in 153 patients over a 4-year period [75]. Hemodialysis patients with AVF have lower mortality and that seems to be attributed not only to decreased incidence of infections and VA dysfunctions but also to other factors, such as LVEF increase and blood pressure and arterial stiffness reduction, as Korsheed et al. [76] showed.

Based on the way of their creation, three types of AVFs can be identified. The first type belongs to the AVFs where an artery and a vein are connected in their natural position, with a side-to-side or side-artery-to-vein-end anastomosis. In the second type, a vein is connected to an artery in end-to-side form, after its metathesis, to connect a further distance or surface the vein to facilitate cannulation; a tunnel creation is required for vein's new positioning. When a vein is connected to an artery end-to-end after it is removed from its anatomical location, we have the third type of AVF [77] (Figures 6–9). The end-to-end technique is abandoned nowadays since it leads to advanced risk for ischemia and thrombosis. Vein end to artery side anastomosis is the most common technique. The first option for the primary AVF is the radial-cephalic. Distal forearm ulnar-basilic has similar secondary patency rate to it and is the best alternative when the first one is not feasible [78]. Stenosis due to technical problems like false surgical cut of vein leads to dysfunctional VA. Complications such as heart failure or steal syndrome may result from a more proximal, big arterial anastomosis [77]. Local anesthesia is usually effective for AVF creation, and the morbidity of the procedure is low. AVF requires time after its creation for maturation before cannulation for at least 14 days according to DOPPS (Data from the Dialysis Outcomes and Practice Patterns Study). During the period of maturation, the blood flow and the vessel size increase over time in 8–12 weeks, and the initial blood flow is in a range of 200–300 ml/min [64].

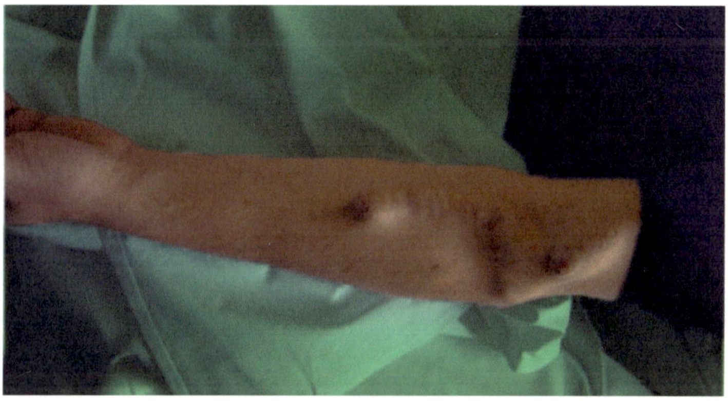

Figure 6. Forearm AVF.

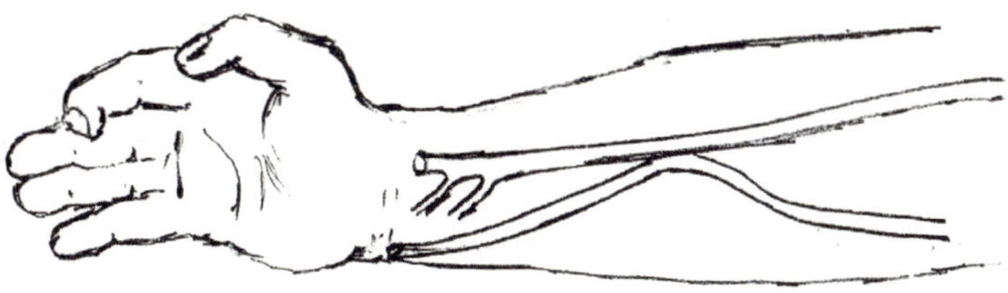

Figure 7. Side-to-side forearm AVF.

The placement of AVFs should be initiated when the patient reaches CKD stage 4, or within 1 year of the anticipated start of dialysis. In their recent study, Hod et al. [79] suggested that

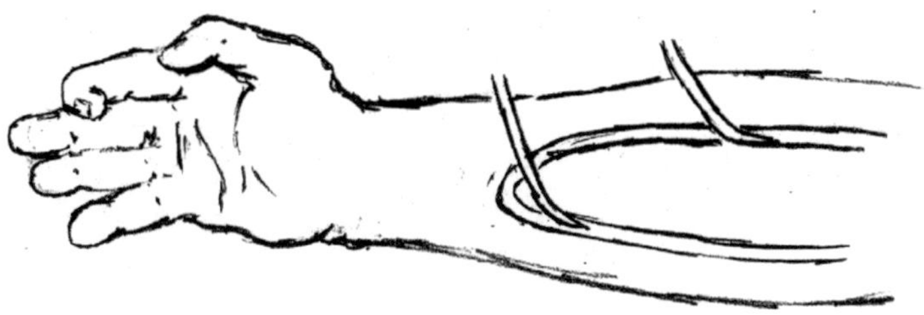

Figure 8. End-to-end forearm AVF.

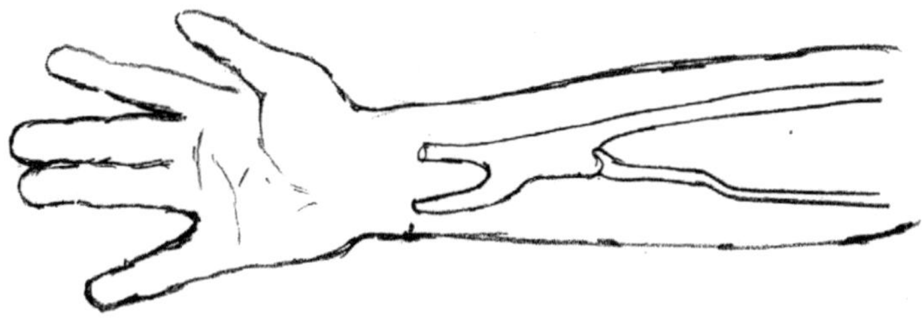

Figure 9. Side-to-end forearm AVF.

creating AVF more than 6 to 9 months before initiating dialysis in elderly may not associate with better AVF success rate. In order to increase the possibilities of a well-functioning AVF's creation and to minimize the complication, a physical examination must be done prior to procedure to identify any differences in blood pressure between the upper extremities [80] and the presence or lack of a well-developed palmar arch to avoid steal syndrome in case of using the dominant artery for AVF creation [81].

Additional information before the creation of AVF can be given with ultrasound of the vessels; their diameter is closely correlated with surgery success with a size of 2 mm and more leads with fruitful maturation [80], in contrast of a size of 1.6 mm and less, which predispose to failure [82]. The upper extremity AVF is the preferred access for hemodialysis, the duplex ultrasound identifies suitable arteries and veins for its successful creation, while early detection and intervention can save the fistula when complications occur [83]. Uzun et al. [84] showed that autologous saphenous vein can be preferably chosen as a prosthetic hemodialysis access graft due to its higher primary and secondary patency and lower complication rate and cost when compared with PTFE grafts. According to the vascular access guidelines of KDOQI, a well-functioning AVF has blood flow over 600 ml/min, with a diameter greater than 6 mm, and is lying less than 6 mm from the surface in a depth between 5 and 10 mm. When an AVF's maturation progresses successfully, then rapidly after surgery blood flow increases from baseline values of 30 to 50 ml/min, reaching 200 to 800 ml/min within 1 week; after 8 weeks, blood flow is over 480 ml/min [85, 86]. The AVFs must be evaluated 4–6 weeks after placement; experienced examiners (e.g., dialysis nurses) can identify nonmaturing fistulas with 80% accuracy [87]. Patients with newly placed AVF are advised for hand squeezing exercises to increase the rate of fistula maturation, such as squeezing a ball, bicep curls, and finger tips

http://dx.doi.org/10.5772/59464

touches resulting to fistulae dilation [88, 89]. Far Infrared therapy, which is a form of heat therapy, has been implicated in improvement of endothelial function and hemodynamics in coronary arteries, probably through up-regulating endothelial nitric oxide synthase (eNOS) expression in arterial endothelium, leading to improved cardiac function in patients with chronic heart diseases. Repeated leg hyperthermia using FIR has been shown to reduce oxidative stress in bed-ridden type II diabetics and may positively influence the complex process of AVF maturation, improving both primary and secondary patency rates [90, 91]. Jennings et al. [92] published a trial, which showed that Venous Window Needle Guide, a subcutaneously placed hemodialysis cannulation device, is safe and effective in facilitating AVF cannulation for patients with an otherwise mature but noncannulatable access. Strozecki et al. described a case report of a 65-year-old female patient who had several hemodialysis sessions by cannulation of dilated collateral abdominal veins with dialysis needles, as an unconventional vascular access for HD in case of central vein occlusion [93]. Humerobasilic and radiocephalic AVF are the two VA types with the most functioning longevity, although in radiocephalic AVF, there is high initial failure rate [94]. It is the preferable VA due to its longevity, low incidence of complications, and easy cannulation [95–97]. In case of failure of radiocephalic AVF creation, the second most preferable VA is brachiocephalic AVF, which comes first in diabetic patients, in whom the inadequacy of vessels for radiocephalic AVF is usually found [98] with a reported 4-year patency of 80% [99]. According to a study of Rondriguez et al., brachiocephalic AVF has a lower survival than radiocephalic. Four years after its creation, just over 50% of the patients have patent AVF and about 30% after 8 years. Failure at first VA increases the risk for following failure, while successful development of the first VA, at about 60% of patients, does not lead to subsequent failure. Diabetes and female gender seem to be risk factors to VA failure [94].

3.2.2. *Arteriovenous graft*

In the USA, AVGs (Figures 10–12) are the most common type of VA that is used for hemodialysis [100]. However, they last less than AVFs and have more complications such as infections and thromboses [70]. Recent technological advances using tissue-engineered AVGs have shown promise for patients receiving hemodialysis and their potential to provide an attractive, viable option for vascular access [101]. Grafts present a second choice of VA when AVF is not possible to be performed because of vascular problems [102]. AVGs have lower risk of nonmaturation in lower time [103]. They can be placed in the forearm, the upper arm and the thigh, when upper-extremity options are exhausted [104] and they can have a straight, curved or loop configuration. Axillary loop arm graft yields acceptable early patency rates in specific patients with vascular problems [105]. Another advantage is that AVGs may offer a large surface for cannulation. Some types of AVGs such as PTFE AVGs can be cannulated immediately after their placement, according to some studies, although it is preferable to wait for about 2 to 3 weeks for the first cannulation [106, 107]. However, the usual time for a functional graft is 2 to 3 weeks in order to reduce the post surgical edema and the perigraft hematoma and seroma [108]. Karatepe et al. [109] presented a novel polycarbonate urethane nanofabric graft, produced by electrospinning technology, which had self-healing features that avoid seroma formation and allow puncturing within 48 hours. It had good 12-month primary and secondary patency rates and substantially lowers infection rates. Early experience with GORE Acuseal is encouraging with patency and bacteremia rates at least comparable to standard polytetrafluoroethylene grafts, permitting cannulation within 24 hours of insertions and line avoidance in the majority of patients [110].

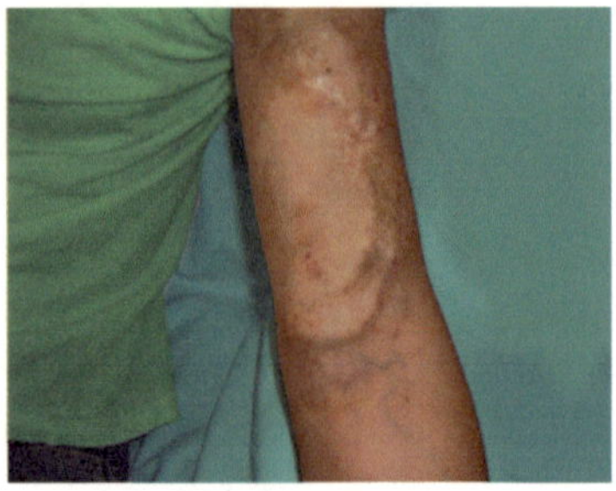

Figure 10. Upper arm AVG.

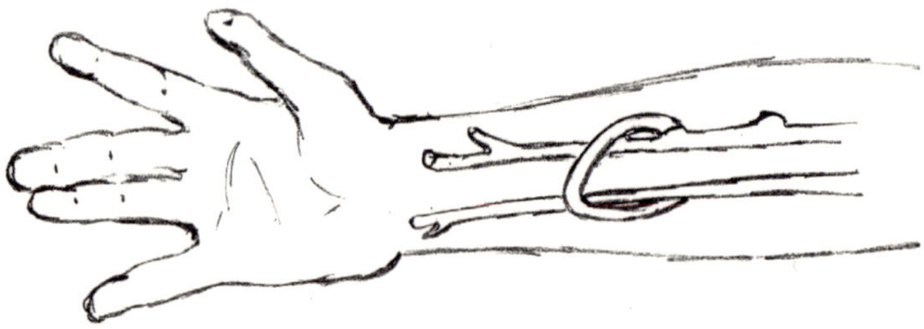

Figure 11. Looped forearm AVG.

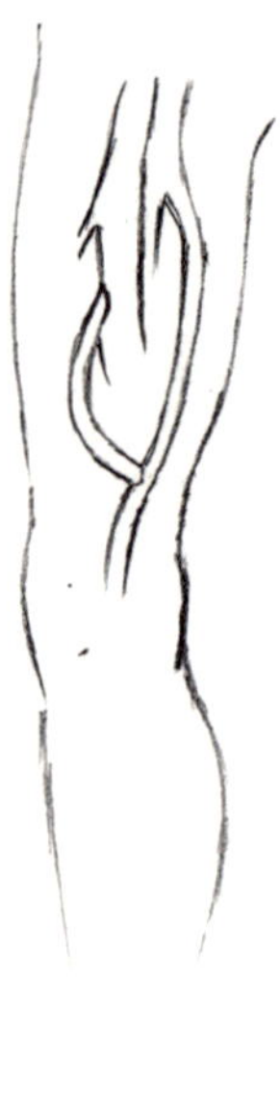

Figure 12. Straight femoral AVG.

3.2.3. Tunneled hemodialysis catheter

TCs (Figures 2 and 3) have higher mortality risk than AVFs or AVGs; thus, they are used when the creation of the latter is not feasible [111]. There are several reasons that lead to the inability for AVF or AVG creation, such as multiple vascular surgeries, which lead to vascular thrombosis, or when patients have severe peripheral vascular disease or very low cardiac output. TCs are more frequently encountered in pediatric and very old patients. They can also be used as a bridge until AVF or AVG maturation [111]. Their use remains very high during the first year of HD care and is associated with high mechanical and infection rates [112]. The incidence of AVFs has been effectively increased since the "fistula first" has been developed [113], although it is accompanied with an increase in TCs, especially those used as a bridge until the maturation of an AVF [100]. Nonetheless, DOPPS shows an increasing use of TCs for the period 1996 to 2006 in many countries [114], which is in accordance with our data of 2011, which showed increased prevalence of TCs in female hemodialysis patients [115]. It is also signified that it is more likely for a patient to have permanent VA (AVF or AVG) than TC if he is at a center with experienced vascular surgery department successfully creating permanent VA in diabetic, older women and early AVF cannulation practice (within 4 weeks from its formation) [114].

They do not last as much as the others types of VA, and they have higher complication rates such as infections. There are studies revealing that CVCs are colonized within the first 10 days of placement; however, the catheter's lumen colonization does not equal to positive blood cultures or clinical signs of bacteremia [116]. The guide-wire change or the complete removal of catheter does not affect the outcome of the infection treatment [117]. Power et al. [118] with their study of 759 TCs showed that the appropriate management of catheters can give functional and complication results similar to AVGs. In their study, survival rates were 85%, 72%, and 48% at 1, 2, and 5 years, respectively, while the infection rate was 0.34 per 1000 catheter-days. Although earlier studies showed a lower risk of catheter-related bloodstream infections with internal jugular TCs compared to femoral, recent studies show no difference between the three sites [119, 120].

Transhepatic hemodialysis catheters seem to be a viable alternative option with low morbidity rates [121]. Another safe and effective long-term access is translumbar inferior vena cava [122]. Retrograde femoral vein catheter insertion is a newly applied lifesaving HD vascular access approach for selected ESRD patients with no available HD vascular access at the ordinary sites with accepted HD adequacy, but it needs more evaluation and studies [123].

4. Children's hemodialysis vascular access

Renal replacement treatment in children varies. According to North American Pediatric Renal Trials and Collaborative Studies (NAPRTCS) registry of patients reaching ESRD in pediatric centers, 25% submitted preemptive renal transplantation, 50% joined in peritoneal dialysis, and 25% started hemodialysis [124, 125]. The preferable therapy is transplantation and in perspective of a rather short time on HD, children receive maintenance HD through an indwelling CVC [126]. In the USA, no more than 800 pediatric patients receive maintenance HD therapy, while the majority of smaller patients, less than 10 kg or 2 years old, receive peritoneal dialysis [127–129].

However, hemodialysis can be performed successfully in infants and very young children, as well [130]. An evaluation of the vasculature of children who will undergo hemodialysis will indicate the appropriate vascular access. Because of the size of their vessels, there is limited use of AVF in children, although there is an effort to make nephrology society to consider AVF as the best access in pediatric HD patients [131]. According to a 2008 pediatric registry (NAPRTCS) annual report, vascular access for hemodialysis included external percutaneous catheter in 78% of patients, internal AV fistula in 12%, and internal and external AV shunt in 7.3 and 0.7%, respectively [125]. K/DOQI has encouraged greater use of AV fistulas in larger children receiving hemodialysis who are not likely to receive a transplant within 12 months, with a goal of achieving more effective dialysis with fewer complications than the ones occurring with catheters. Patient's size determines catheter size. An 8-F dual lumen catheter is well tolerated in 4- to 5-kg children, and as the child's size increases, a vascular access of larger volume can be placed [132]. Blood flow in pediatric patients varies due to the catheter size, which depends on the child's size. In most of the patients, a recommended blood flow of 3 to 5 ml/kg/min is acceptable [133], providing adequate dialysis with Kt/V equal or greater than 1.2. A recent study by Fadel et al. found a significant correlation between serum soluble vascular cell adhesion molecule 1 and ESA doses in thrombosed AVF, and this could have clinical significance after further investigation [134].

5. Vascular access morbidity and mortality

Studies have shown a mortality risk dependent on access type, with the highest risk associated with central venous dialysis catheters, followed by AVGs and then AVFs [135–137]. Recently Hicks et al. [137] stated that this benefit of AVG over TCs may not apply to younger (18–48 years) or older (over 89 years) age-groups. Additionally, patients who had a catheter as the first VA had more complications and higher mortality [138]. The same results have been presented by Ng et al. [139], who examined hospitalization burden related to VA type among 2635 incident patients. The risk for vascular access complications is increased in intensive HD, with overall reported rates being lower in patients with AVF [140]. The CHOICE study examined mortality based on access type in 616 hemodialysis patients for up to 3 years of follow-up. Increased mortality was observed in CVCs and AVGs compared to AVFs in a rate of 50% and 26%, respectively, with greater prevalence in male and elderly patients [141, 142]. Despite these findings and the KDOQI recommendations, dialysis access data from 2002 to 2003 showed that only 33% of prevalent hemodialysis patients in the USA were being dialyzed via AVFs. On the contrary, in Europe and Canada, the majority of the patients [74% and 53%, respectively) were being dialyzed via AVFs [143], but a decreasing trend in the use of AVF seems to take place accompanied by an increasing trend in the use of TCs at the start and after the start of HD [144].

Vascular access admissions continue to fall, with more procedures now performed in an outpatient setting, and are 45% below than in 1993. Among African American patients, the relative risk of an all-cause hospitalization or one related to infection is almost equal to that of Caucasians; the risk of a vascular access hospitalization, however, is 24% higher [145]. Thrombotic occlusion remains a major event, leading to permanent failure in 10% of AVFs and 20% of grafts each year. Interventional (percutaneous transluminal angioplasty and/or stent implantation) or surgical revision of thrombosed accesses has similar outcomes with a high rate of reinterventions. Diabetic elderly patients suffering from peripheral arteriosclerotic obstructive disease are particularly prone to angioaccess-induced hand ischemia [146]. Patients with TCs and AVGs have higher chronic inflammation levels than those with AVFs and increased requirements in epoetin [147]. In our previous work with 149 hemodialysis patients with 202 vascular access procedures (177 Cimino-Brescia AVFs and 25 PTFE AVGs), Cimino–Brescia fistula was used in all patients as the first choice vascular access, except for one patient in the elderly group. Fifteen patients in the elderly group and 7 younger than 65 years old had PTFE AVGs as the third or second choice of VA, respectively. Vascular thrombosis was the only reason of technique failure in both groups. Other complications were aneurysms (10/48 and 14/101), infections (0/48 and 2/101) and edema (0/48 and 6/101) (Table 1). AVF had a 5-year technique survival in two groups of 35% and 45%, respectively (Figure 13). According to our findings, there was no difference in VA complications across age-groups and the first AVF survival was independent of age [6]. Swindlehurst et al. [148] have published similar results, according to which the creation of AVF in the elderly is not only possible but also proved to have a short hospital stay, high patency rates, and an acceptable rate of further intervention. The outcome of AVF benefits more from acknowledging individual vascular conditions rather than age of the patient and therefore AVF creation should not be denied to elderly patients [149]. Among patients over 80 years of age, the AVF as vascular access for HD at the time of dialysis initiation was among the factors that benefit their survival [150].

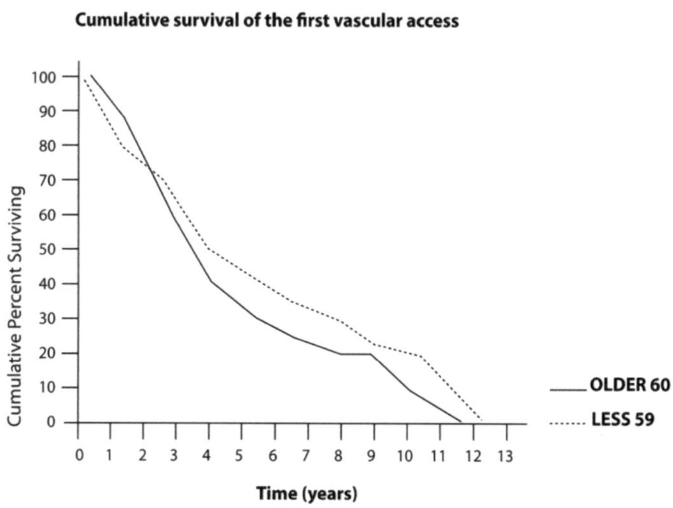

Figure 13. Cumulative survival of first VA according to the patients' age.

	Group A (age>60)	Group B(age<60)	*P*
Thrombosis	14/48	39/101	N.S.
Aneurysm	10/48	14/101	N.S.
Edema	0/48	6/101	N.S.
Infection	0/48	2/101	N.S.

Table 1. Complications of vascular access

According to the 2010 USRDS Annual Data Report, in 2008, hospitalizations increased, to a point of 46% over 1993. Women on hemodialysis were 16% more likely to be hospitalized than men, overall, in 2007–2008. Also, they had a greater risk than men of cardiovascular, infectious and vascular access hospitalizations 11%, 14%, and 29%, respectively. Recently, in a retrospective single-center analysis, our data varies to those we published in 1998. In 145 patients on HD, we found that female had more possibilities to start HD with double lumen catheter than male and also patients with heart failure independent of gender [115]. Patibandla et al. [151] in their logistic regression model found that increasing age, female sex, black race, lower body mass index, urban location, certain comorbidities and shorter pre-end-stage renal disease nephrology care are all associated with a significantly lower like hood of AVF placement as initial access predialysis. Additionally, there are geographic disparities in AVF creation with decreased rates of AVF placement as the first access in metropolitan, but not rural, populations compared with micropolitan communities [152]. Improvement in standardization of care according to practice guidelines is necessary. AVF rate could be increased by improving access to surgical resources and patients education [153]. Enhancing patient self-care abilities and working together with patients on proper vascular access care can prolong vascular access site viability [154]. Intraoperative blood flow measurements greater than 120 ml/min in AVF and less than 320 ml/min in AVGs may be predictive factors of early failure and fistulography is essential to access patency [155]. In addition to the clinical examination, there are numerous radiological assessments of vascular access pre- and postoperative that enrich our diagnostic armamentarium [156]. Recently, Remuzzi and Manini [157] presented a numerical model that in the clinical setting should allow to reduce the incidence of AVF nonmaturation as well as incidence of VA complications. Cannulation of VA is a crucial part of its management in HD patients and the proper use of the rotating site technique might still be the best approach to cannulation [158]. Evidence do not support the preferential use of buttonhole over rope-ladder cannulation [159]. However, according to systematic review of Muir et al. [160], buttonhole cannulation is associated with higher rates of infectious events, staff support requirements and no reduction in surgical AVF interventions compared with rope ladder in home HD patients.

6. Nontunneled double lumen catheters complications

The nontunneled double lumen catheters' complications concern the early ones during the insertion and the late ones such as infection and thrombosis of the vessels.

http://dx.doi.org/10.5772/59464

The severity of acute complications varies with the site of insertion. The lowest rate is in the femoral position. A significant complication is perforation of the femoral artery. Bleeding usually resolves within minutes of direct compression and large femoral or retroperitoneal hematomas occur occasionally [161]. Subclavian insertion complications are more serious. The overinsertion of guide wire can occasionally lead to atrial or ventricular arrhythmias, but they are frequently transient [162]. The penetration or cannulation of the subclavian artery can lead to hemothorax, which may require a thoracotomy tube. The incidence of pneumothorax varies from less than 1% to more than 10% of insertions, depending on the skill and experience of the physician. Pericardial rupture and tamponade also have been described [163, 164]. There is less likelihood of arterial puncture or pneumothorax in ultrasound-guided catheter insertion [165]. Subclavian insertion from the left has an increased risk of pneumothorax and atrial perforation, which can be presented with acute hemopericardium upon initiation of dialysis. Internal jugular vein is the preferred site of insertion because of subclavian stenosis and loss of the ipsilateral arm for future hemodialysis access. This complication appears to occur more often with subclavian (40–50%) than with internal jugular insertions (up to 10%) [166, 167]. At internal jugular insertions, a carotid artery penetration may occur, but there is also a lower risk of pneumothorax (0.1%). Post procedural chest X-ray is taken for confirmation of position of catheter tip and to detect early complications, but delayed complications can occur after catheterization. Thus, the patient should be monitored carefully and managed appropriately according to the presenting signs and symptoms [168].

Prevention and treatment of catheter thrombosis are important clinical issues. To prevent formation of thrombus, both lumens of the double lumen catheter are instilled with heparin following hemodialysis [46]. Lytic agents such as urokinase and alteplase are effective in treatment of catheter thrombosis. Alteplase has effectiveness rates in thrombosis treatment comparable to the ones observed with urokinase [169]. Central vein catheters are associated with the development of central vein stenosis [170]. The K/DOQI guidelines therefore recommend avoiding placement in the subclavian vein, unless no other options are available. If central venous thrombosis is detected early, it responds well to directly applied thrombolytic therapy [170] or to percutaneous transluminal angioplasty when the fibrotic stenosis can be crossed with a guide wire [171]. The infection risks associated with temporary double lumen catheters include local exit site infection and systemic bacteremia, both of which require prompt removal of the catheter and appropriate intravenous antibiotic therapy [48, 172, 173]. Bacteremia generally results from either contamination of the catheter lumen or migration of bacteria from the skin through the entry site, down the hemodialysis catheter into the blood stream [174–176]. It seems that prevention strategies should target the first 6 months after access placement or a remedial access-related procedure as over time the risk decline [177]. Skin flora, *Staphylococcus* and *Streptococcus* species, are responsible for the majority of infections. It has been reported that surface modification with bismuth film reduces bacterial colonization of nontunneled HD catheters [178]. Guidelines have been proposed by working group with O'Grady et al. [179], with major areas of emphasis such as educating and training healthcare personnel, who insert and maintain catheters, maximal sterile barrier precautions during CVC insertion, using >0.5% chlorexidine. The use of prophylactic gentamicin/citrate lock seems to be associated with a substantial reduction in catheter-related bloodstream than heparin [180]. Nurse is also a key figure in the preventions of such infections with the adoption of standard precautions such as washing hands, managing HD rooms and other medical devices, managing vascular access, and providing educational support to patient [181].

There is conflicting evidence concerning the risk of infection based on the site of insertion [172, 182, 183]. Coagulase-negative staphylococci, *Staphylococcus aureus*, aerobic gram-negative bacilli, and *Candida albicans* most commonly cause catheter-related bloodstream infection. In most cases of nontunneled CVC-related bacteremia and fungemia, the CVC should be removed. The decision should be based on the severity of the patient's illness, documentation that the vascular-access device is infected, assessment of the specific pathogen involved and presence of complications, such as endocarditis, septic thrombosis, tunnel infection, or metastatic seeding [184].

Overall, compared with the subclavian vein, the internal jugular vein remains the preferred access site in ambulatory patients. In the intensive care unit, either femoral or internal jugular vein placement is satisfactory, with the use of ultrasound making internal jugular vein placement safer.

The best solution is to prevent the infection by proper placement technique, optimal exit site care and management of the catheter within the HD facility [46, 185]. It is generally believed that CVC can adversely affect permanent VA ipsilateral placement outcomes due to central vein stenosis that they cause, but it seems that the primary failure rate of AVF and AVG is not affected by the presence of an ipsilateral catheter, but cumulative access survival is inferior [186].

7. Arteriovenous fistulas complications

Early causes include inflow problems due to small or atherosclerotic arteries, or juxta-anastomotic stenosis, so a preoperative evaluation for suitable access sites has to be performed [187]. Selective use of duplex ultrasonography appears to enhance AVF success rate, although agreed vessels criteria are needed [188]. It seems that the type of anesthesia plays a role in the fistula surgery, with regional anesthesia having a beneficial sympathectomy like effect that causes vasodilation with increased blood flow during surgery and in the AVF postoperatively that may prevent early thrombosis and potentially improve outcome [189], but more evidence are expected to establish this [190].

The etiology of this acquired lesion is not entirely clear but may be related to manipulating the free end of the vein, torsion, poor angulation or loss of the vasa vasorum during anatomic dissection. More often than not, this lesion can be effectively managed with angioplasty [191, 192] or surgical revision [193].

Accessory veins that divert blood flow from the intended superficial vessels to deeper conduits or central venous stenoses due to prior TCs placements may cause outflow problems. Vessels, smaller than one-fourth of the fistula diameter, are usually not hemodynamically relevant. Juxta-anastomotic stenosis and accessory veins are the most common causes for early failure

AVFs when preoperative evaluations for suitable access sites have been performed [187]. In elderly population, there is an association of older age, female gender, black race, diabetes, cardiac failure and shorter pre-ESRD nephrology care with predialysis AVF failure [194].

A rather rare complication secondary to bleeding from a catheter-related puncture of an AVF is an acute forearm compartment syndrome [195].

Venous stenosis, thrombosis and attained arterial lesions like aneurysms or stenoses constitute late causes of AVFs' failure.

As blood flow decreases due to venous stenosis, weekly Kt/V ([dialyzer clearance time]/body volume) decreases and/or recirculation increases, constituting great clinical signs of VA dysfunction. AVF salvage surgery is of paramount importance in order to increase the patency rate, which prolongs survival and increases the patient's quality of life [196]. Balloon angioplasty followed with stenting maintains the vessel lumen shape over time, as the stent is likely to reduce the risk of restenosis that can otherwise occur after balloon angioplasty because of the viscoelastic recoil of the vessel [197]. According to Aftab et al. [198], for AVF stenosis resistant to conventional percutaneous transluminal angioplasty (PTA), cutting balloon angioplasty may be a better second line treatment given its superior patency rates. It seems that the deficiency of circulating endothelial progenitor cells is associated with early and frequent restenosis after angioplasty of HD VA [199].

Native fistulas will not typically thrombose until flow is severely diminished. The thrombectomy of fistulas, although technically more challenging than in AVGs, is often successful and if flow is reestablished, primary patency is longer than in grafts [200]. Antiplatelet treatment protects fistula from thrombosis or loss of patency but has little or no effect on graft patency and uncertain effects on vascular access maturation for dialysis and major bleeding [201]. Elective repair of subclinical stenosis in AVFs with blood flow >500 ml/min cost-effectively reduces the risk of thrombosis and access loss [202]. Reconstructing the AVF by surgically removing venous neointimal hyperplasia is an effective technique for late hemodialysis access failure which preserves patients' vessels [203].

As AVF's size increases over time with increased blood flow, aneurysms may be formed, constituting rather a cosmetic than functional concern, unless stenotic lesions accompany them. If the overlying skin is atrophic or blanching, or there are signs of ulceration or bleeding, a surgical evaluation must be performed urgently [204]. Also, if there is a high association of venous outflow stenosis and AVF aneurysms, comprehensive therapy should encompass treatment of any venous outflow stenosis before open AVF aneurysm repair. A two-stage repair may decrease tunneled HD catheter use in patients with multiple aneurysms [205]. In order to maintain an autogenous access while conserving future dialysis sites, partial aneurysmectomy is recommended as a first-line choice for managing aneurysm associated complications [206]. Also, autologous surgical reconstruction is feasible in the majority of AVF aneurysms. It preserves fistula function and keeps the advantages of an autogenous access [207]. The rupture of such aneurysms in high-flow fistulas can lead to exsanguination and death (Figure 14).

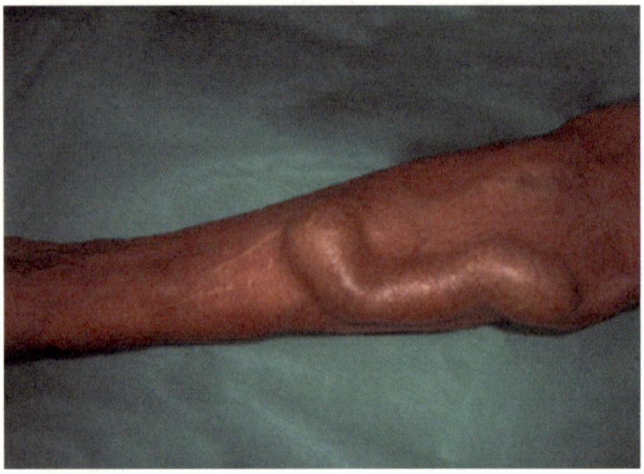

Figure 14. Aneurysm in forearm AVF.

Infections of AVFs are rare but must be treated properly due to patients' impaired immunologic status. Very rare infections of the AV anastomosis require surgery with resection of the infected tissue. More often, infections occur at cannulation sites and then the arm should be rested and cannulation cease [208]. In all cases of AVF infection, antibiotic therapy is initiated with broad-spectrum vancomycin plus an aminoglycoside and converting to appropriate one based on results of culture and sensitivities. Infections of primary AVFs should be treated for a total of 6 weeks, analogous to subacute bacterial endocarditis [209].

8. Arteriovenous graft complications

AVGs have a functional life much shorter than AVFs. Neointimal hyperplasia causes venous stenosis, which leads to thrombosis, and this is the natural course of AVGs. The principal cause of thrombosis is the increased production of smooth muscle cells, myofibroblasts and vascularization within the neointima. Around the graft, there is also angiogenesis and numerous macrophages in the tissue [210, 211]. Growth factors (GF) such as VEGF (vascular endothelial), PDGF (platelet derived) and basic FGF (fibroblast) are present within the neointimal lesion [211]. The presence of shear stress regulates vascular endothelium [212, 213] and that flow within AVGs is likely to be different from native veins. Understanding the pathophysiology of neointimal hyperplasia could lead to targeted therapy. Current studies are evaluating the role of radiation [214], decoy peptides against transcription factors [215, 216] and local delivery of drugs with cell-cycle inhibitory effects (e.g., paclitaxel [217] and sirolimus). Cell-based strategies seek to take advantage of endothelial progenitor cells that release endogenous inhibitors of proliferation and thrombosis, such as nitric oxide (NO) and prostacyclin [218]. Venous stenosis in AVGs leads to decreased blood flow and thrombosis, at a rate of 1–1.5 times/patient/year [70]. Thrombosis is associated with anatomical stenosis, in most cases, which is located in the venous anastomosis (60%), followed by the peripheral vein (37%) and within the graft (38%) [219]. Stenosis and closure by venous anastomoses are the most frequent causes of failure of AVG for hemodialysis. AVG closure can be addressed surgically and endovasc-

http://dx.doi.org/10.5772/59464

ularly (amenable to thrombectomy by radiological or surgical means) [220]. Percutaneous angioplasty is safe and effective in treating venous stenosis [221], with a success rate of 80% to 94% and primary patency around 60% at 6 months and 40% at 1 year. The placement of self-expanding nitinol stents at the venous anastomosis appears to prolong patency in cases where focal lesions are resistant to repeated angioplasty and recur and improve PTFE grafts longevity in selected cases of older grafts [222]. Central stenosis is technically more difficult to treat, and stenotic lesions often recur within 6 months [77]. Recently, a modular anastomotic valve device (MAVD) has been in preliminary use in order to isolate the graft from the circulation between dialysis sessions, decreasing the flow disturbances this way and as a result the intimal hyperplasia [223]. During the last decades, percutaneous techniques became increasingly important for the treatment of AVG failure [224]. Cutting balloon angioplasty is a safe and effective treatment of graft to vein anastomotic stenosis, with significantly higher patency than that of conventional balloon angioplasty [225]. From the point of view of Troisi et al. [226], the combined simultaneous hybrid (open and endovascular) approach in urgency maximizes the use of different available techniques, improving overall success rate to save a thrombosed graft.

As described above, AVGs' thromboses are usually the result of multiple factors; such as stenosis, hypotension and excessive compression for hemostasis. Hemodialysis nurses have to be careful in order to avoid these factors. Thrombosis risk increases as blood flow (BF) decreases, as May et al. [227] showed in their study. AVG thrombosis can be managed in an outpatients' basis endovascularly. Angiography for venous stenosis is always required and is often accompanied by an angioplasty.

Prompt pharmaceutical thrombolysis or mechanical removal of the thrombus with a Fogarty catheter and thromboaspiration or thrombectomy with a mechanical device [228] may avoid a new catheter placement.

Infections of AVGs are severe complications and the second cause of vascular access loss. Hemodialysis-related bacteraemia is 10-fold more often in AVGs than AVFs: 2.5 incidents every 1000 HD sessions versus 0.2 [229]. It seems that the most significant modifiable risk factor is patients' hygiene [230].

A referral to surgeon of pseudoaneurysms for resection is imposed when they are increasing rapidly in size, their width is more than 2-fold bigger than the graft, or the overlying skin seems under duress (thin, bleeding, blanching) [231].

Ischemia, as a result of access placement, is more common for AVGs than AVFs: vascular steal syndrome and ischemic monomelic neuropathy are two important clinical entities to distinguish.

"Physiological" steal phenomenon occurs in 73% of AVFs and 90% of AVGs. Thus, in a radiocephalic fistula, arterial blood from the palmar arch may also deliver blood into the fistula. Unless there is the capacity for collateralization, this can lead to ischemia in the hand, ranging from complaints about cold hands to necrotic fingertips. Most of these complaints improve over time, but 1% of AVFs and up to 4% of AVGs require surgical revision [232]. Doppler ultrasonography is a useful adjunctive tool to determine the etiology of chronic hemodialysis access-induced distal ischemia (HAIDI). Conservative measures combined with close follow-up can be used as the first step in the management of chronic HAIDI patients with mild symptoms [233]. Ischemic monomelic neuropathy is characterized by warm hands with a good pulse, but the hands are tender and swollen, usually immediately after surgery, and there is muscle weakness [234]. The cause is likely ischemia of the nerves, and rapid surgical reevaluation is needed. Wound and skin complications and greater incidence of thrombosis of VA associated with recombinant human erythropoietin have been reported (rHuEPO) [235].

9. Tunneled catheter complications

Early or late catheter dysfunctions are the functional complications of TCs. Kinking and unsuitable positioning of the catheter tip may be the cause of early dysfunction and can be managed under fluoroscopic guidance. Around or at the catheter tip, fibrin sheaths and thrombi can be formed constituting late causes of failure. Balloon angioplasty can disrupt fibrinous sheaths, improving flow through a new catheter in the same location. Valliant et al. [236] have demonstrate in their study that there is no significant increase in bacteraemia and subsequent catheter dysfunction rates after fibrin sheath disruption by balloon procedure compared to simple over the wire exchange. Symptomatic occlusions of the central veins usually require the removal of the catheter and system anticoagulation and must be weighed in the context of a continued need for dialysis and other available access options. Yoon et al. recently referred a novel two-stage hemodialysis reliable outflow (HeRO) graft implantation technique that avoids the use of a femoral bridging hemodialysis catheter in internal jugular vein (IJV) catheter-dependent patients with contralateral central venous occlusion and thus lowering the risk of infection related to a femoral catheter [237]. The use of catheter is related to a higher incidence of infection and could compromise dialysis adequacy [238, 239]. Catheter-related infections (CRI) are linked with increased all cause morbidity and mortality. The 8–10% of MRSA bacteraemia in the UK occurs in patients receiving long-term hemodialysis. It appears that the catheter locking with appropriate antimicrobial lock solutions (ALS) decrease the infections' incidence in HD patients [180, 240, 241]. It seems that prophylaxis with gentamicin of the catheter lumens reduces bacterial infection morbidity and mortality-related bacteremia of catheter without obvious bacterial resistance, making such use advisable [242]. Even taurolidine–citrate–heparin catheter lock solution reduces staphylococcal bacteraemia rates in HD patients [243] and improves the inflammatory profile in HD patients with TCs [244]. Del Pozo et al. [245] in their prospective study showed that an evaluation of tunneled catheters with intracatheter leukocyte culture helps in the early colonization of HD catheters, giving the possibility to eradicate biofilm without the removal of catheter. Recent studies have demonstrate that the "shower and no-dressing" technique appears to be a safe TC option that improves quality of life [246, 247], although there is skepticism and uncertainty about the appropriate dressing [248].

10. Final conclusions and remarks

Unfortunately, there are no revolutionary changes in the field of vascular access for hemodialysis in the last years. According to the guidelines, AVFs are still the best choice. Luckily, AVGs' survival has been increased, but still TCs are used in a great portion of ESDRD patients.

http://dx.doi.org/10.5772/59464

As a result, humerobasilic and radiocephalic AVFs are the two VA types with the most functioning longevity. However, AVFs' primary patency rates at 1 year vary considerably between USA and Europe. Hemodialysis patients with AVF seem to have lower mortality.

The incidence of AVFs has been effectively increased since the "fistula first" has been developed, although it is accompanied with an increase in TCs.

AVGs as a second choice remain a good solution for patients without the possibility of AVF and the survival of grafts has been improved.

TCs seem to be a new reality in most American and European dialysis units because of the increase of number of elderly patients and with heart failure. Early referral to nephrologists and patient's education has an important role for a successful VA.

Additionally, the cannulation of VA is a crucial part of its management in HD patients and the proper use may improve the survival of VA.

Summarized from the international literature and our experience, when there are suitable vessels, the creation of AVF is of top priority. When this is not feasible or there is an AVF failure, AVGs or TCs are the first choice alternative or the second best, respectively. Female and old patients are more likely to initiate HD treatments via TC. A well-matured and functioning permanent vascular access is of great importance for its longevity and thus early referral to a nephrologist is mandatory.

Author details

Eirini Grapsa[1*] and Konstantinos Pantelias[2]

*Address all correspondence to: grapse@otenet.gr

1 National and Kapodistrian University of Athens, Aretaieio, University Hospital, Athens, Greece

2 Protypo Nefrologiko Kentro Athinon, Athens, Greece

References

[1] Gilbertson DT, Liu J, Xue JL, Louis TA, Solid CA, Ebben JP, et al. Projecting the number of patients with end-stage renal disease in the United States to the year 2015. J Am Soc Nephrol. 2005;16(12):3736–41.

[2] Schieppati A, Remuzzi G. Chronic renal diseases as a public health problem: epidemiology, social, and economic implications. Kidney Int Suppl. 2005(98):S7–S10.

[3] Eggers PW. Has the incidence of end-stage renal disease in the USA and other countries stabilized? Curr Opin Nephrol Hypertens. 2011.

[4] Grassmann A, Gioberge S, Moeller S, Brown G. ESRD patients in 2004: global overview of patient numbers, treatment modalities and associated trends. Nephrol Dial Transplant. 2005;20(12):2587–93.

[5] Santoro A, Canova C, Freyrie A, Mancini E. Vascular access for hemodialysis. J Nephrol. 2006;19(3):259–64.

[6] Grapsa EJ, Paraskevopoulos AP, Moutafis SP, Vourliotou AJ, Papadoyannakis NJ, Digenis GE, et al. Complications of vascular access in hemodialysis (HD)—aged vs adult patients. Geriatr Nephrol Urol. 1998;8(1):21–4.

[7] III. NKF-K/DOQI Clinical Practice Guidelines for Vascular Access: update 2000. Am J Kidney Dis. 2001;37(1 Suppl 1):S137–81.

[8] Schwab SJ, Oliver MJ, Suhocki P, McCann R. Hemodialysis arteriovenous access: detection of stenosis and response to treatment by vascular access blood flow. Kidney Int. 2001;59(1):358–62.

[9] Feldman HI, Kobrin S, Wasserstein A. Hemodialysis vascular access morbidity. J Am Soc Nephrol. 1996;7(4):523–35.

[10] System USRD. 2002 Annual Data Report. Bethesda, National Institutes of Health, National Institute of Diabetes and Digestive Diseases. 2002.

[11] Roy-Chaudhury P, Duncan H, Barrett W, Elson H, Narayana A, Foley J, et al. Vascular brachytherapy for hemodialysis vascular access dysfunction: exploring an unmet clinical need. J Invasive Cardiol. 2003;15 (Suppl A):25A–30A.

[12] Lee H, Manns B, Taub K, Ghali WA, Dean S, Johnson D, et al. Cost analysis of ongoing care of patients with end-stage renal disease: the impact of dialysis modality and dialysis access. Am J Kidney Dis. 2002;40(3):611–22.

[13] Allon M. Implementing a vascular access program: improved outcomes with multidisciplinary approaches. In: Gray RJ, Sands JJ, editors. Dialysis Access: A Multidisciplinary Approach. Philadelphia: Lippincott Williams & Wilkins; 2002. pp. 6–9.

[14] Haas G. Versuche der Blutauswaschung am Lebenden mit Hilfe der Dialyse. Klin Wochenschr. 1925;4:13–4.

[15] Kolff WJ. The artificial kidney. J Mt Sinai Hosp N Y. 1947;14(2):71–9.

[16] Vienken J. 'Bioengineering for life': a tribute to Willem Johan Kolff. Nephrol Dial Transplant. 2009;24(8):2299–301.

[17] Kolff WJ. First clinical experience with the artificial kidney. Ann Intern Med. 1965;62:608–19.

http://dx.doi.org/10.5772/59464

[18] Aubaniac R. A new route for venous injection or puncture: the subclavicular route, subclavian vein, brachiocephalic trunk. Sem Hop. 1952;28(85):3445–7.

[19] Quinton W, Dillard D, Scribner BH. Cannulation of blood vessels for prolonged hemodialysis. Trans Am Soc Artif Intern Organs. 1960;6:104–13.

[20] Seldinger SI. Catheter replacement of the needle in percutaneous arteriography; a new technique. Acta Radiol. 1953;39(5):368–76.

[21] Shaldon S, Chiandussi L, Higgs B. Hemodialysis by percutaneous catheterisation of the femoral artery and vein with regional heparinization. Lancet. 1961. 278(7207): 857–9.

[22] Cimino JE, Brescia MJ. Simple venipuncture for hemodialysis. N Engl J Med. 1962;267:608–9.

[23] Fogarty TJ, Cranley JJ, Krause RJ, Strasser ES, Hafner CD. A method for extraction of arterial emboli and thrombi. Surg Gynecol Obstet. 1963;116:241–4.

[24] Brescia MJ, Cimino JE, Appel K, Hurwich BJ. Chronic hemodialysis using venipuncture and a surgically created arteriovenous fistula. N Engl J Med. 1966;275(20):1089–92.

[25] Sperling M, Kleinschmidt W, Wilhelm A, Heidland A, Klutsch K. [Subcutaneous arteriovenous shunt for intermittent hemodialysis treatment]. Dtsch Med Wochenschr. 1967;92(10):425–6.

[26] Stolic RV, Trajkovic GZ, Krstic NJ, Stolic DZ, Subaric-Gorgieva G. Correlation of mortality and location of arteriovenous fistula in hemodialysis patients. Int J Artif Organs. 2011;34(1):26–33.

[27] Konner K, Nonnast-Daniel B, Ritz E. The arteriovenous fistula. J Am Soc Nephrol. 2003;14(6):1669–80.

[28] Rohl L, Franz HE, Mohring K, Ritz E, Schuler HW, Uhse HG, et al. Direct arteriovenous fistula for hemodialysis. Scand J Urol Nephrol. 1968;2(3):191–5.

[29] Girardet RE, Hackett RE, Goodwin NJ, Friedman EA. Thirteen months experience with the saphenous vein graft arteriovenous fistula for maintenance hemodialysis. Trans Am Soc Artif Intern Organs. 1970;16:285–91.

[30] Brittinger WD SM, Huber W et al. 16 months experience with the subcutaneously fixed superficial femoral artery for chronic haemodialysis. Proc EDTA. 1970;7:408–12.

[31] Brittinger W-D vHG, Twittenhoff W-D et al. Implantation of a plastic valve into the superficialised femoral artery. Proc EDTA. 1971;8:521–5.

[32] Buselmeier TJ, Kjellstrand CM, Simmons RL, Duncan DA, von Hartitzsch B, Rattazzi LC, et al. A totally new subcutaneous prosthetic arterio-venous shunt. Trans Am Soc Artif Intern Organs. 1973;19:25–32.

[33] Baker LD, Jr., Johnson JM, Goldfarb D. Expanded polytetrafluoroethylene (PTFE) subcutaneous arteriovenous conduit: an improved vascular access for chronic hemodialysis. Trans Am Soc Artif Intern Organs. 1976;22:382–7.

[34] Mindich BP, Silverman MJ, Elguezabal A, Levowitz BS. Umbilical cord vein fistula for vascular access in hemodialysis. Trans Am Soc Artif Intern Organs. 1975;21:273–80.

[35] Dardik H, Ibrahim IM, Dardik I. Arteriovenous fistulas constructed with modified human umbilical cord vein graft. Arch Surg. 1976;111(1):60–2.

[36] Erben J KJ, Bastecky J, Vortel V. Experience with routine use of sucblavian vein cannulation in haemodialysis. Proc EDTA. 1969;6:59–64.

[37] Schillinger F, Schillinger D, Montagnac R, Milcent T. Post catheterisation vein stenosis in haemodialysis: comparative angiographic study of 50 subclavian and 50 internal jugular accesses. Nephrol Dial Transplant. 1991;6(10):722–4.

[38] Dotter CT, Judkins MP, Rosch J. Nonoperative treatment of arterial occlusive disease: a radiologically facilitated technique. Radiol Clin North Am. 1967;5(3):531–42.

[39] Gracz KC, Ing TS, Soung LS, Armbruster KF, Seim SK, Merkel FK. Proximal forearm fistula for maintenance hemodialysis. Kidney Int. 1977;11(1):71–5.

[40] Konner K. Primary vascular access in diabetic patients: an audit. Nephrol Dial Transplant. 2000;15(9):1317–25.

[41] Golding AL, Nissenson AR, Raible D. Carbon transcutaneous access device (CTAD). Proc Clin Dial Transplant Forum. 1979;9:242–7.

[42] Shapiro FL, Keshaviah PR, Carlson LD, Ilstrup KM, Collins AJ, Andersen RC, et al. Blood access without percutaneous punctures. Proc Clin Dial Transplant Forum. 1980;10:130–7.

[43] Canaud B. DS. Vascular access for hemodialysis. In: Horl HW, Lindsay BR, Ronco C, Winchester FJ, editors. Replacement of Renal Function by Dialysis. Kluwer Academic Publishers; 2004. pp. 203–30.

[44] Randolph AG, Cook DJ, Gonzales CA, Pribble CG. Ultrasound guidance for placement of central venous catheters: a meta-analysis of the literature. Crit Care Med. 1996;24(12):2053–8.

[45] Work J. Vascular access for renal replacement therapy. In: Murray PT, Hall JB, editors. Intensive Care in Nephrology. Taylor & Francis; 2006. pp. 157–64.

[46] Schwab SJ, Beathard G. The hemodialysis catheter conundrum: hate living with them, but can't live without them. Kidney Int. 1999;56(1):1–17.

[47] Fan PY, Schwab SJ. Vascular access: concepts for the 1990s. J Am Soc Nephrol. 1992;3(1):1–11.

[48] Clinical practice guidelines for hemodialysis adequacy, update 2006. Am J Kidney Dis. 2006;48 (Suppl 1):S2–90.

[49] Oliver MJ, Edwards LJ, Treleaven DJ, Lambert K, Margetts PJ. Randomized study of temporary hemodialysis catheters. Int J Artif Organs. 2002;25(1):40–4.

[50] Little MA, Conlon PJ, Walshe JJ. Access recirculation in temporary hemodialysis catheters as measured by the saline dilution technique. Am J Kidney Dis. 2000;36(6): 1135–9.

[51] Cheesbrough JS, Finch RG, Burden RP. A prospective study of the mechanisms of infection associated with hemodialysis catheters. J Infect Dis. 1986;154(4):579–89.

[52] Contreras G, Liu PY, Elzinga L, Anger MS, Lee J, Robert N, et al. A multicenter, prospective, randomized, comparative evaluation of dual- versus triple-lumen catheters for hemodialysis and apheresis in 485 patients. Am J Kidney Dis. 2003;42(2):315–24.

[53] Konner K. The initial creation of native arteriovenous fistulas: surgical aspects and their impact on the practice of nephrology. Semin Dial. 2003;16(4):291–8.

[54] Drew DA, Lok CE, Cohen JT, Wagner M, Tangri N, Weiner DE. Vascular access choice in incident hemodialysis patients: a decision analysis. J Am Soc Nephrol. 2014.

[55] Sidawy AN, Gray R, Besarab A, Henry M, Ascher E, Silva M, Jr., et al. Recommended standards for reports dealing with arteriovenous hemodialysis accesses. J Vasc Surg. 2002;35(3):603–10.

[56] de Almeida E, Dias L, de Sousa FT, Mil-Homens MC, Pataca I, Prata MM. Survival in haemodialysis: is there a role for vascular access? Nephrol Dial Transplant. 1997;12(4):852.

[57] Stehman-Breen CO, Sherrard DJ, Gillen D, Caps M. Determinants of type and timing of initial permanent hemodialysis vascular access. Kidney Int. 2000;57(2):639–45.

[58] Sesso R, Yoshihiro MM. Time of diagnosis of chronic renal failure and assessment of quality of life in haemodialysis patients. Nephrol Dial Transplant. 1997;12(10):2111–6.

[59] Arora P, Obrador GT, Ruthazer R, Kausz AT, Meyer KB, Jenuleson CS, et al. Prevalence, predictors, and consequences of late nephrology referral at a tertiary care center. J Am Soc Nephrol. 1999;10(6):1281–6.

[60] Roubicek C, Brunet P, Huiart L, Thirion X, Leonetti F, Dussol B, et al. Timing of nephrology referral: influence on mortality and morbidity. Am J Kidney Dis. 2000;36(1):35–41.

[61] Pena JM, Logrono JM, Pernaute R, Laviades C, Virto R, Vicente de Vera C. Late nephrology referral influences on morbidity and mortality of hemodialysis patients. A provincial study. Nefrologia. 2006;26(1):84–97.

[62] Pisoni RL, Young EW, Dykstra DM, Greenwood RN, Hecking E, Gillespie B, et al. Vascular access use in Europe and the United States: results from the DOPPS. Kidney Int. 2002;61(1):305–16.

[63] Ravani P, Brunori G, Mandolfo S, Cancarini G, Imbasciati E, Marcelli D, et al. Cardiovascular comorbidity and late referral impact arteriovenous fistula survival: a prospective multicenter study. J Am Soc Nephrol. 2004;15(1):204–9.

[64] Rayner HC, Pisoni RL, Gillespie BW, Goodkin DA, Akiba T, Akizawa T, et al. Creation, cannulation and survival of arteriovenous fistulae: data from the Dialysis Outcomes and Practice Patterns Study. Kidney Int. 2003;63(1):323–30.

[65] Ethier J, Mendelssohn DC, Elder SJ, Hasegawa T, Akizawa T, Akiba T, et al. Vascular access use and outcomes: an international perspective from the Dialysis Outcomes and Practice Patterns Study. Nephrol Dial Transplant. 2008;23(10):3219–26.

[66] Aitken E, Jackson AJ, Kasthuri R, Kingsmore DB. Bilateral central vein stenosis: options for dialysis access and renal replacement therapy when all upper extremity access possibilities have been lost. J Vasc Access. 2014;0(0):0.

[67] Kudlaty EA, Pan J, Allemang MT, Kendrick DE, Kashyap VS, Wong VL. The end stage of dialysis access: femoral graft or HeRO vascular access device. Ann Vasc Surg. 2014.

[68] Santoro D, Benedetto F, Mondello P, Pipito N, Barilla D, Spinelli F, et al. Vascular access for hemodialysis: current perspectives. Int J Nephrol Renovasc Dis. 2014;7:281–94.

[69] Ganie FA, Lone H, Dar AM, Lone GN, Wani ML. Native arterio-venous fistula is the vascular access of choice for hemodialysis in end stage renal disease. Int Cardiovasc Res J. 2013;7(2):67–70.

[70] Lameire N, Mehta RL. Complications of Dialysis. New York: M. Dekker; 2000. xiv, 877 p. p.

[71] Sommer G, Bruce HM. Vascular Access for Hemodialysis II. 1991. pp. 145–57.

[72] Leapman SB, Boyle M, Pescovitz MD, Milgrom ML, Jindal RM, Filo RS. The arteriovenous fistula for hemodialysis access: gold standard or archaic relic? Am Surg. 1996;62(8):652–6; discussion 6-7.

[73] Hodges TC, Fillinger MF, Zwolak RM, Walsh DB, Bech F, Cronenwett JL. Longitudinal comparison of dialysis access methods: risk factors for failure. J Vasc Surg. 1997;26(6):1009–19.

[74] Konner K, Hulbert-Shearon TE, Roys EC, Port FK. Tailoring the initial vascular access for dialysis patients. Kidney Int. 2002;62(1):329–38.

[75] Fassiadis N, Morsy M, Siva M, Marsh JE, Makanjuola AD, Chemla ES. Does the surgeon's experience impact on radiocephalic fistula patency rates? Semin Dial. 2007;20(5):455–7.

[76] Korsheed S, Eldehni MT, John SG, Fluck RJ, McIntyre CW. Effects of arteriovenous fistula formation on arterial stiffness and cardiovascular performance and function. Nephrol Dial Transplant. 2011.

[77] Hentschel MD. Vascular access for hemodialysis. Nephrology Rounds. 2008;6(1).

[78] Shintaku S, Kawanishi H, Moriishi M, Bansyodani M, Tsuchiya S. Distal ulnar-basilic fistula as the first hemodialysis access. J Vasc Access. 2014;15(2):83–7.

[79] Hod T, Patibandla BK, Vin Y, Brown RS, Goldfarb-Rumyantzev AS. Arteriovenous fistula placement in the elderly: when is the optimal time? J Am Soc Nephrol. 2014.

[80] Silva MB, Jr., Hobson RW, 2nd, Pappas PJ, Jamil Z, Araki CT, Goldberg MC, et al. A strategy for increasing use of autogenous hemodialysis access procedures: impact of preoperative noninvasive evaluation. J Vasc Surg. 1998;27(2):302–7; discussion 7-8.

[81] Beatherd GB. A Practitioner's Resource Guide to Hemodialysis Arteriovenous Fistulas. ESRD Network of Texas; 2003.

[82] Wong V, Ward R, Taylor J, Selvakumar S, How TV, Bakran A. Factors associated with early failure of arteriovenous fistulae for haemodialysis access. Eur J Vasc Endovasc Surg. 1996;12(2):207–13.

[83] Lew SQ, Nguyen BN, Ing TS. Hemodialysis vascular access construction in the upper extremity: a review. J Vasc Access. 2014;0(0):0.

[84] Uzun A, Diken AI, Yalcinkaya A, Hanedan O, Cicek OF, Lafci G, et al. Long-term patency of autogenous saphenous veins vs. PTFE interposition graft for prosthetic hemodialysis access. Anadolu Kardiyol Der. 2014;14(6):542–6.

[85] Yerdel MA, Kesenci M, Yazicioglu KM, Doseyen Z, Turkcapar AG, Anadol E. Effect of haemodynamic variables on surgically created arteriovenous fistula flow. Nephrol Dial Transplant. 1997;12(8):1684–8.

[86] Malovrh M. Non-invasive evaluation of vessels by duplex sonography prior to construction of arteriovenous fistulas for haemodialysis. Nephrol Dial Transplant. 1998;13(1):125–9.

[87] Robbin ML, Chamberlain NE, Lockhart ME, Gallichio MH, Young CJ, Deierhoi MH, et al. Hemodialysis arteriovenous fistula maturity: US evaluation. Radiology. 2002;225(1):59–64.

[88] Oder TF, Teodorescu V, Uribarri J. Effect of exercise on the diameter of arteriovenous fistulae in hemodialysis patients. ASAIO J. 2003;49(5):554–5.

[89] Rus RR, Ponikvar R, Kenda RB, Buturovic-Ponikvar J. Effect of local physical training on the forearm arteries and veins in patients with end-stage renal disease. Blood Purif. 2003;21(6):389–94.

[90] Bashar K, Healy D, Browne LD, Kheirelseid EA, Walsh MT, Moloney MC, et al. Role of far infra-red therapy in dialysis arterio-venous fistula maturation and survival: systematic review and meta-analysis. PLoS One. 2014;9(8):e104931.

[91] Lin CC, Yang WC, Chen MC, Liu WS, Yang CY, Lee PC. Effect of far infrared therapy on arteriovenous fistula maturation: an open-label randomized controlled trial. Am J Kidney Dis. 2013;62(2):304–11.

[92] Jennings WC, Galt SW, Shenoy S, Wang S, Ladenheim ED, Glickman MH, et al. The Venous Window Needle Guide, a hemodialysis cannulation device for salvage of uncannulatable arteriovenous fistulas. J Vasc Surg. 2014.

[93] Strozecki P, Flisinski M, Serafin Z, Wiechecka-Korenkiewicz J, Manitius J. Abdominal collateral vein as an unconventional vascular access for hemodialysis in patient with central vein occlusion. Semin Dial. 2014;27(4):E48–50.

[94] Rodriguez JA, Armadans L, Ferrer E, Olmos A, Codina S, Bartolome J, et al. The function of permanent vascular access. Nephrol Dial Transplant. 2000;15(3):402–8.

[95] Kinnaert P, Vereerstraeten P, Toussaint C, Van Geertruyden J. Nine years' experience with internal arteriovenous fistulas for haemodialysis: a study of some factors influencing the results. Br J Surg. 1977;64(4):242–6.

[96] Reilly DT, Wood RF, Bell PR. Prospective study of dialysis fistulas: problem patients and their treatment. Br J Surg. 1982;69(9):549–53.

[97] Windus DW. Permanent vascular access: a nephrologist's view. Am J Kidney Dis. 1993;21(5):457–71.

[98] Hakaim AG, Nalbandian M, Scott T. Superior maturation and patency of primary brachiocephalic and transposed basilic vein arteriovenous fistulae in patients with diabetes. J Vasc Surg. 1998;27(1):154–7.

[99] Bender MH, Bruyninckx CM, Gerlag PG. The brachiocephalic elbow fistula: a useful alternative angioaccess for permanent hemodialysis. J Vasc Surg. 1994;20(5):808–13.

[100] USRDS. 2007 Annual Data Report. 2007.

[101] Dukkipati R, Peck M, Dhamija R, Hentschel DM, Reynolds T, Tammewar G, et al. Biological grafts for hemodialysis access: historical lessons, state-of-the-art and future directions. Semin Dial. 2013;26(2):233–9.

[102] Gowda A, Pavan M, Babu K. Vascular access profile in maintenance hemodialysis patients. Iran J Kidney Dis. 2014;8(3):218–24.

[103] Disbrow DE, Cull DL, Carsten CG, 3rd, Yang SK, Johnson BL, Keahey GP. Comparison of arteriovenous fistulas and arteriovenous grafts in patients with favorable vas-

http://dx.doi.org/10.5772/59464

cular anatomy and equivalent access to health care: is a reappraisal of the Fistula First Initiative indicated? J Am Coll Surg. 2013;216(4):679–85; discussion 85-6.

[104] Ong S, Barker-Finkel J, Allon M. Long-term outcomes of arteriovenous thigh grafts in hemodialysis patients: a comparison with tunneled dialysis catheters. Clin J Am Soc Nephrol. 2013;8(5):804–9.

[105] Hunter JP, Nicholson ML. Midterm experience of ipsilateral axillary–axillary arteriovenous loop graft as tertiary access for haemodialysis. J Transplant. 2014;2014:908738.

[106] Schild AF, Schuman ES, Noicely K, Kaufman J, Gillaspie E, Fuller J, et al. Early cannulation prosthetic graft (FlixeneTM) for arteriovenous access. J Vasc Access. 2011.

[107] Hakaim AG, Scott TE. Durability of early prosthetic dialysis graft cannulation: results of a prospective, nonrandomized clinical trial. J Vasc Surg. 1997;25(6):1002–5; discussion 5-6.

[108] Quinn B, Cull LD, Carsten G. Hemodialysis access: placement and management of complications. In: Comprehensive Vascular and Endovascular Surgery, 2nd ed. [Internet]. Mosby ELSEVIER; 2009. pp. 429–62].

[109] Karatepe C, Aitinay L, Yetim TD, Dagli C, Dursun S. A novel electrospun nano-fabric graft allows early cannulation access and reduces exposure to central venous catheters. J Vasc Access. 2013;14(3):273–80.

[110] Aitken EL, Jackson AJ, Kingsmore DB. Early cannulation prosthetic graft (Acuseal) for arteriovenous access: a useful option to provide a personal vascular access solution. J Vasc Access. 2014;0(0):0.

[111] Donati G, Cianciolo G, Mauro R, Rucci P, Scrivo A, Marchetti A, et al. PTFE grafts versus tunneled cuffed catheters for hemodialysis: which is the second choice when arteriovenous fistula is not feasible? Artificial Organs. 2014.

[112] Xue H, Ix JH, Wang W, Brunelli SM, Lazarus M, Hakim R, et al. Hemodialysis access usage patterns in the incident dialysis year and associated catheter-related complications. Am J Kidney Dis. 2013;61(1):123–30.

[113] Beasley C, Rowland J, Spergel L. Fistula first: an update for renal providers. Nephrol News Issues. 2004;18(11):88, 90.

[114] Rayner HC, Pisoni RL. The increasing use of hemodialysis catheters: evidence from the DOPPS on its significance and ways to reverse it. Semin Dial. 2010;23(1):6–10.

[115] Grapsa E, Pantelias K, Vourliotou A, Tseke P, Pipili C, Deda E, et al. Patients with cardiac failure and female gender are most likely to start hemodialysis using a double lumen catheter. Minerva Urol Nefrol. 2014.

[116] Raad I, Costerton W, Sabharwal U, Sacilowski M, Anaissie E, Bodey GP. Ultrastructural analysis of indwelling vascular catheters: a quantitative relationship between luminal colonization and duration of placement. J Infect Dis. 1993;168(2):400–7.

[117] Troidle L, Finkelstein FO. Catheter-related bacteremia in hemodialysis patients: the role of the central venous catheter in prevention and therapy. Int J Artif Organs. 2008;31(9):827–33.

[118] Power A, Singh SK, Ashby D, Cairns T, Taube D, Duncan N. Long-term Tesio catheter access for hemodialysis can deliver high dialysis adequacy with low complication rates. J Vasc Interv Radiol. 2011.

[119] Marik PE, Flemmer M, Harrison W. The risk of catheter-related bloodstream infection with femoral venous catheters as compared to subclavian and internal jugular venous catheters: a systematic review of the literature and meta-analysis. Crit Care Med. 2012;40(8):2479–85.

[120] Timsit JF, Bouadma L, Mimoz O, Parienti JJ, Garrouste-Orgeas M, Alfandari S, et al. Jugular versus femoral short-term catheterization and risk of infection in intensive care unit patients. Causal analysis of two randomized trials. Am J Respir Crit Care Med. 2013;188(10):1232–9.

[121] Younes HK, Pettigrew CD, Anaya-Ayala JE, Soltes G, Saad WE, Davies MG, et al. Transhepatic hemodialysis catheters: functional outcome and comparison between early and late failure. J Vasc Interv Radiol. 2011;22(2):183–91.

[122] Power A, Singh S, Ashby D, Hamady M, Moser S, Gedroyc W, et al. Translumbar central venous catheters for long-term haemodialysis. Nephrol Dial Transplant. 2010;25(5):1588–95.

[123] Gouda Z. Retrograde femoral vein catheter insertion. A new approach for challenging hemodialysis vascular access. J Vasc Access. 2014;0(0):0.

[124] Seikaly M, Ho PL, Emmett L, Tejani A. The 12th Annual Report of the North American Pediatric Renal Transplant Cooperative Study: renal transplantation from 1987 through 1998. Pediatr Transplant. 2001;5(3):215–31.

[125] NAPRTCS. NAPRTCS: 2008 Annual Report 2008. Available from: https://web.emmes.com/study/ped/announce.htm.

[126] USRDS: the United States Renal Data System. Am J Kidney Dis. 2003;42(6 Suppl 5):1–230.

[127] Verrina E, Cappelli V, Perfumo F. Selection of modalities, prescription, and technical issues in children on peritoneal dialysis. Pediatr Nephrol. 2009;24(8):1453–64.

[128] Fischbach M, Edefonti A, Schroder C, Watson A. Hemodialysis in children: general practical guidelines. Pediatr Nephrol. 2005;20(8):1054–66.

[129] Carey WA, Talley LI, Sehring SA, Jaskula JM, Mathias RS. Outcomes of dialysis initiated during the neonatal period for treatment of end-stage renal disease: a North

American Pediatric Renal Trials and Collaborative Studies special analysis. Pediatrics. 2007;119(2):e468–73.

[130] Sadowski RH, Harmon WE, Jabs K. Acute hemodialysis of infants weighing less than five kilograms. Kidney Int. 1994;45(3):903–6.

[131] Chand DH, Geary D, Patel H, Greenbaum LA, Nailescu C, Brier ME, et al. Barriers, biases, and beliefs about arteriovenous fistula placement in children: a survey of the International Pediatric Fistula First Initiative (IPFFI) within the Midwest Pediatric Nephrology Consortium (MWPNC). International Symposium on Home Hemodialysis. 2014.

[132] Goldstein SL JK. Pediatric hemodialysis. In: Avner ED, Niaudet P, editors. Pediatric Nephrology, 5th ed. Lippincott Williams & Wilkins; 2003. pp. 1395–410.

[133] Donckerwolcke RA, Bunchman TE. Hemodialysis in infants and small children. Pediatr Nephrol. 1994;8(1):103–6.

[134] Fadel FI, Elshamaa MF, Nabhan MM, Essam RG, Kantoush N, El Sonbaty MM, et al. Soluble adhesion molecules as markers of native arteriovenous fistula thrombosis in children on uremia. Blood Coagul Fibrinolysis. 2014;25(7):675–82.

[135] Pastan S, Soucie JM, McClellan WM. Vascular access and increased risk of death among hemodialysis patients. Kidney Int. 2002;62(2):620–6.

[136] Xue JL, Dahl D, Ebben JP, Collins AJ. The association of initial hemodialysis access type with mortality outcomes in elderly Medicare ESRD patients. Am J Kidney Dis. 2003;42(5):1013–9.

[137] Hicks CW, Canner JK, Arhuidese I, Zarkowsky DS, Qazi U, Reifsnyder T, et al. Mortality benefits of different hemodialysis access types are age dependent. J Vasc Surg. 2014.

[138] El Minshawy O, Abd El Aziz T, Abd El Ghani H. Evaluation of vascular access complications in acute and chronic hemodialysis. J Vasc Access. 2004;5(2):76–82.

[139] Ng LJ, Chen F, Pisoni RL, Krishnan M, Mapes D, Keen M, et al. Hospitalization risks related to vascular access type among incident US hemodialysis patients. Nephrol Dial Transplant. 2011.

[140] Cornelis T, Usvyat LA, Tordoir JH, Wang Y, Wong M, Leunissen KM, et al. Vascular access vulnerability in intensive hemodialysis: a significant Achilles' heel? Blood Purif. 2014;37(3):222–8.

[141] Astor BC, Eustace JA, Powe NR, Klag MJ, Fink NE, Coresh J. Type of vascular access and survival among incident hemodialysis patients: the Choices for Healthy Outcomes in Caring for ESRD (CHOICE) Study. J Am Soc Nephrol. 2005;16(5):1449–55.

[142] Ocak G, Halbesma N, le Cessie S, Hoogeveen EK, van Dijk S, Kooman J, et al. Haemodialysis catheters increase mortality as compared to arteriovenous accesses especially in elderly patients. Nephrol Dial Transplant. 2011.

[143] Mendelssohn DC, Ethier J, Elder SJ, Saran R, Port FK, Pisoni RL. Haemodialysis vascular access problems in Canada: results from the Dialysis Outcomes and Practice Patterns Study (DOPPS II). Nephrol Dial Transplant. 2006;21(3):721–8.

[144] Noordzij M, Jager KJ, van der Veer SN, Kramar R, Collart F, Heaf JG, et al. Use of vascular access for haemodialysis in Europe: a report from the ERA-EDTA Registry. Nephrol Dial Transplant. 2014.

[145] System USRD. 2010 Annual Data Report. Bethesda, National Institutes of Health, National Institute of Diabetes and Digestive Diseases. 2010.

[146] Tordoir JH, Van Der Sande FM, De Haan MW. Current topics on vascular access for hemodialysis. Minerva Urol Nefrol. 2004;56(3):223–35.

[147] Movilli E, Brunori G, Camerini C, Vizzardi V, Gaggia P, Cassamali S, et al. The kind of vascular access influences the baseline inflammatory status and epoetin response in chronic hemodialysis patients. Blood Purif. 2006;24(4):387–93.

[148] Swindlehurst N, Swindlehurst A, Lumgair H, Rebollo Mesa I, Mamode N, Cacciola R, et al. Vascular access for hemodialysis in the elderly. J Vasc Surg. 2011;53(4):1039–43.

[149] Watorek E, Golebiowski T, Kusztal M, Letachowicz K, Letachowicz W, Augustyniak Bartosik H, et al. Creation of arteriovenous fistulae for hemodialysis in octogenarians. Hemodial Int. 2014;18(1):113–7.

[150] Sladoje-Martinovic B, Mikolasevic I, Bubic I, Racki S, Orlic L. Survival of chronic hemodialysis patients over 80 years of age. Clin Interv Aging. 2014;9:689–96.

[151] Patibandla BK, Narra A, Desilva R, Chawla V, Vin Y, Brown RS, et al. Disparities in arteriovenous fistula placement in older hemodialysis patients. Hemodial Int. 2014;18(1):118–26.

[152] Goldfarb-Rumyantzev AS, Syed W, Patibandla BK, Narra A, Desilva R, Chawla V, et al. Geographic disparities in arteriovenous fistula placement in patients approaching hemodialysis in the United States. Hemodial Int. 2014;18(3):686–94.

[153] Trepanier P, Quach C, Gonzales M, Fortin E, Kaouache M, Desmeules S, et al. Survey of infection control practices in hemodialysis units: preventing vascular access-associated bloodstream infections. Infect Control Hosp Epidemiol. 2014;35(7):833–8.

[154] Bai YL, Hung SY, Chiou CP. Vascular access management and education for hemodialysis patients. Hu Li Za Zhi. 2014;61(1):93–8.

[155] Saucy F, Deglise S, Holzer T, Salomon L, Engelberger S, Corpataux JM. Intraoperative assessment of vascular access. J Vasc Access. 2014;15 (Suppl 7):S6–9.

[156] Kamper L, Frahnert M, Grebe SO, Haage P. Radiological assessment of vascular access in haemodialysis patients. J Vasc Access. 2014;15 (Suppl 7):S33–7.

[157] Remuzzi A, Manini S. Computational model for prediction of fistula outcome. J Vasc Access. 2014;15 (Suppl 7):S64–9.

[158] Gallieni M, Brenna I, Brunini F, Mezzina N, Pasho S, Fornasieri A. Which cannulation technique for which patient. J Vasc Access. 2014;15 (Suppl 7):S85–90.

[159] Wong B, Muneer M, Wiebe N, Storie D, Shurraw S, Pannu N, et al. Buttonhole versus rope-ladder cannulation of arteriovenous fistulas for hemodialysis: a systematic review. Am J Kidney Dis. 2014.

[160] Muir CA, Kotwal SS, Hawley CM, Polkinghorne K, Gallagher MP, Snelling P, et al. Buttonhole cannulation and clinical outcomes in a home hemodialysis cohort and systematic review. Clin J Am Soc Nephrol. 2014;9(1):110–9.

[161] Raja RM, Fernandes M, Kramer MS, Barber K, Rosenbaum JL. Comparison of subclavian vein with femoral vein catheterization for hemodialysis. Am J Kidney Dis. 1983;2(4):474–6.

[162] Fan PY. Acute vascular access: new advances. Adv Ren Replace Ther. 1994;1(2):90–8.

[163] Vanholder R, Lameire N, Verbanck J, van Rattinghe R, Kunnen M, Ringoir S. Complications of subclavian catheter hemodialysis: a 5 year prospective study in 257 consecutive patients. Int J Artif Organs. 1982;5(5):297–303.

[164] Edwards H, King TC. Cardiac tamponade from central venous catheters. Arch Surg. 1982;117(7):965–7.

[165] Geddes CC, Walbaum D, Fox JG, Mactier RA. Insertion of internal jugular temporary hemodialysis cannulae by direct ultrasound guidance—a prospective comparison of experienced and inexperienced operators. Clin Nephrol. 1998;50(5):320–5.

[166] Hernandez D, Diaz F, Rufino M, Lorenzo V, Perez T, Rodriguez A, et al. Subclavian vascular access stenosis in dialysis patients: natural history and risk factors. J Am Soc Nephrol. 1998;9(8):1507–10.

[167] Cimochowski GE, Worley E, Rutherford WE, Sartain J, Blondin J, Harter H. Superiority of the internal jugular over the subclavian access for temporary dialysis. Nephron. 1990;54(2):154–61.

[168] Zadeh MK, Shirvani A. The role of routine chest radiography for detecting complications after central venous catheter insertion. Saudi J Kidney Dis Transpl. 2014;25(5): 1011–6.

[169] Daeihagh P, Jordan J, Chen J, Rocco M. Efficacy of tissue plasminogen activator administration on patency of hemodialysis access catheters. Am J Kidney Dis. 2000;36(1):75–9.

[170] Schwab SJ, Quarles LD, Middleton JP, Cohan RH, Saeed M, Dennis VW. Hemodialysis-associated subclavian vein stenosis. Kidney Int. 1988;33(6):1156–9.

[171] Newman GE, Saeed M, Himmelstein S, Cohan RH, Schwab SJ. Total central vein obstruction: resolution with angioplasty and fibrinolysis. Kidney Int. 1991;39(4):761–4.

[172] Oliver MJ, Callery SM, Thorpe KE, Schwab SJ, Churchill DN. Risk of bacteremia from temporary hemodialysis catheters by site of insertion and duration of use: a prospective study. Kidney Int. 2000;58(6):2543–5.

[173] Ishani A, Collins AJ, Herzog CA, Foley RN. Septicemia, access and cardiovascular disease in dialysis patients: the USRDS Wave 2 study. Kidney Int. 2005;68(1):311–8.

[174] Dahlberg PJ, Yutuc WR, Newcomer KL. Subclavian hemodialysis catheter infections. Am J Kidney Dis. 1986;7(5):421–7.

[175] Nielsen J, Kolmos HJ, Espersen F. *Staphylococcus aureus* bacteraemia among patients undergoing dialysis—focus on dialysis catheter-related cases. Nephrol Dial Transplant. 1998;13(1):139–45.

[176] Nielsen J, Ladefoged SD, Kolmos HJ. Dialysis catheter-related septicaemia—focus on *Staphylococcus aureus* septicaemia. Nephrol Dial Transplant. 1998;13(11):2847–52.

[177] Ravani P, Gillespie BW, Quinn RR, MacRae J, Manns B, Mendelssohn D, et al. Temporal risk profile for infectious and noninfectious complications of hemodialysis access. J Am Soc Nephrol. 2013;24(10):1668–77.

[178] Schindler R, Heemann U, Haug U, Stoelck B, Karatas A, Pohle C, et al. Bismuth coating of non-tunneled haemodialysis catheters reduces bacterial colonization: a randomized controlled trial. Nephrol Dial Transplant. 2010;25(8):2651–6.

[179] O'Grady NP, Alexander M, Burns LA, Dellinger EP, Garland J, Heard SO, et al. Summary of recommendations: Guidelines for the Prevention of Intravascular Catheter-related Infections. Clin Infect Dis. 2011;52(9):1087–99.

[180] Moore CL, Besarab A, Ajluni M, Soi V, Peterson EL, Johnson LE, et al. Comparative effectiveness of two catheter locking solutions to reduce catheter-related bloodstream infection in hemodialysis patients. Clin J Am Soc Nephrol. 2014;9(7):1232–9.

[181] Grimaldi R. The centrality of the nurse in the prevention of the infections in hemodialysis. G Ital Nefrol. 2014;31(3).

[182] Parienti JJ, Thirion M, Megarbane B, Souweine B, Ouchikhe A, Polito A, et al. Femoral vs jugular venous catheterization and risk of nosocomial events in adults requiring acute renal replacement therapy: a randomized controlled trial. JAMA. 2008;299(20):2413–22.

[183] Kairaitis LK, Gottlieb T. Outcome and complications of temporary haemodialysis catheters. Nephrol Dial Transplant. 1999;14(7):1710–4.

[184] Mermel LA, Farr BM, Sherertz RJ, Raad, II, O'Grady N, Harris JS, et al. Guidelines for the management of intravascular catheter-related infections. J Intraven Nurs. 2001;24(3):180–205.

[185] George A, Tokars JI, Clutterbuck EJ, Bamford KB, Pusey C, Holmes AH. Reducing dialysis associated bacteraemia, and recommendations for surveillance in the United Kingdom: prospective study. BMJ. 2006;332(7555):1435.

[186] Shingarev R, Barker-Finkel J, Allon M. Association of hemodialysis central venous catheter use with ipsilateral arteriovenous vascular access survival. Am J Kidney Dis. 2012;60(6):983–9.

[187] Beathard GA. Strategy for maximizing the use of arteriovenous fistulae. Semin Dial. 2000;13(5):291–6.

[188] Bashar K, Clarke-Moloney M, Walsh SR. Pre-operative ultrasonography and arteriovenous fistulae maturation. J Vasc Access. 2014;15 (Suppl 7):S60–3.

[189] Shemesh D, Raikhinstein Y, Orkin D, Goldin I, Olsha O. Anesthesia for vascular access surgery. J Vasc Access. 2014;15 (Suppl 7):S38–44.

[190] Macfarlane AJ, Kearns RJ, Aitken E, Kinsella J, Clancy MJ. Does regional compared to local anaesthesia influence outcome after arteriovenous fistula creation? Trials. 2013;14:263.

[191] Beathard GA, Settle SM, Shields MW. Salvage of the nonfunctioning arteriovenous fistula. Am J Kidney Dis. 1999;33(5):910–6.

[192] Beathard GA, Arnold P, Jackson J, Litchfield T. Aggressive treatment of early fistula failure. Kidney Int. 2003;64(4):1487–94.

[193] Romero A, Polo JR, Garcia Morato E, Garcia Sabrido JL, Quintans A, Ferreiroa JP. Salvage of angioaccess after late thrombosis of radiocephalic fistulas for hemodialysis. Int Surg. 1986;71(2):122–4.

[194] Hod T, Desilva RN, Patibandla BK, Vin Y, Brown RS, Goldfarb-Rumyantzev AS. Factors predicting failure of AV "fistula first" policy in the elderly. Hemodial Int. 2014;18(2):507–15.

[195] Lin CT, Dai NT, Chen SG, Chang SC. Acute forearm compartment syndrome following haemodialysis access fistula puncture in uraemia. ANZ J Surg. 2014.

[196] Belli S, Yabanoglu H, Aydogan C, Parlakgumus A, Yildirim S, Haberal M. Surgical interventions for late complications of arteriovenous fistulas. Int Surg. 2014;99(4): 467–74.

[197] Decorato I, Kharboutly Z, Legallais C, Salsac AV. Comparison of two endovascular treatments of a stenosed arteriovenous fistula: balloon-angioplasty with and without stenting. Int J Artif Organs. 2014;0(0):0.

[198] Aftab SA, Tay KH, Irani FG, Gong Lo RH, Gogna A, Haaland B, et al. Randomized clinical trial of cutting balloon angioplasty versus high-pressure balloon angioplasty in hemodialysis arteriovenous fistula stenoses resistant to conventional balloon angioplasty. J Vasc Interv Radiol. 2014;25(2):190–8.

[199] Wu CC, Huang PH, Lai CL, Leu HB, Chen JW, Lin SJ. The impact of endothelial progenitor cells on restenosis after percutaneous angioplasty of hemodialysis vascular access. PLoS One. 2014;9(6):e101058.

[200] Turmel-Rodrigues L, Pengloan J, Baudin S, Testou D, Abaza M, Dahdah G, et al. Treatment of stenosis and thrombosis in haemodialysis fistulas and grafts by interventional radiology. Nephrol Dial Transplant. 2000;15(12):2029–36.

[201] Palmer SC, Di Micco L, Razavian M, Craig JC, Ravani P, Perkovic V, et al. Antiplatelet therapy to prevent hemodialysis vascular access failure: systematic review and meta-analysis. Am J Kidney Dis. 2013;61(1):112–22.

[202] Tessitore N, Bedogna V, Poli A, Lipari G, Pertile P, Baggio E, et al. Should current criteria for detecting and repairing arteriovenous fistula stenosis be reconsidered? Interim analysis of a randomized controlled trial. Nephrol Dial Transplant. 2014;29(1): 179–87.

[203] Lu FP, Liu LP, Lu ZX. One-year patency rate of native arteriovenous fistulas reconstructed by vascular stripping in hemodialysis patients with venous neointimal hyperplasia. J Vasc Surg. 2014.

[204] Beathard GA. Physical examination: the forgotten tool. In: Gray RJ, Sands JJ, editors. Dialysis Access: A Multidisciplinary Approach. Lippincott Williams & Wilkins; 2002. pp. 111–228.

[205] Patel MS, Street T, Davies MG, Peden EK, Naoum JJ. Evaluating and treating venous outflow stenoses is necessary for the successful open surgical treatment of arteriovenous fistula aneurysms. J Vasc Surg. 2014.

[206] Hossny A. Partial aneurysmectomy for salvage of autogenous arteriovenous fistula with complicated venous aneurysms. J Vasc Surg. 2014;59(4):1073–7.

[207] Sigala F, Kontis E, Sassen R, Mickley V. Autologous surgical reconstruction for true venous hemodialysis access aneurysms-techniques and results. J Vasc Access. 2014;0(0):0.

[208] KDOQI. Guideline 5. Treatment of Fistula Complications. 2006.

[209] Stevenson KB. Management of hemodialysis vascular access infection. In: Gray RJ, Sands JJ, editors. Dialysis Access: A Multidisciplinary Approach Philadelphia, PA: Lippincott Williams & Wilkins; 2002. pp. 98–106.

[210] Swedberg SH, Brown BG, Sigley R, Wight TN, Gordon D, Nicholls SC. Intimal fibromuscular hyperplasia at the venous anastomosis of PTFE grafts in hemodialysis pa-

tients. Clinical, immunocytochemical, light and electron microscopic assessment. Circulation. 1989;80(6):1726–36.

[211] Roy-Chaudhury P, Kelly BS, Miller MA, Reaves A, Armstrong J, Nanayakkara N, et al. Venous neointimal hyperplasia in polytetrafluoroethylene dialysis grafts. Kidney Int. 2001;59(6):2325–34.

[212] Paszkowiak JJ, Dardik A. Arterial wall shear stress: observations from the bench to the bedside. Vasc Endovascular Surg. 2003;37(1):47–57.

[213] Corpataux JM, Haesler E, Silacci P, Ris HB, Hayoz D. Low-pressure environment and remodelling of the forearm vein in Brescia–Cimino haemodialysis access. Nephrol Dial Transplant. 2002;17(6):1057–62.

[214] Misra S, Bonan R, Pflederer T, Roy-Chaudhury P. BRAVO I: a pilot study of vascular brachytherapy in polytetrafluoroethylene dialysis access grafts. Kidney Int. 2006;70(11):2006–13.

[215] Cai X, Freedman NJ. New therapeutic possibilities for vein graft disease in the post-edifoligide era. Future Cardiol. 2006;2(4):493–501.

[216] Conte MS, Bandyk DF, Clowes AW, Moneta GL, Seely L, Lorenz TJ, et al. Results of PREVENT III: a multicenter, randomized trial of edifoligide for the prevention of vein graft failure in lower extremity bypass surgery. J Vasc Surg. 2006;43(4):742–51; discussion 51.

[217] Melhem M, Kelly B, Zhang J, Kasting G, Li J, Davis H, et al. Development of a local perivascular paclitaxel delivery system for hemodialysis vascular access dysfunction: polymer preparation and in vitro activity. Blood Purif. 2006;24(3):289–98.

[218] Rotmans JI, Heyligers JM, Verhagen HJ, Velema E, Nagtegaal MM, de Kleijn DP, et al. In vivo cell seeding with anti-CD34 antibodies successfully accelerates endothelialization but stimulates intimal hyperplasia in porcine arteriovenous expanded polytetrafluoroethylene grafts. Circulation. 2005;112(1):12–8.

[219] Beathard GA. Angioplasty for arteriovenous grafts and fistulae. Semin Nephrol. 2002;22(3):202–10.

[220] Bachleda P, Utikal P, Kocher M, Cerna M, Fialova J, Kalinova L. Arteriovenous graft for hemodialysis, graft venous anastomosis closure—current state of knowledge. Minireview. Biomedical papers of the Medical Faculty of the University Palacky, Olomouc, Czechoslovakia. 2014.

[221] Vesely TM. Endovascular intervention for the failing vascular access. Adv Ren Replace Ther. 2002;9(2):99–108.

[222] Sreenarasimhaiah VP, Margassery SK, Martin KJ, Bander SJ. Salvage of thrombosed dialysis access grafts with venous anastomosis stents. Kidney Int. 2005;67(2):678–84.

[223] McNally A, Akingba AG, Robinson EA, Sucosky P. Novel modular anastomotic valve device for hemodialysis vascular access: preliminary computational hemodynamic assessment. J Vasc Access. 2014;0(0):0.

[224] Planken RN, van Kesteren F, Reekers JA. Treatment of hemodialysis vascular access arteriovenous graft failure by percutaneous intervention. J Vasc Access. 2014;15 (Suppl 7):S114–9.

[225] Saleh HM, Gabr AK, Tawfik MM, Abouellail H. Prospective, randomized study of cutting balloon angioplasty versus conventional balloon angioplasty for the treatment of hemodialysis access stenoses. J Vasc Surg. 2014;60(3):735–40.

[226] Troisi N, Chisci E, Frosini P, Romano E, Setti M, Mingardi G, et al. Hybrid simultaneous treatment of thrombosed prosthetic grafts for hemodialysis. J Vasc Access. 2014;0(0):0.

[227] May RE, Himmelfarb J, Yenicesu M, Knights S, Ikizler TA, Schulman G, et al. Predictive measures of vascular access thrombosis: a prospective study. Kidney Int. 1997;52(6):1656–62.

[228] Vesely TM. Mechanical thrombectomy devices to treat thrombosed hemodialysis grafts. Tech Vasc Interv Radiol. 2003;6(1):35–41.

[229] Taylor G, Gravel D, Johnston L, Embil J, Holton D, Paton S. Prospective surveillance for primary bloodstream infections occurring in Canadian hemodialysis units. Infect Control Hosp Epidemiol. 2002;23(12):716–20.

[230] Kaplowitz LG, Comstock JA, Landwehr DM, Dalton HP, Mayhall CG. Prospective study of microbial colonization of the nose and skin and infection of the vascular access site in hemodialysis patients. J Clin Microbiol. 1988;26(7):1257–62.

[231] KDOQI. Guideline 27:Treatment do pseuoaneurysm of dialysis AV grafts.

[232] Schanzer H, Schwartz M, Harrington E, Haimov M. Treatment of ischemia due to "steal" by arteriovenous fistula with distal artery ligation and revascularization. J Vasc Surg. 1988;7(6):770–3.

[233] Modaghegh MH, Kazemzadeh G, Pezeshki Rad M, Ravari H, Hafezi S, El-Husheimi A, et al. Chronic hemodialysis access-induced distal ischemia (HAIDI): distinctive form of a major complication. J Vasc Access. 2014;0(0):0.

[234] Hye RJ, Wolf YG. Ischemic monomelic neuropathy: an under-recognized complication of hemodialysis access. Ann Vasc Surg. 1994;8(6):578–82.

[235] Grapsa Irene OD. Dialysis in the elderly. In: Horl HW, Lindsay BR, Ronco C, Winchester FJ, editors. Replacement of Renal Function by Dialysis. 5th ed. Kluwer Academic Publishers; 2004.

[236] Valliant AM, Chaudhry MK, Yevzlin AS, Astor B, Chan MR. Tunneled dialysis catheter exchange with fibrin sheath disruption is not associated with increased rate of bacteremia. J Vasc Access. 2014;0(0):0.

[237] Yoon WJ, Lorelli DR. Two-stage hemodialysis reliable outflow (HeRO) graft implantation technique that avoids the use of a femoral bridging dialysis catheter. J Vasc Access. 2014;0(0):0.

[238] Hoen B, Kessler M, Hestin D, Mayeux D. Risk factors for bacterial infections in chronic haemodialysis adult patients: a multicentre prospective survey. Nephrol Dial Transplant. 1995;10(3):377–81.

[239] Combe C, Pisoni RL, Port FK, Young EW, Canaud B, Mapes DL, et al. Dialysis outcomes and practice patterns study: data on the use of central venous catheters in chronic hemodialysis. Nephrologie. 2001;22(8):379–84.

[240] Jaffer Y, Selby NM, Taal MW, Fluck RJ, McIntyre CW. A meta-analysis of hemodialysis catheter locking solutions in the prevention of catheter-related infection. Am J Kidney Dis. 2008;51(2):233–41.

[241] Zhao Y, Li Z, Zhang L, Yang J, Yang Y, Tang Y, et al. Citrate versus heparin lock for hemodialysis catheters: a systematic review and meta-analysis of randomized controlled trials. Am J Kidney Dis. 2014;63(3):479–90.

[242] Fdez-Gallego J, Martin M, Gutierrez E, Cobelo C, Frias P, Jironda C, et al. Prophylaxis with gentamicin reduces bacterial infection morbidity and mortality related to permanent tunneled central venous catheter and does not cause bacterial resistance. Nefrologia. 2011.

[243] Murray EC, Deighan C, Geddes C, Thomson PC. Taurolidine-citrate-heparin catheter lock solution reduces staphylococcal bacteraemia rates in haemodialysis patients. QJM. 2014;107(12):995–1000.

[244] Fontsere N, Cardozo C, Donate J, Soriano A, Muros M, Pons M, et al. Tunneled catheters with taurolidine–citrate–heparin lock solution significantly improve the inflammatory profile of hemodialysis patients. Antimicrob Agents Chemother. 2014;58(7): 4180–4.

[245] Del Pozo JL, Aguinaga A, Garcia-Fernandez N, Hernaez S, Serrera A, Alonso M, et al. Intra-catheter leukocyte culture to monitor hemodialysis catheter colonization. A prospective study to prevent catheter-related bloodstream infections. Int J Artif Organs. 2008;31(9):820–6.

[246] Lawrence JA, Seiler S, Wilson B, Harwood L. Shower and no-dressing technique for tunneled central venous hemodialysis catheters: a quality improvement initiative. Nephrol Nurs J. 2014;41(1):67–72; quiz 3.

[247] Evans EC, Hain D, Kear TM, Dork LA, Schrauf C. Hemodialysis catheter outcomes pilot study: no dressing coverage with prescribed showering. Nephrol Nurs J 2014;41(1):53–64; 72; quiz 65.

[248] Gillies D, O'Riordan L, Carr D, Frost J, Gunning R, O'Brien I. Gauze and tape and transparent polyurethane dressings for central venous catheters. Cochrane Database Syst Rev. 2003(4):CD003827.